Government Procedures and Operations

snova
New York

Government Procedures and Operations

Putting an End to Surprise Medical Billing
Danial E. Tackett (Editor)
2022. ISBN: 979-8-88697-296-2 (Hardcover)
2022. ISBN: 979-8-88697-327-3 (eBook)

Abortion Rights, Access, and Legislative Response
Jorge P. Sandford (Editor)
2022. ISBN: 979-8-88697-258-0 (Softcover)
2022. ISBN: 979-8-88697-294-8 (eBook)

Review of Capitol Police Procedures During the Capitol Attack
Rafael B. Phillips (Editor)
2022. ISBN: 979-8-88697-260-3 (Hardcover)
2022. ISBN: 978-1-53617-478-6 (eBook)

Sanctions in Response to the Russian Invasion of Ukraine
Eric Freitag (Editor)
2022. ISBN: 979-8-88697-154-5 (Hardcover)
2022. ISBN: 979-8-88697-280-1 (eBook)

Is the U.S. Postal Service Sustainable?
Malissa R. Rojas (Editor)
2020. ISBN: 978-1-53618-505-8 (Hardcover)
2020. ISBN: 978-1-53618-551-5 (eBook)

More information about this series can be found at https://novapublishers.com/product-category/series/government-procedures-and-operations/

John S. Gill
Editor

The Significance of the COVID Pandemic in Nursing Homes

snova
New York

Library of Congress Cataloging-in-Publication Data

ISBN: 979-8-88697-660-1

Published by Nova Science Publishers, Inc. † New York

Contents

Preface

The COVID-19 pandemic has had a disproportionate impact on the 1.4 million elderly or disabled residents in the nation's more than 15,000 Medicare- and Medicaid-certified nursing homes. Over 175,000 long-term care residents and workers, including 130,000 living and working in federally certified nursing homes, have died of COVID-19. They were at the center of a collision of mismanagement.

Chapter 1

A National Tragedy: COVID–19 in the Nation's Nursing Homes*

Committee on Finance

Wednesday, March 17, 2021
U.S. Senate, Committee on Finance,
Washington, DC.

The hearing was convened, pursuant to notice, at 10 a.m., via Webex, in the Dirksen Senate Office Building, Hon. Ron Wyden (chairman of the committee) presiding.

Present: Senators Stabenow, Cantwell, Menendez, Cardin, Brown, Bennet, Casey, Warner, Whitehouse, Hassan, Cortez Masto, Crapo, Grassley, Thune, Portman, Toomey, Cassidy, Lankford, Daines, Young, and Barrasso.

Also present: Democratic staff: Peter Gartrell, Investigator; Kristen Lunde, Health Policy Advisor; and Joshua Sheinkman, Staff Director. Republican staff: Gregg Richard, Staff Director; Erin Dempsey, Deputy Health Policy Director; and Stuart Portman, Senior Health Policy Advisor.

Opening Statement of Hon. Ron Wyden, a U.S. Senator from Oregon, Chairman, Committee on Finance

The CHAIRMAN. This morning, the Finance Committee is holding the second of three hearings that we will be holding this week. And this is a particularly important hearing, because our country is now a full year into the COVID–19 pandemic.

And let me just give a brief kind of process statement with respect to how we are going to do this. We have two votes at 11:30, and we are going to do everything we can to keep this moving. We have been working with the ranking member, Senator Crapo, on this. And if we

---

* This is an edited, reformatted and augmented version of Hearing before the Committee on Finance, United States Senate, One Hundred Seventeenth Congress, First Session, Publication No. S. HRG. 117–280, dated March 17, 2021.

In: The Significance of the COVID Pandemic in Nursing Homes
Editor: John S. Gill
ISBN: 979-8-88697-660-1

do not do that, we will probably be here until 3 o'clock. So we are going to do our best to keep this moving.

As I indicated, we are a year in, and vaccinations are up. Americans are beginning to feel encouraged, and yet so many families— hundreds of thousands spread across the country—are unable to share in the sense of uplift because they are mourning loved ones whom they have lost.

Over the last year, more than 175,000 long-term care residents and workers, including 130,000 living and working in federally certified nursing homes, have died of this terrible disease. They were at the center of a collision of mismanagement. In too many nursing homes—even before the pandemic—there was chronic understaffing, slipshod plans for infection control, and abuse and neglect of vulnerable patients.

When COVID–19 arrived, the Trump administration came up small by withholding data, failing to distribute protective equipment, and issuing guidance that put seniors in harm's way. This was a systemic, nationwide failure, and it will be challenging to fix. Members can start by agreeing on basic facts.

First, what is true of the overall population is true in our nursing homes. Blacks, Latinos, and Native Americans are suffering the worst of COVID–19. A recent study authored by Professor Konetzka, one of the witnesses joining the committee, found that the loss of life was more than three times higher in nursing homes with the highest proportions of black and Latino residents compared to facilities with mostly white residents.

Black Americans and immigrants also make up a disproportionate share of nursing home staff. Often, they get paid low wages. More than half a million of them have had confirmed cases of COVID–19, and thousands have died. There is also real concern that COVID–19 will continue to circulate among those communities where vaccines are not readily available, or where uptake is lower.

These disparities in COVID–19 deaths are the result of generations of inequity in society and in health care. Undoing it is going to take a lot of work by this committee, and I know colleagues feel very strongly about getting it done.

Second, the previous administration actively impeded efforts to address long-running problems in nursing homes. You could fill a library with the watchdog reports calling public attention to these issues: incidents of abuse and neglect, chronic under-staffing, horrendous living conditions, inadequate emergency preparedness. This was an industry-wide failure also when it came to inspection control.

Instead of addressing these questions, the Trump administration dramatically reduced the penalties for failing to meet basic protective Federal standards. They went out of their way to undermine a chance for real accountability. When States rushed to develop COVID policies, some followed Trump administration guidance that encouraged nursing homes to accept patients regardless of whether they had tested positive for the virus.

When the pandemic was spreading and nursing homes desperately needed PPE, the Trump administration sent out shipments that reportedly included loose, unusable gloves, hospital gowns that resembled trash bags, and defective masks.

The Trump administration did not want people to know about what was going on in nursing homes. Our colleague, Senator Casey, and I spent months pressuring and pleading with them to release comprehensive data. The Trump administration stonewalled. They dithered, and they delayed before they finally began to relent. As of now, there still is no reliable data on COVID in nursing homes before May 1st of last year because of the Trump administration's stonewalling.

One final point. The terrible impact of COVID–19 on seniors in long-term care is not a red State or a blue State issue. It is a nationwide tragedy. Specifically, if you look at the 10 States where nursing homes have been hit the hardest, it is five Republican-led States and five Democratic-led States.

So the reality is, long-term care residents in all 50 States are incredibly vulnerable to a pandemic like COVID–19 for longstanding reasons, but the Trump administration worked harder to protect their unscrupulous friends in management than to improve the safety of residents.

The Biden administration is working to turn things around. It starts with ramping up vaccinations and creating strike teams of highly trained workers who will go into nursing homes and identify the safety risks.

This hearing is not the first or the last time the committee is going to be digging into nursing home safety. We are going to continue to work with members, all members of this committee, because looking after the well-being of America's seniors is at the heart of our jurisdiction.

Personally, I feel strongly about this after my 7 years as co-director of the Oregon Gray Panthers, and I look forward to working with colleagues on both sides of the aisle.

We will start with our panelists, and an introduction, right after Senator Crapo's opening statement.

[The prepared statement of Chairman Wyden appears in the appendix.]

Opening Statement of Hon. Mike Crapo, a U.S. Senator from Idaho

Senator CRAPO. Thank you, Mr. Chairman.

At the national, State, and local levels the pandemic has challenged our sense of normalcy. It has tested every institution of daily life we know, threatening the physical and economic health of our Nation.

Americans from all walks of life have experienced a full year of tremendous hardship and tragedy. It is the people living and working in our Nation's nursing homes, however, who bore an outsized burden.

More than 174,000 people died as COVID–19 ravaged our long-term care facilities. That number represents almost one-third of all U.S. deaths that have occurred during the pandemic.

Both long-stay nursing homes and short-stay post-acute skilled nursing facilities rely on direct-care workers—such as licensed practical nurses, Certified Nursing Assistants, and personal care aides—to provide most hands-on care.

These workers are in close physical contact with residents, assisting with bathing, dressing, and eating. Current data shows that long-term care workers are typically female, and a disproportionate share are women of color. Many of these direct-care workers live paycheck to paycheck. Over the past year, they have put their lives on the line. We owe them a debt of gratitude. Thank you to the dedicated nursing home workers like Adelina Ramos, one of our witnesses.

These workers hear Americans calling them heroes, but they are often under-appreciated when on the job. To these front-line workers, please know that the sacrifices you are making every day do not go unnoticed or unappreciated.

Today we will hear from a number of expert witnesses who will provide key insights into nursing home conditions over the past year. This testimony will help us better understand exactly what happened, when it happened, and why it happened. It will give us insight into policies that produce results, as well as areas that need improvement.

Hearings are just oversight tools this committee uses to hold government agencies, the health-care industry, and individual providers accountable. Another key part of oversight is securing reliable and accurate data.

Transparent data reporting brings accountability and helps drive decision-making. Transparent data reporting brings tremendous support to the system. As we look to the future, it is vital that all States report accurate COVID–19 data. That is the only way for economists, researchers, advocacy organizations, and policy-makers to tackle the challenges facing the nursing home sector head-on.

This is not a job for the Federal Government alone. Multiple Federal, State, and local programs and partnerships work to support the health-care needs of our Nation's most vulnerable populations. We must work together—in an honest and transparent manner— to safeguard our nursing home residents and the workers who care for them.

Over the weekend, *The New York Times* published the results of an investigation into the Centers for Medicare and Medicaid Services' nursing home five-star rating system. The investigation questions the objectivity and accuracy of the CMS star ratings system. This rating system, which was first implemented during the Obama administration, is designed to help beneficiaries, their families, and caregivers compare nursing home quality more easily.

Care Compare is another online tool available to help seniors, the disabled, and their families find out if a particular nursing home facility meets Federal health and safety standards, staffing levels, and quality performance metrics.

After several bipartisan hearings held by the Finance Committee during 2019, CMS implemented changes to Nursing Home Compare that specifically denote nursing homes that have been cited for incidents of abuse, neglect, or exploitation.

That may have been a start, but clearly there is a lot more work that needs to be done. I am grateful to each of our witnesses for the work they are doing, and for taking the time to join us today. Their expertise will help us advance public policies that slow the spread of COVID–19 and lessen its devastating impacts on our Nation's elderly and the disabled.

And, Mr. Chairman, before I conclude, Senator Scott will not be able to make his statement, or be participating today, but he is one of the leaders in our Senate on trying to deal with and address this issue properly. And he has asked that I request a statement of his be entered into the record.

I ask unanimous consent that his statement be entered into the record.

The CHAIRMAN. Without objection, so ordered.

[The prepared statement of Senator Scott appears in the appendix.]

Senator CRAPO. Thank you very much, Mr. Chairman.

[The prepared statement of Senator Crapo appears in the appendix.]

The CHAIRMAN. Okay. We are now going to go to our panel. Senator Whitehouse has requested to introduce Ms. Ramos. We are very glad that you could be here and have known of your efforts for quite some time, Ms. Ramos. So we are glad you are here.

Senator Whitehouse?

Senator WHITEHOUSE. Thank you, Mr. Chairman.

Rhode Island lost more than 1,000 nursing home residents to COVID. Nationwide, as Senator Crapo pointed out, there have been more than 174,000 nursing home residents and caretakers who have died.

Nearly a quarter of Rhode Island's nursing homes reported shortages of nurses and nursing aides during the pandemic. So I am very pleased and grateful that the committee will be hearing from Rhode Islander Adelina Ramos today.

She lived this crisis as a Certified Nursing Assistant at the Greenville Nursing Center in Greenville, RI. She is a proud SEIU member, and I am grateful to her and to her union.

From late April to Memorial Day, Ms. Ramos witnessed 20 residents at her 160-bed facility perish. She watched a colleague die. In one harrowing moment, she and a team of just three staffers cared for over two dozen critically ill COVID patients.

Eventually, she caught the virus herself, and feared spreading it to her family, for whom she also provides care at home. At last, Ms. Ramos is fully vaccinated and hopeful for the future.

Senator Casey and I worked to provide our nursing homes emergency funding for staffing and testing and PPE, and for nursing home strike teams to boost capacity at facilities in need. We finally got much of this support into the American Rescue Plan, but it had been blocked in all the previous COVID bills.

It would have served Adelina and her colleagues better if we had done this earlier, but at least we got it done at last.

So I am pleased to welcome Ms. Ramos here to our committee. Thank you, Mr. Chairman, and thank you, Ranking Member.

The CHAIRMAN. Thank you very much, Senator Whitehouse. At this point, I am just going to give brief introductions for our other guests.

Denise Bottcher is here. She is a State director of AARP in Louisiana. She has worked for AARP since 2010, and previously was with Governor Kathleen Blanco.

Then we will have a very important presentation from a Long-Term Care Ombudsman, Quiteka Moten. She is from Tennessee. She is based in Nashville. She works with the Alzheimer's Association now, establishing rural senior networks, training first responders, and managing early-stage engagement programs.

And then Tamara Konetzka, Louis Block professor of public health in the Department of Public Health Sciences at the University of Chicago. She serves on a number of Federal boards. She received her Ph.D. from the University of North Carolina. We are very glad to have her because we have seen her renowned scholarship, and we look forward to her presentation.

So, let's begin with Ms. Ramos.

Statement of Adelina Ramos, Certified Nursing Assistant, Seiu District 1199 New England, Greenville, RI

Ms. RAMOS. Thank you, Mr. Chairman, Ranking Member Crapo, and the members of the Senate community. My name is Adelina Ramos. I am a CNA at a nursing home in Greenville, RI. I am a proud immigrant from the Cape Verde Islands off the western coast of Africa.

At my facility, I work with Alzheimer's patients. To be trusted by families to care for their loved ones is a great honor. But over the past year, my days have been filled with fear and sadness.

I do not think anyone in my small community thought that COVID–19 would arrive at our doorstep. But it did, and nursing homes were not prepared. When COVID first hit, we lost over 20 residents in just over a month—and a CNA died too.

We confronted management to let them know we did not have enough PPE or enough training to keep our residents safe and to prevent the virus from spreading in our facility.

We are extremely short-staffed too. At one point, I was caring for 26 critically ill residents with the help of only one other CNA, a nurse, and a housekeeper. They could not eat, drink, or move by themselves. Some of them required oxygen changes every 15 minutes. And because they had Alzheimer's, sometimes they would get scared.

I was horrified. We begged management for more staff on each shift, but they said they could not find anyone. And so our residents and staff kept getting sick and dying.

The day after Mother's Day, I realized I could not smell my ginger tea. I thought it was because of my mask. But a few weeks later, I got symptoms and I had COVID. I did not have other symptoms, so I did not know, and I put those around me at risk. I never thought I would have to tell my son to stay away from me, don't touch me, don't hug me, don't get too close. I would never be able to forgive myself if I infected him, so I did what I had to do to keep him safe.

Today, I am COVID-free and vaccinated, and I am holding my family close. And I am working to educate others about how important it is to get vaccinated. Things are looking up, but the physical and emotional trauma this pandemic caused cannot be cured with a shot in the arm.

When I started working at a nursing home, I understood I would have residents pass away. In their final moments, our job is to make sure they are comfortable, cared for, and surrounded by loved ones. The family members could not come into our facility. The funeral homes could not come either, because they did not have enough PPE. So we became the mortician and had to put bodies into body bags.

My residents deserved so much better than what we were able to provide them, with few staff and resources. As they took their final, difficult breath, I hope they knew that we tried our best.

The starting wage for Rhode Island nursing home workers is just $12.34. Some of us have to work multiple jobs to meet our basic needs. Because of these actions, we do not have time to spend with the residents when they need us.

My worst day during COVID was when one of my residents was dying and wanted me to sit and hold her hand, but I could not stay because I had 20-plus other residents who also needed me.

I feel a calling to do this job and care for others, but passion cannot pay bills. I am fortunate that I am a member of my union, SEIU 1199 New England. We negotiated higher wages and pandemic pay. We were able to advocate for ourselves and residents, but not every nursing home worker has a union.

This issue existed before COVID. COVID–19 just exposed the most tragic and deadly part of nursing home work. It is why I keep fighting for a $15 minimum wage in the union for all workers.

This pandemic has shown us what happens when we are not prepared to meet the demands for care. We must build back better so that when the time comes when your loved one needs care—and that time will come for all of us—someone like me will be there to answer your call.

[The prepared statement of Ms. Ramos appears in the appendix.]

The CHAIRMAN. Ms. Ramos, thank you. And we wanted you to speak first because we felt that you could really give us a sense of what this was like on the floor where patients lived, and the challenge. And we knew you were going to give us an important presentation. And thank you, thank you, thank you, because you are speaking for so many this morning.

Our next speaker will be Denise Bottcher, and, let's see, there is Ms. Bottcher. Please proceed.

Statement of Denise Bottcher, State Director, AARP Louisiana, Baton Rouge, LA

Ms. BOTTCHER. Good morning, Chairman Wyden, Ranking Member Crapo, and members of the committee. My name is Denise Bottcher, and I am State director for AARP of Louisiana. On behalf of our 38 million members—including over 425,000 in Louisiana— and all older Americans nationwide, AARP appreciates the opportunity to provide testimony at today's hearing.

The situation in our Nation's nursing homes and other long-term care facilities has been alarming since the first COVID outbreak in Washington State. AARP has heard from thousands of people who have lost loved ones, and that is why, across the Nation, AARP has advocated for the health, safety, and well-being of residents and staff.

As has been mentioned, over 175,000 long-term care facility residents and staff have died. And that includes almost 3,000 in Louisiana. This represents about 35 percent of deaths nationwide. While there may be a sense of relief with vaccines rolling out and infection rates declining, much more is needed to protect nursing home residents.

The consequence of not acting is that someone's mother or father dies. One resounding message I have received from families across Louisiana is this: if 175,000 deaths does not inspire bold action, then nothing will.

AARP has urged action in a five-point plan to protect the health and safety of residents.

First, ensure facilities have adequate personal protective equipment for everyone at the facility, and ensure its consistent and proper use, as well as prioritizing testing.

Yesterday I had the opportunity to visit with Mark Ferguson in Lake Charles, LA. His 86-year-old dad and 63-year-old brother lived in the same nursing home. And every week he visited with his dad and brother through a window. And each time, he observed staff not wearing masks or gloves.

He told me he felt helpless in this moment because it was a matter of life and death. The only thing he could do was call and report it to the administrator. The following week, he would again visit, and the staff were not properly wearing PPE. He eventually lost his dad to COVID, and he still fights this battle today.

I asked him what keeps him up at night, and he told me the health and safety of his brother Scott. It is unacceptable for facilities to have PPE shortages a year into the pandemic.

AARP's second point: continue to improve transparency. We believe care facilities should publicly report cases and deaths daily, rather than weekly. That reporting should include demographic data such as race and ethnicity.

Information about the number and percentage of residents and staff who have been vaccinated should be available by facility and State. We urge the Federal Government to work with States and long-term care facilities to ensure they can access and administer vaccines to new residents and staff as needed.

Finally, millions of taxpayer dollars from the Provider Relief Fund have gone to facilities to fight COVID. AARP strongly urges that the administration and Congress ensure that these funds are directly used for the health, safety, and care of residents and staff. AARP's third point is to ensure safe access to in-person visitation, following Federal and State guidelines, and to require continued access to facilitated virtual visitation for all residents.

Our fourth point is to ensure quality care for residents through adequate staffing and oversight. We are deeply concerned about staffing shortages at facilities—and even before the pandemic. According to AARP's Nursing Home Dashboard, over 25 percent of nursing homes across the Nation have reported a staffing shortage since June of 2020. Residents' health and safety are at continued risk without adequate staffing.

Finally, oversight and enforcement are a shared responsibility between Federal and State agencies. Oversight from CMS and State survey agencies, including regular annual surveys, is vital now more than ever.

AARP 's final point is to reject immunity and hold long-term care facilities accountable when they fail to provide adequate care to residents.

You know, when I speak to folks, young and old, about how they want to live their lives, an overwhelming majority tell me they want to live at home for as long as possible with the support of family and friends. Helping people to remain in their homes and communities would help alleviate some of the challenges we are facing in our Nation's nursing homes. This includes supporting family caregivers who make it possible.

Families across the country are looking to Congress and the administration for swift action to protect the health and safety of their loved ones living in long-term care facilities now, and well into the future. We cannot wait any longer.

Thank you.

[The prepared statement of Ms. Bottcher appears in the appendix.]

The CHAIRMAN. Thank you.

Let's go next to Ms. Moten, the Ombudsman. Ms. Moten, welcome.

Statement of Quiteka Moten, MPH, CDP, State Long-Term Care Ombudsman, Commission on Aging and Disability, State of Tennessee, Nashville, TN

Ms. MOTEN. Thank you. Good morning.

Thank you, Chairman Wyden, Ranking Member Crapo, and distinguished members of the committee. I am Teka Moten, State Long-Term Care Ombudsman for Tennessee.

I am honored to discuss my experiences, challenges, and lessons learned while serving residents during COVID. I want to first thank you for CARES funding and American Recovery

Act funding. It has greatly assisted in the provision of programs and activities, as well as the procurement of equipment and PPE in this time.

I sit before you as a Certified Dementia Practitioner, trainer, and coach, as well as a former volunteer Ombudsman. I have spent the entirety of my career in public service—specifically, Asian programs and policies.

I began as State Ombudsman of Tennessee January 17, 2020. I had less than 60 days to learn my role, staff, and major stakeholders prior to the lockdown. Coincidentally enough, there was also a tornado that affected the Nashville area and the upper Cumberland region, and this affected a number of long-term care homes.

Swedish for the term "representative of the people," the Ombudsman Program is an essential component to the oversight of long-term care facilities. We operate as a community-based at-the-bedside advocacy program for the rights of residents.

We handle complaint investigations as laid out by the CMP State Operations Manual. The major components of the Ombudsman Program, fortified by the Older Americans Act, include a mandated quarterly visit to our nursing homes by staff Ombudsmen, and regular visits to communities by trained and designated volunteer Ombudsmen who, at the average age of 70, are very much a vital and integral part of our program.

COVID, alongside ensuing policies, disrupted the Ombudsman Program's immediate access to residents. The inability to have face-to-face meetings made it difficult to verify complaints, assure confidentiality, and to readily gain consent for the medical surrogates or POAs.

In addition, it made it difficult for us to advocate on behalf of residents being discharged against their wishes, oftentimes leaving them in behavioral health or medical centers with the risk of losing their Medicaid. Particularly affected by these major barriers are people living with dementia, those who are aphasic or unable to speak, those who are deaf or hard of hearing but have assisted technology needs, those without the manual dexterity to pick up the phone, and those with that ability who were without a phone or had to purchase their own.

Residents in fact were not silent. Lack of staffing and inability to be with their families silenced them. But staffing issues were nothing new in the most-regulated industry in this country.

Nursing homes were already dealing with a workforce shortage, and COVID exacerbated that issue further. Staff members got sick, as you have already heard. Many had to quarantine, and some faced a lack of child care options.

What resulted was an overall decline in the quality of care that our residents received. Throughout the country, Ombudsmen received complaints of dehydration, unanswered call lights, a lack of basic care and assistance—cleaning, bathing, feeding—but most identifiable probably, a lack of repositioning, which left residents in the bed, resulting in an exponential increase in bed sores.

Unchanged catheters and pressure sores resulted in sepsis, and sometimes death, for our residents. There are issues of dignity and hygiene stemming from residents having to sit in their own feces and urine for hours on end, delayed discharges to hospitals for serious conditions, access and transport issues to dialysis and other appointments, and an uptake in facility-initiated hospice.

Residents dealing with COVID, its reoccurrence, testing, and room changes had to deal with resident isolation. This led to emotional distress and physical decline.

I can remember, vividly, calls from skilled rehab residents who would recount their experience in facilities. For me, the toughest part was knowing that if we received calls to our hotline on the weekend and the evenings, it was more than likely it was a resident who knew that there were going to be less staff in the building.

Worried family members also shared their concerns for unkempt residents as they looked on in discontentment at disheveled hair, unbrushed teeth, and filthy fingernails. This added to our task of helping family caregivers adapt to a different type of caregiver's role, especially for those moving into a facility in the midst of COVID.

But for those who would take their final breaths in nursing homes, the term "compassionate care" altogether presented another set of challenges for us in dealing with the discretion of facilities.

Ombudsmen have worked tirelessly throughout the last year. Ideally, the worst has subsided, yet the fact remains that residents of long-term care make up less than 1 percent of the U.S. population, but as of March 4, 2021, they account for 34 percent of all deaths in America.

As we move forward, it is my hope that we can lean on a few actionable items: for facilities, a comprehensive plan for recruiting and retaining staff; for the Ombudsman Program, consideration as an essential part of a system that responds to and supports the safety and welfare of residents, regardless of any status the State may bestow upon them; and last but not least, for the residents remaining in our facilities, the loving embrace of family, friends, pets, and a return to some version of normalcy.

[The prepared statement of Ms. Moten appears in the appendix.]

The CHAIRMAN. Thank you, very much.

Our final two witnesses will be John Dicken, Director of Health Care at the Government Accountability Office, where he has worked since 1991. He oversees a portfolio of audits on health-care questions, and he has been before us before, and we appreciate it.

And then we will close with Dr. David Gifford, an M.D. and a master of public health, chief medical officer of the American Health Care Association and a geriatrician.

But first, let us proceed now to Dr. Konetzka.

Statement of R. Tamara Konetzka, Ph.D., Louis Block Professor, Department of Public Health Sciences, Biological Sciences Division, University of Chicago, Chicago, IL

Dr. KONETZKA. Chairman Wyden, Ranking Member Crapo, and distinguished members of the committee, thank you for holding this hearing.

My name is Tamara Konetzka. I am a professor of health economics at the University of Chicago, and I have been conducting research on long-term and post-acute care for more than 25 years. I have intensely studied COVID–19 in nursing homes during this pandemic. I will focus my remarks on what we have learned from research, followed by recommendations.

First, what do we know about the predictors of nursing home cases and deaths? A large body of evidence shows that the two strongest and most consistent predictors of worst COVID–19 outcomes are larger nursing home size and COVID–19 prevalence in the surrounding community.

Given two similar nursing homes with an outbreak, being in a virus hotspot is associated with five more deaths. Equally important are nursing home attributes that are not linked with COVID–19 outcomes.

Multiple rigorous studies have found no meaningful association between COVID–19 outcomes and standard quality metrics. Even prior infection control citations were not associated with COVID–19 outcomes. These results suggest that high quality and good infection control are not enough in this pandemic.

The numbers bear this out. At this point, more than 99 percent of nursing homes in the Nation have had at least one COVID–19 case. And more than 80 percent have had at least one death. This is clearly not a bad apples problem, and no subset of nursing homes has found a magic bullet to keep the virus out.

The single most important thing we could have done as a Nation to reduce the tragedy in nursing homes over the past year was to use public health measures to control the spread of the virus in the general population.

Second, what about disparities? As Chairman Wyden mentioned, our research found striking disparities by race. Nursing homes serving more residents of color experienced more than three times as many COVID–19 cases and deaths as those serving primarily white residents.

Why? Most of the disparity can be explained by what race is correlated with. Residents of color are more likely to live in larger facilities in neighborhoods where COVID–19 is prevalent.

Third, are there any predictors of bad outcomes that are more amenable to change? In the often-contentious world of nursing home policy, it is difficult to find things that everyone agrees on, but here is one. On average, nursing homes lack sufficient numbers of staff to provide the quality of care we would all like to receive.

In our research, we found that having more staff did not reduce the probability of a COVID–19 outbreak, but nursing homes with the most staff hours experienced fewer deaths and cases once an outbreak occurred.

The effects of staffing are still dwarfed by the effect of community spread. But increasing staffing represents a clear intervention that could improve care and save lives during this pandemic and beyond.

This evidence base suggests several policy recommendations moving forward.

First, policies implemented during the past year that reward or fine facilities based on COVID deaths are not appropriate in a crisis. Instead, I strongly support the allocation of American Rescue Plan funds to provide strike teams to rapidly fill staffing gaps during an outbreak.

Second, we must provide greater assistance to large facilities in communities of color. Such facilities do not typically earn performance bonuses, but may be most in need of resources.

Third, the American Rescue Plan put substantial funding into improving infection control. Although improvement is certainly necessary, we should recognize that this is a solution to a relatively narrow set of problems, a solution that would not have avoided the tragedy of the past year.

Fourth, CMS should immediately release facility-specific data on vaccination dates and rates and demographics, including race and ethnicities, essential for both research and policy. Consumers who are considering nursing home care also have a right to know what percent of residents and staff have been vaccinated.

Finally, direct-care staffing in nursing homes needs to be increased. Addressing this challenge requires resources, which is where the agreement about staffing ends and the harder problems begin.

Many argue—and I largely agree—that America's long-term care system is grossly underfunded. At the same time, the growing role of related-party transactions and private-equity ownership makes it difficult to see where taxpayer money is being spent, and what profit margins truly are. Greater transparency about the flow of money is urgently needed.

We will never achieve adequate nursing home quality unless we find a way to support the workforce. In addition to low pay and few benefits, the job of direct-care nursing staff is difficult, often dangerous, and emotionally and physically taxing. Add the risk of a potentially fatal infectious disease, and it is amazing they show up. Addressing this challenge is the best way to honor the memory of the more than 1,900 nursing home workers and all the residents who have died from COVID thus far. We cannot turn back the clock to prevent the tragedy of the past year. We can at least take steps to learn from it.

Thank you.

[The prepared statement of Dr. Konetzka appears in the appendix.]

The CHAIRMAN. Thank you very much.

Our next speaker will be John Dicken.

Statement of John E. Dicken, Director, Health Care, Government Accountability Office, Washington, DC

Mr. DICKEN. Well, good morning, Chairman Wyden, Ranking Member Crapo, and members of the committee. Thank you for the opportunity to discuss with you findings and recommendations on the Federal response to COVID–19 in nursing homes.

As characterized in the title of today's hearing, and as we have heard this morning, the last year has indeed been a national tragedy for nursing home residents and their loved ones. Just over a year ago, a Washington State nursing home was battling one of the first major outbreaks of COVID in the United States.

Today, the pandemic has reached nearly all nursing homes in the country. More than 130,000 nursing home residents have died from COVID–19, representing nearly 30 percent of all COVID–19 deaths recorded by the CDC as of early February.

Even for those nursing home residents not infected, nearly all have faced increased isolation and restrictions from loved ones. The pandemic has also posed tremendous challenges to the homes and their staffs. Notably, more than half a million nursing home staff themselves have contracted COVID–19.

In response to this unprecedented national emergency, HHS has taken a series of actions. These include providing guidance to States and nursing homes, developing targeted inspections to focus on infection control practices, and distributing testing devices and vaccines to homes.

GAO continues to evaluate the Federal response to the pandemic in nursing homes as part of a series of comprehensive reports to Congress on the government-wide response. My statement states a few key findings and recommendations from these reviews during the pandemic, as well as our longer-term work examining nursing home oversight prior to the pandemic.

With the ongoing administration of vaccines to nursing home residents and staff, nursing homes may be beginning to see a reprieve, as cases and deaths declined by more than 80 percent as of February from their peaks in December.

Just last week, CMS updated its guidance to expand resident visitations. This issue has posed an ongoing challenge in providing residents the ability to have visitors—which can benefit their overall mental and physical health—and minimizing further COVID–19 outbreaks.

Other challenges nursing homes have faced in battling COVID– 19 include obtaining personal protective equipment and conducting COVID–19 tests. Although these challenges are still notable, they have generally shown signs of improvement.

Some new challenges have also emerged, such as reluctance among some staff to receive a COVID–19 vaccine, and the need for continuous vigilance with the emergence of more highly transmittable virus variants.

GAO has made two recommendations specific to HHS's response to nursing homes to date. The first recommendation is for HHS to develop a strategy for having more complete data on COVID cases and deaths in nursing homes, which were only voluntarily reported until last May.

The second recommendation is to more systematically develop a plan detailing if and how the Centers for Medicare and Medicaid Services will respond to remaining recommendations from a commission appointed by former Administrator Verma and publicly reported last September.

To date, CMS has not yet implemented these recommendations. We maintain the importance of these recommendations to better inform the government's continued response.

We also made a number of recommendations to improve nursing home oversight, as work completed prior to the pandemic, that have yet to be implemented. For example, less than 2 years ago I testified before this committee regarding GAO's report on the abuse occurring in nursing homes. That report made six recommendations to CMS, including that CMS require State surveyor agencies to immediately notify law enforcement of any reasonable suspicion of a crime against a resident.

These recommendations are particularly relevant during the COVID–19 pandemic because, with reduced visitors, Ombudsmen, and State surveyor presence, there may be a higher risk of abuse going unreported.

In closing, GAO's recommendations could help address some of the challenges nursing homes continue to face, and fill important gaps in the Federal Government's understanding of, and transparency around, data on COVID–19 in nursing homes.

Going forward, the spotlight that COVID–19 has placed on the vulnerability of nursing home residents may be best used to inform future pandemic responses and refocus on longstanding challenges that place nursing home residents' health and safety at risk.

This completes my prepared statement.

[The prepared statement of Mr. Dicken appears in the appendix.] The CHAIRMAN. Thank you very much, Mr. Dicken.

Dr. Gifford?

Statement of David Gifford, M.D., MPH, Chief Medical Officer, American Health Care Association/National Center for Assisted Living, Washington, DC

Dr. GIFFORD. Chairman Wyden, Ranking Member Crapo, and distinguished members of the Senate, thank you for making long-term care providers a priority as you examine how COVID–19 has impacted the Nation, and for providing our association the opportunity to share our members' challenges during the pandemic.

AHCA represents over 14,000 nursing homes and assisted living communities across the country, including not-for-profit, for-profit, and government facilities. As a geriatrician, I can attest that COVID–19 is the greatest tragedy ever to impact our residents and their families.

Over 635,000 residents have been infected, and more than 130,000 have died, worse than any other infection or disease we have faced. This virus has also affected health-care workers, with over half a million becoming infected, and thousands dying.

As you know, our residents are at the highest risk for COVID– 19 complications. More than half are over the age of 85 and suffer from multiple chronic diseases. Residents depend on our nurses, our aides, support staff—including housekeepers—to help them with their daily activities that require close one-on-one contact like eating, getting dressed, and bathing.

COVID–19 has impacted every aspect of long-term care. For nearly a year, family members were unable to visit. Residents could not leave their room. They could not see the smiles of the nurses and aides caring for them, hidden behind their masks.

Our dedicated staff did everything they could to keep residents safe, engaged, and happy. Meanwhile, they constantly worried about becoming ill or infecting their family, as Ms. Ramos clearly described.

Our hearts go out to the residents, their families, and the healthcare workers who have suffered through the past year, separated from each other, in some cases forever.

Why did such devastation happen in long-term care? The timeline in my written testimony demonstrates how our knowledge of this virus continually evolved, but the public health advice could not keep up, and as a result, it was typically too late.

For example, initial guidance was focused on a symptom-based approach that we know is ineffective, since half the people spreading the virus do not have symptoms. But guidance for mask-wearing for all staff did not come until June, 4 months into the pandemic.

Compounding these challenges was the failure to make nursing homes a priority. Despite numerous calls for help, it took months to receive much-needed PPE. In many circumstances, staff had to use their ingenuity to make their own masks, gowns, and face shields.

I recall getting a call one weekend asking if rain ponchos worked better as gowns than trash bags. As we now know, COVID–19 outbreaks in nursing homes are principally driven by how many people in the surrounding community have COVID, as Dr. Konetzka testified.

But testing kits needed to detect asymptomatic carriers of the virus were not provided to nursing homes until almost 6 months into the pandemic. As a result, staff in these communities, often unwittingly, brought COVID–19 in the building.

With these delays, even the best nursing homes with the most rigorous infection control practices could not stop this highly contagious virus. The long-term care community was left behind, forgotten, and even blamed. This further demoralized the staff, who were risking their lives and trying their best—with inadequate support.

It is critical that we determine what we can do to keep this from ever happening again. We must reflect on the challenges within the long-term care profession that this pandemic has exposed and exacerbated.

We recognize that providers can and must do better to meet the needs of the elderly. Prior to COVID–19—and only made worse by the pandemic—the long-term care facilities struggled to attract and retain a highly dedicated workforce, particularly registered nurses, who are most in need during an infectious disease outbreak. Our ability to find nurses and other caregivers is correlated with the lack of availability and proper funding.

As many academic experts have highlighted, chronic Medicaid under-funding makes it a challenge for providers to compete with hospitals for nurses and make infrastructure changes.

What we have learned from this tragedy is that it will take considerable investment to make meaningful changes. We stand ready to work with policy-makers and others to take bold action. Earlier this week, AHCA and LeadingAge together announced the Care for Our Seniors Act, a set of proposals focused on clinical improvements, strengthening and supporting our workforce, improving oversight—particularly for chronically poor-performing facilities— and modernizing our physical structures.

The good news is that nursing home residents and staff were made a priority to receive the remarkably safe and effective COVID–19 vaccine. As a result, cases and deaths have declined dramatically since mid-December. Making them a priority for the vaccine demonstrates the power of putting long-term care and our Nation's seniors first during emergencies.

On behalf of the staff and the residents in nursing homes around the country, I would like to thank the Senate and the members of this committee for your dedication and leadership during this pandemic.

We look forward to working with you on implementing constructive solutions to combat COVID–19 and usher in a strong long-term care system.

[The prepared statement of Dr. Gifford appears in the appendix.]

The CHAIRMAN. Thank you, Dr. Gifford. And all of you have been excellent.

I am going to begin my questioning with you, Ms. Ramos, because I was listening to what you said, and it was clear you too are at the center of this collision of mismanagement. You talked about the under-staffing issue. You talked about the problems getting PPE, protective equipment. You mentioned the fact that you all were in the dark with respect to getting information.

And I think, apropos of information, I heard you say that there was concern among health-care workers—and you, initially—about getting vaccinated. Do you think getting more good information out, particularly in communities of color, about the success of vaccinations, would really be helpful?

Ms. RAMOS. Yes. I had to do my own research. I was scared to get vaccinated. I talked to my union rep about the vaccine, and I got the information. But I think most of my co-workers, they felt the same way I did. They did not want to be guinea pigs of the system, because what we went through was horrible. We did not get the help that we needed, and we felt like the companies just wanted us to be the guinea pigs.

But if there is more information in the community—because we all have different backgrounds, we all speak different languages, and we come from everywhere—so if there are more resources in the community that they trust, it would be easier for them to get vaccinated.

So they should talk to the church members, or somebody who speaks their language, to the leaders of the communities, to help them out.

The CHAIRMAN. You know, your point is so logical, it is almost like you are being too logical for Washington, DC, because you should not have to be a private eye to get this information. So we are going to follow up with you on that. And again, I just so appreciate your leadership.

Dr. Konetzka, let me turn to you. I am very appreciative of the fact you mentioned the strike teams, because I think they are extraordinarily important in bringing the expertise to this issue. We had a floor fight during our 24-hour day where we had to defend it, and fortunately we prevailed.

I would like you to amplify on your concern, because I share it, about private equity getting more involved in the field. Because my concern is—and I heard Ms. Ramos make another point, that she is concerned that all they are interested in is money and the like. This trend towards more private equity looks to me like something that the Finance Committee should be digging into. And I thought maybe you could amplify on your statement.

Dr. KONETZKA. I agree. I think it would be a good thing if the Finance Committee could look into this. The increasing role of private equity in nursing homes, along with other complex arrangements like the related-party transactions, is a problem.

There is really interesting recent research showing that nursing homes bought by private equity subsequently have higher revenues, but lower staffing and worse patient outcomes. And when those revenues are coming from public funds, this is not acceptable. And I think regulators have been reluctant to interfere with ownership transactions in the industry, an industry that is mostly for-profit, but it may be time to do so—at least in the sense of transparency.

So we should think about assistance, or potentially increasing reimbursement rates so that we at least know where the money is going, even the current reimbursement rates.

The CHAIRMAN. We are going to be calling on you again on this issue, because it seems to me this is an area that has not gotten the oversight and the accountability that is needed. And I am glad that you have lit this concern up in front of the Senate Finance Committee.

A question for you, Ms. Moten, and I so appreciate your Ombudsman role. When I was director of the Gray Panthers, we worked with the Ombudsmen. And dollar for dollar, you all make such a big difference.

We have been reading about how these rating systems are not doing a particularly good job of rating. What would you do with these and have, as counsel for the Finance Committee, some direction at improving them?

Ms. MOTEN. You know, honestly I am not exactly certain what I would do to change the rating system. I think that a lot of what we see as Ombudsmen is that facilities are on their best behavior when help is in the building oftentimes.

And so I think that some more impromptu approaches to that will probably be the best way to work through those issues.

The CHAIRMAN. Well, three cheers for getting us started on that because, when I was on the nursing home board, if they knew you were coming, everything was perfect. And that is a very important suggestion. We will call on you again.

All right, I am over my time. And our next member, we see our friend, Senator Crapo.

Senator CRAPO. Thank you very much, Mr. Chairman.

And I will start with you, Mr. Dicken. In your testimony, you mentioned a statistic, if I got it right, that the deaths in nursing homes had gone down by 80 percent by February. Could you give me that correct statistic again? And if that is generally correct, could you tell me, do you have an idea as to what we can attribute that reduction to?

Mr. DICKEN. Yes. Thank you, Ranking Member Crapo. And you do have it correct. What we have seen from reporting from HHS is that, from the peak of cases and deaths in nursing homes in December until reporting early last month, the cases and rates have declined by 80 percent. And we are pleased that that decline has continued even beyond early February.

Certainly, you know, we are continuing to evaluate kind of what those factors are. There is still a need for continued vigilance. That is a sharper rate of decline than we have seen throughout the broader community. There have been declines in cases and rates outside of nursing homes, and while it does seem to be sharper, certainly the prioritization of vaccinations of nursing home residents and staff is a key thing to look at in why it is an even faster decline in the rates recently for nursing homes.

Senator CRAPO. Well, thank you. It seems to me that something must be being very helpful. Something is working. And we need to identify exactly what that is. And so I would appreciate your assistance in that.

GAO has issued at least four reports regarding the Federal and State response to COVID–19 in nursing homes. And I do not want to use up all my time on this, because I have a few other questions for others, but you mentioned that Seema Verma had issued some recommendations that have not yet been implemented. And I believe that GAO has made a number of recommendations in its report.

Could you pick just a couple, like one or two of the most important recommendations you think are yet to be implemented and need to be?

Mr. DICKEN. Yes, and I will be brief. As you noted, the former CMS Administrator had a commission that made over 27 recommendations on ways, both short-term and long-term, that CMS could help respond to the pandemic.

CMS took a number of steps, but we have recommended that they do a more systematic plan on how they can more fully continue to draw from the expertise of the commission that was appointed, and we would recommend that that would help improve the Federal response.

The other one I would highlight is that the data is very important for oversight, and for transparency, and that prior to May, that was voluntary. And we recommend that CMS identify a strategy to have more complete data for the early months of the pandemic. That is very important not only for ongoing response, but for understanding lessons from the pandemic over the course of time.

Senator CRAPO. Well, thank you. We want to work with you, and with all of our witnesses. I know our Ombudsman—and I will not be able to get to you in my questioning—but there are a lot of recommendations out there from all of you.

We need to know what is working and what needs to be done better, and I encourage you to give us that information.

I would like to move quickly to Dr. Gifford. Doctor, how did the AHCA respond to certain State directives mandating that long-term care facilities admit active COVID–19 cases?

Dr. GIFFORD. Well, thank you, Senator Crapo, for that. I think, as we heard from Ms. Ramos and others, there was just chaos in May and April. The nursing homes were terrified of this COVID. Families were terrified. Staff were terrified. And hospitals were terrified.

We saw in some cities, you know, lines forming in hospitals, and creating intensive care units in the parking lot in tents. And so there was sort of a lot of trying to figure out what was going on out there. And as a result, we saw variations and different recommendations that were out there.

Nursing homes typically play an important role in emergencies in that they take on patients out of the hospital to free up hospital beds to deal with the emergencies. In this situation, though, freeing up the beds and taking people out of the hospital could potentially lead to further spread, and so that was sort of a worrying concern that we had. But we realized we needed to play a role in the health-care decision, because any decision that was going to be made was going to have dire consequences.

If you decide not to move people out of the hospitals, you move people into parking lots. If you move people into nursing homes, you might create spread. And our position was to try to create special units and make sure there was enough PPE and enough staff that were out there that was really lacking. And I think you have heard that from the testimony that was out here so far.

Senator CRAPO. Well, thank you. I see my time has run out. It runs out quickly. For those of you whom I did not get to, I will submit some written questions to you. And I would really welcome your responses to these. Thank you very much.

Thanks, Mr. Chairman.

The CHAIRMAN. Thank you, Senator Crapo.

Senator Stabenow?

Senator STABENOW. Well, thank you very much, Mr. Chairman, for doing this very, very important hearing. And I think we all know this last year has been a horrible situation. And we have to say this started with a lack of seriousness by the former President and the lack of action by the administration. And certainly that has been something that we have seen where, in nursing homes, it has played itself out in a very, very serious way.

High-quality staff are what make high-quality nursing homes. And a recent report, as has been said, found that the average yearly turnover rate for nursing home staff was 128 percent. So 128 percent means the average staff completely turned over in a year. And some nursing homes had staff that changed over every few months, which is a very, very serious issue, obviously.

Ms. Ramos, first of all I want to thank you for your incredible work, particularly over the past year. I am really in awe of your courage and your resolve, as well as the colleagues that you work with.

You said at one point you were caring for 26 critically ill patients. Can you talk a little bit more about the impact of staff turnover on patient care?

Ms. RAMOS. Thank you for your question. So on the Mother's Day of last year, we had critically ill patients with COVID. They were all in bed. So there was me and another aide for 26 residents, and a nurse and a housekeeper.

We had to, you know, check their temperature, check their oxygen every 15 minutes. I was in an Alzheimer's unit, so it was very challenging, because our residents kept taking off their masks. So we kept going to their rooms because the oxygen was dropping, because they could not keep their masks on.

So the quality of care, it was horrible. We were only two CNAs. And most of our residents were in bed. We could not sit there with them and talk to them while they were dying. We could not keep them hydrated when we knew that that was a part of it, that you had to keep them hydrated because they could not hold a glass of water.

So we had to pick and choose, which is a thing that we have to do all the time—this did not start with COVID. So sometimes we have to pick and choose who are the critical residents for us to assist first. And that is a thing we do every day. And I do not think we should be put in that position where we constantly have to pick and choose what resident to care for, because we love them. We care for them. And the quality of care that they deserve is not there right now.

Senator STABENOW. Well, and from your perspective—this sounds horrible, trying to figure this out when you can, and I am sure you are doing everything you can to care for people. From your perspective and your experience, what are the main reasons that nurses and CNAs leave their jobs at nursing homes?

Ms. RAMOS. Well, we do not want to leave our jobs. I had a thought, you know, during this pandemic. I was like, "I cannot do this anymore." But then I said to myself, "You know, right now is when they need me the most." So why would I leave them when the family members cannot come in? So I got up, sticking it out, and went back to work, because they need me.

The reason why a lot of CNAs and nurses leave nursing homes is because the workload is a lot. We are constantly working short-staffed, and we, the CNAs, we make low wages. And we have to work in multiple nursing homes to pay our bills.

So we do not want to leave nursing homes, but we have to do what we have to do for our families.

Senator STABENOW. Of course. And I hear over and over again from our nursing homes that are really doing quality work as well, that not having enough nurses, right, and CNAs, is also, along with pay structure, really an issue.

One of the things right now is, staff turnover information is not made public, and it seems to me that that would be important for patients and families.

So if I might ask, Dr. Konetzka—you are on the Technical Expert Panel that advises CMS. Do you agree this information should be made public?

Dr. KONETZKA. Yes. I think turnover information is really important. There is a large body of literature tying higher turnover to worse patient outcomes in nursing homes. So I think that information could be useful.

I think there are bigger gaps in terms of what we report, such as quality of life and customer satisfaction. But knowing turnover could be helpful to consumers.

Senator STABENOW. Thank you. And then just finally—I know I am running out of time—but, Dr. Konetzka, in your opening statement you included recent findings that nursing homes with higher proportions of non-white residents experienced death counts three times higher than those facilities with higher proportions of white residents.

So, like in many other areas, we have seen longstanding racial disparities put under bright lights, under COVID, certainly. But could you, based on your research—what would your recommendations be to address this?

Dr. KONETZKA. I would divide that into short-term and long-term recommendations. I think in the short term, we need to make sure the assistance gets to those facilities and communities of color, because they are the ones experiencing the worst outcomes. So strike teams, for example—we have to make sure they get to those facilities.

I would say also with vaccinations, we do not have the data to know this. The data need to be released. But we need to make sure that vaccination is equitable, and that people in nursing homes in communities of color, and people out in the community in those same neighborhoods, get vaccinated.

The CHAIRMAN. This is an incredibly important topic, and we are going to return to it. We just have to move on because we have so many other Senators waiting.

Senator STABENOW. Thank you.

The CHAIRMAN. Our next Senator is Senator Grassley.

[No response.]

The CHAIRMAN. No Senator Grassley.

Senator Cantwell is next.

Senator CANTWELL. Thank you, Mr. Chairman. Thank you for holding this important hearing.

The State of Washington was one of the first States to record the impact of the COVID–19 virus. And many people may remember, on February 10th the Life Care Center in Kirkland, WA reported an outbreak of COVID–19 within the facility that ultimately would claim 46 lives.

In the State of Washington, nearly half of the reported deaths have been in long-term care facilities. That is why in the American Rescue Plan there is included $750 million of support for nursing homes and skilled nursing facilities, including $500 million for strike teams and $200 million for infection control. This was something my colleague, Senator Casey, in his leadership made part of the COVID–19 Nursing Home Protection Act, which I also co-sponsored with him, which was very important legislation.

This, I believe, is critical, so I would like to ask Dr. Konetzka how this utilization of both strike teams and staffing issues can help protect nursing home residents during these times of major outbreaks?

Dr. KONETZKA. Thank you for that question. I think the strike teams are essential. I think they have been a good tool all along for States that have decided to do that. The problem is that nursing homes, even prior to the pandemic, were often under-staffed. And the pandemic exacerbated that, for all the reasons we have been talking about.

Staff were sometimes getting sick, or afraid to bring the virus home to their families, or needed to stay home with kids who were learning online. And so you really could not implement the best practices that we now know can address a COVID outbreak, such as testing all residents as soon as there is a case in the facility, such as separating residents and assigning dedicated staff to COVID-positive versus COVID-negative residents so they do not have to go back and forth between the two.

All of those things take staff. And in the short run, we cannot incentivize facilities into finding more staff and hiring them in the middle of a crisis, in the middle of an outbreak. And so the strike teams are really essential to fill those gaps. Time is essential. Once you have an outbreak, you really need to deal with it immediately. And that is what the strike teams enable.

Senator CANTWELL. Well, my question is, what else can you do in the coordination? I think in this case the pandemic was new to the United States. We were at the very first impact; Life Care Center of Kirkland was at the very first initial impact. In fact, I think the University of Washington stepped in and tried to help, both in identifying and testing, but it was almost that, at that point, we needed more leadership beyond just the facility itself.

So what else should we be doing to consider the coordination with the strike teams of almost, if not global technically, but theoretically global input to help on these crises?

Dr. KONETZKA. Yes, to me this is about policy leadership as well. I think the strike teams have mostly been facilitated through States. And the strike teams need to come, of course, with some coordination and technical assistance.

There needs to be State leadership to identify which nursing homes really need this help, and coordination in getting them there and filling the necessary gaps.

Senator CANTWELL. Do you think we have these protocols in place now?

Dr. KONETZKA. I think it is unclear. I think there are still some things that need to be worked on in terms of overall coordination.

Senator CANTWELL. I think you are right too. That is why I asked the question. I think we really need to think about this in the sense of protocols that need to be established, because this is such a painful experience for everyone. And I think knowing how we could improve upon it in, not just the strike teams but the larger coordinated effort in marrying everything together, I think that would be great.

Thank you so much. Thank you, Mr. Chairman.

The CHAIRMAN. Thank you, Senator Cantwell.

And our next questioner will be Senator Thune.

[No response.]

The CHAIRMAN. Senator Thune, are you out there?

[No response.]

The CHAIRMAN. Senator Menendez?

[No response.]

The CHAIRMAN. Senator Portman?

[No response.]

The CHAIRMAN. Senator Cardin?

[No response.]

The CHAIRMAN. Senator Toomey?

[No response.]

The CHAIRMAN. Senator Brown?

[No response.]

The CHAIRMAN. And I see Senator Cassidy.

Senator CASSIDY. Super. Am I up?

The CHAIRMAN. Yes.

Senator CASSIDY. Good. Let me ask this, because when I speak to providers—I will probably go first with you, Dr. Gifford. I spoke to folks back home who ran nursing homes. They had an incredible problem with staffing during the pandemic. And what they told me is that the initial stimulus checks that were as generous as they were—as we know, about 80 percent of folks were making more money on stimulus checks than they were working—killed their ability to recruit staffing.

Now this does not address the longer-term staffing issues, but it does beg the question of whether or not the decrease in staffing associated with the pandemic could have been associated with government policies which in effect paid more to folks not to work than to work.

Dr. Gifford, any thoughts on that? And then I will probably come back to you, Dr. Konetzka.

Dr. GIFFORD. Thank you, Senator Cassidy. You know, we have heard, I think from all of us, that the workforce is a challenge, and it was exacerbated with COVID. A lot of health-care workers were home sick and could not come in, so that even made it worse.

We did put together a training to train many of the unemployed who were out there, and we had over 200,000 people come through training to be temporary aides, whom we would love to see get into permanent aide positions and move on to become nurses out there.

So there was a lot of demand for people coming in and helping to work. I think a lot of it was more around the licensure and the bureaucratic aspects of getting health-care workers into this sector. That was the biggest challenge that we faced, and we are really thankful for many of the States and the Federal Government for some 1135 waivers to make that more effective.

Senator CASSIDY. And, Dr. Konetzka, it does seem intuitive to me though, that if somebody can make 20 percent more on transfer payments as opposed to working—and if you are doing so, by the way, it suggests that you are kind of economically challenged to begin with—that there was an incentive for folks to retire from the workforce in order to do this.

You are the economist. What are your thoughts?

Dr. KONETZKA. Nobody has collected data on that. I think what I have found anecdotally from talking to people who work in nursing homes is that that really was not a major reason why nursing homes were under-staffed.

And I think when you look at people who work in nursing homes, some of whom are on this panel, people generally have different motivations for doing that work. And you really cannot be in it for the economics solely, if you work in a nursing home for low wages, take care of people, endure sometimes really physically and emotionally taxing work.

So I would guess—although we do not have data on it—that a lot of the workforce shortage had to do with pandemic-related reality—getting sick, having family at home that you do not want to bring the virus to, or having kids at home—plus competition from other sectors. Hospitals were also competing for these same workers——

Senator CASSIDY. So let me ask you——

Dr. KONETZKA [continuing]. So I don't think incentives were a major force.

Senator CASSIDY. Got it. Let me ask you this. Again, if I speak to folks from the industry, they will say that many of them—and we noticed the racial disparity among those affected—that the racial disparity suggests—we do not know for sure—that the nursing homes most impacted were those which are most likely to have Medicaid as a primary payer.

Now to what extent do low reimbursement rates affect the ability of someone to have that extra resiliency required to handle something like a pandemic? I will stay with you, Doctor.

Dr. KONETZKA. Okay. Are you asking about the resiliency of the workers themselves?

Senator CASSIDY. No, the nursing home. The ability to have that kind of redundancy of systems, the extra supplies on hand, the kind of—and really now, I am a doctor. So I walk into an older nursing home, and the rooms are smaller. The halls are more narrow. If you walk into something built for assisted living in which there is a payer mix, in which there is not just Medicaid but there is also private pay, you end up having better facilities, frankly, newer, better kept-up.

So to what degree do low Medicaid reimbursement rates impact the ability of a nursing home to be better prepared for an incident such as we have seen?

Dr. KONETZKA. I think it is a big problem. There is a lot of controversy here. I think that the long-term care system in this country is generally underfunded, and a lot of that is because we depend on Medicaid. And the Medicaid rates in nursing homes in many States are really quite low.

When we look at the high Medicaid facilities, they tend to have the lowest staffing ratios. They tend to have very little slack. They are always putting out yesterday's fires. And when you are hit with something like a pandemic, they are the least likely to be able to deal with it.

Senator CASSIDY. We are over time, so I will ask you a question for the record. If you did a regression analysis controlling for your payer mix being predominantly Medicaid, how much does that obviate the racial aspect of this, knowing that there is somewhat of a correlation between race and being on Medicaid as a primary payer? We are out of time.

And I just want to give a shout-out to Denise from Louisiana. Denise, good to see you. It is always wonderful to see a friend as a panelist.

I yield back.

The CHAIRMAN. I thank my colleague.

Next is Senator Portman.

Senator PORTMAN. Thank you, Mr. Chairman, and thanks for fitting me in. I want to talk a little bit about home and community-based services, and get the reaction from this great panel of witnesses.

In Ohio, about 40 percent of our COVID deaths were in nursing homes. And that is not atypical, unfortunately, around the country. We tend to have a little higher percentage of people in nursing homes than in other States—but 40 percent. This makes it really the focus, and really the worst part of our crisis: 7,000 nursing home residents in Ohio lost their lives over the past year.

It has improved recently, dramatically, because of the vaccinations, and I am excited about that. But in the meantime, it has been a huge problem.

Long-term care of course is really important to ensuring seniors, and people with disabilities, can live meaningful lives. And while nursing homes are essential to our country, as is a long-term care system, they are not the only ones who offer this care.

For years, I championed this push towards home and community-based services, or HCBS, where we can offer long-term care in residential settings that are more personalized and allow beneficiaries to live in their own homes, near to their family and their friends and their familiar surroundings.

This is what we know about HCBS care: it costs less than nursing home care; it produces similar or better outcomes; and people are happier in it. Furthermore, Ohio data has shown that only .3 percent of all beneficiaries with severe disabilities receiving HCBS died of COVID this past year, or about 120 deaths. So it was more successful in avoiding the fatalities with regard to COVID.

Because it works, last year we passed two major efforts that the chair and ranking member and others have supported. I appreciate that. We passed the Ensuring Access to DSPs Act, which allows people on Medicaid to use direct support professionals for HCBS care, to have them assist with their hospital care, to help improve outcomes, and to get them back home quicker.

That was really important, particularly for the disabilities community, and Medicaid helps cover that. We also passed the EMPOWER Care Act, which authorizes the Money Follows the Person program for 3 additional years. I would like to have gone further on that, and again many colleagues on the other side of the aisle have helped on this. But it helped transition people from nursing homes to HCBS care.

My question to the panel is this: when the pandemic was beginning, what could we have done to have better utilized HCBS services to have potentially prevented some of these deaths?

And second, what policy changes should we now consider in order to further promote such services?

And it is open to the panel.

Dr. KONETZKA. I will start. I think it is a—I thank you for your efforts to expand home and community-based care. I dream of a system where the funding mechanisms are smooth between nursing homes and home and community-based care, and people and policy-makers can decide how to target that care appropriately, and people can get care where they would like.

I only caution that it is not a panacea, that we probably will always need nursing homes. And there are some cases in which home and community-based care can lead to worse outcomes. I think we have to be very careful about targeting, but I think that expansion of home and community-based care in a pandemic, or beyond, is critical.

Senator PORTMAN. Thank you.

Mr. Dicken, have you looked into this for GAO?

Mr. DICKEN. Yes; thank you. It is certainly a really important question. I certainly agree that it is important, especially in the sense to make sure that, at any time, people are getting appropriate long-term care in the appropriate setting.

In this area, there is much less Federal information and data on what is occurring in home and community-based settings, or assisted living and nursing homes. I know that today's hearing is focused on some of the limitations on what is known within nursing homes.

You were able to indicate some Ohio-specific information, and there is information at the State level. But many of the same vulnerabilities exist for the population that is at risk, that needs direct support.

And we have heard similar types of challenges, of things like having adequate protective equipment, staffing challenges. So similar types of challenges may be less of a problem in a congregate setting, in some other settings. But also there is much less information at the Federal level on what is occurring in settings outside of nursing homes.

Senator PORTMAN. So more data is needed. And if we had that data, we would have a better understanding of what the different outcomes are.

Mr. DICKEN. That would be helpful, yes.

Senator PORTMAN. Ms. Ramos, or Dr. Gifford, any thoughts?

Dr. GIFFORD. Go ahead, Ms. Ramos.

Ms. RAMOS. I think that, in the nursing homes, we need oversight. And Congress is the only one that can have that law passed. Right now, we are fighting on the State level, but it is not just in our State that we have these issues in the nursing homes. It is across the country.

And our union is fighting really hard for us to pass the bill so that everyone in the State, and in this country, will have a law that will support the staff and the patients' quality of care.

Senator PORTMAN. Thank you, Mr. Chairman.

Dr. Gifford, if you have additional thoughts, I would love to hear them, maybe with a written response. Thank you, very much. Thank you, Mr. Chairman.

The CHAIRMAN. Senator Cardin was here before Senator Brown. I apologize to my colleagues for the juggling. Senator Cardin is next, and then Senator Brown.

Senator CARDIN. Well, thank you, Mr. Chairman. I appreciate that very much, and I appreciate the panel. This is obviously an extremely important subject. We know that nursing home safety has been a critical part of dealing with COVID–19.

I appreciate the challenges that we have had with personnel, with safety of the personnel as well. I want to talk about an issue that was present before COVID–19, and that is that nursing homes have——

[Pause.]

The CHAIRMAN. Senator Cardin, we seem to have some audio issues on your end. Can you hear me?

[No response.]

The CHAIRMAN. Why don't we go to Senator Brown, and then we will go to Senator Cardin.

Senator BROWN. Thank you, Mr. Chairman.

Just last month researchers from leading institutions across the country published a working paper on private equity investment in health care, specifically nursing homes. They studied Medicare data from 18,000 nursing home facilities over a 12-year period, examining patient outcomes at private, equity-owned facilities.

The results are disturbing. Let me quickly summarize. Researchers found private equity firms tend to shift money away from patient care, cutting the number of hours that front-line nurses spend providing care to patients. They also—and Ms. Ramos, I am sure, is familiar with this, because of the union that she is a part of that represents some of these workers—they also found that patients at private equity-owned facilities were more likely to be given antipsychotic drugs. They found that patients who receive care at private equity-owned facilities are more likely to die. In fact, the researchers found that more than 20,000—20,000—Medicare beneficiaries died as a result of private equity-ownership of nursing homes during that sample period of 12 years. Finally, they found that taxpayer spending per patient episode increased by 11 percent.

To summarize, the study found that when private equity firms acquire nursing homes, they cut staff, they prescribe more dangerous drugs, more patients die, and taxpayers pay more money.

In November 2019, Senator Warren and I sent letters to four private equity firms that invest in nursing home care and other long-term care services to request information on how these private equity firms manage their facilities.

So, Mr. Chairman, I would like to ask unanimous consent to enter this paper by Atul Gupta and his colleagues, as well as the letters that Senator Warren and I sent out to these private equity firms and their responses, into today's record.

The CHAIRMAN. Without objection.

[The documents appear in the appendix beginning on p. 61.]

The CHAIRMAN. And I would note, Senator Brown, I have been asking some of those same questions, so I very much appreciate it. Go ahead.

Senator BROWN. Thank you. We also see this private equity issue—I'm the new chair of the Banking, Housing, and Urban Affairs Committee. We see private equity firms, starting in Iowa, we believe, but all over the country, private equity firms buying up manufactured housing, so-called trailer parks, and squeezing those generally low-income residents.

So we see it throughout our economy. My question—and I have a follow-up question too—Ms. Ramos, two questions for you.

First—and make your answer as short as you can—talk about the difference between what adequate staffing and an under-staffed shift means for your patients, and what it means to you and your colleagues, if you would, Ms. Ramos.

Ms. RAMOS. Thank you for your question. So with more staffing, we can give the residents better care. For example, if a resident asks me—if two residents ask me to go to the bathroom, I have to pick and choose which one of them to take to the bathroom first.

So when we have more staff, another aide can help the other one. But when we are short-staffed, if I am in the bathroom with one of the residents and a patient has fallen, like a patient fell in the dining room, the nurse is calling for help, we have to leave the resident who is in the bathroom and go to help the other resident who just had a fall.

So those are the types of things that we have to do all the time. We have to pick and choose which resident we have to take care of first. And it is a challenge for the nurses and for the CNAs that we deal with every day.

Senator BROWN. Thank you for that good, concise answer. Throughout COVID, higher nurse staffing levels have been associated with fewer COVID–19 cases and deaths. We know that. I have introduced legislation in this committee to require hospitals to maintain safe staffing levels. And I know Chairman Wyden wants to do this and consider ways to improve nurse-to-patient staffing ratios at long-term care facilities.

My last question, Ms. Ramos—I notice your T-shirt, and I know you are a proud member of the Service Employees International Union. Talk to me about how being part of a union has allowed you to better advocate for your patients.

Ms. RAMOS. Being part of my union helps me advocate for and be a voice for the workers who do not have a union, and the patients who do not have the family members who will stick up for them.

And we do that across the country. And also, when we are united and we have power—so with that power, we got hazard pay during the pandemic. And to make our voices heard and really inspire change, that is the reason why I am here today telling you our stories in a nursing home.

Senator BROWN. Thank you, Ms. Ramos. Thanks for your conciseness.

Mr. Chairman, my time has expired. Thanks very much for having this hearing, Chairman Wyden.

The CHAIRMAN. Thank you, Senator Brown.

Our next—we've got Senator Cardin back; wonderful.

Senator CARDIN. I think I am with you now. We changed the connection.

The CHAIRMAN. Perfect.

Senator CARDIN. Thank you very much. First, thanks for this hearing. It is very important.

Ms. Ramos, I want to thank you and all the front-line workers for what you have done during COVID–19. You truly have stepped up to help our community, and we thank all of our front-line workers during this time.

It has been very challenging. We know of the circumstances when personnel become difficult because of getting COVID–19, and protecting our workers, and protecting the residents at nursing homes. It is a real challenge.

We recognized this before COVID–19. And that is why we looked at the issue of infection prevention in nursing homes. In 2016, the Obama administration issued certain regulations in regard to the requirements for nursing homes. The Trump administration reduced some of those requirements.

I guess my question to you is, do we have adequate Federal guideline protection to deal with ongoing issues of infectious diseases? Look, COVID–19—we will get beyond that at some point— but there are going to be other issues that are going to come up that affect the health of the nursing home residents and the personnel who work in nursing homes.

Are we doing enough as far as Federal guidelines to require nursing homes to have adequate protection to deal with infectious diseases? Whoever wants to answer it, I welcome your thoughts.

Mr. DICKEN. This is John Dicken with GAO, and I can just note that certainly even making the point that you made is important, that even before the pandemic we found that the highest source of deficiencies that were found in nursing homes was for infection control.

And so it is essential that there be focus even outside of this pandemic environment on trying to control and prevent infections, and to apply appropriate infection control practices. That is a requirement: that the nursing homes have plans to be able to prevent and control infections. Even before this pandemic, that was the primary type of deficiency that was found in nursing homes.

Senator CARDIN. So I guess my question to all of us is that, obviously, a lot of this can be done administratively, but we in Congress might need to take a look at policies that reflect that.

One of my interests is how we share best practices. We know that nursing homes have come up with creative ways to protect their residents, and to protect their essential workers. Is there an adequate communications system within the nursing home industry itself to implement the best practices that are being used around the Nation? And is there a way that the best practices can make their way to us policy-makers so that if we look at legislation, we look at what is working and what is not working and try to develop the best policies for our country?

Again, I welcome anyone on the panel who wants to talk about that, as to how we can take the best practices that are being used today to keep nursing home residents safe, and the personnel safe, and how we can implement that in Federal policy.

Ms. RAMOS. This is Adelina. From my experience, we need to have oversight in the nursing homes. And the Senate is the only one that can do that.

We tried working on it through the State to have a law passed so we could have safety and better quality care for our residents, because before the pandemic, like you said, we had this problem. And with the pandemic, it made things worse.

So it is not just a State-by-State problem, it is across the whole country. Because my story is not unique. If you ask anybody else in any other States, they have similar stories. They have seen similar things, or worse, of what I have been through.

So I think Congress has the power to change the laws across the country.

Senator CARDIN. And I think the SEIU can play a major part in that. You have people around the country who have seen what works well, and what has not worked, and I think sharing that information with us would certainly be very helpful as we try to deal with this issue moving forward.

We have to look at the lessons learned as a result of COVID–19, recognizing that infectious disease spread within confined nursing homes is going to be an ongoing challenge in regards to the safety of people in this country.

Thank you, Mr. Chairman. I thank our witnesses.

The CHAIRMAN. Thank you, Senator Cardin. Next will be Senator Lankford, and then Senator Casey, and I hope we can get both of them in. We have a vote going on.

Senator Lankford?

Senator LANKFORD. I will hustle, Mr. Chairman. Thank you very much for doing that. I have been a very outspoken advocate for, obviously, safety in facilities, in all of our long-term care facilities, as all of you have been as well. So I appreciate very much what you are doing for this.

But I have also been an advocate to say many individuals in my State—in fact, all the individuals who want it in my State—who are in long-term care facilities have already been vaccinated, both the staff and the individuals. Some of them were vaccinated 5, 6 weeks ago and have been through the full regimen and been on the other side of it.

There is a difficult balance there of trying to provide safety to those individuals, but also to have access to their grandchildren, their families, and other individuals, school groups that want to be able to come in and bless them.

What they have seen is some normal activity in the past around the facility in trying to strike that balance. CDC has put out some guidance. States, including my own State, have put out some guidance on their own. Sometimes they are not lining up.

So my question on this is, based on where we are right now, what would you recommend that we put out as guidance for individuals who are dealing with real depression and real isolation in a very difficult season of life already? What would you recommend we start to do right now for those who have already been vaccinated in the facility? So I open that up. Dr. Gifford, obviously you are going to be the obvious one on this, but I would open it up to anyone else who wants to be able to respond to that as well.

Dr. GIFFORD. Well, I think—I am glad you are raising that point. And I think we have all seen—the families and health-care givers—that when you take a frail elderly person and restrict them from seeing their family, and they cannot participate in activities with the other residents, and really have trouble interacting with the staff as well because many of them have dementia and they do not understand what is going on, it will have dire consequences with them.

And I think the challenge is when you balance the safety of a virus that has a 20-percent mortality risk with the clearly devastating impacts you have had with that. I think we are transitioning out of that, which is good.

I think this raises just a broader question about how do we move to provide the care, activities, and infection control when you have to restrict people's movements around in a building?

Senator LANKFORD. Other comments from other individuals?

Ms. RAMOS. Yes, please, I would like to add to that. I think in large part, on the temporary nurse aides, and how people have gone and gotten the certification to be able to work in facilities but may not have all the credentials, I think from a logistical standpoint, just simply put, we could allow families to take the same type of training for infection control and universal precautions and allow for the designation of essential caregivers, so they are able to be in there, and able to come in and help supplement the care the staff may not be able to provide.

A lot of these people were going to see their families weekly prior to COVID, and so I think it is just one of many solutions that we could look at across the board. And you know, in working through that, they would still be held to the same requirements as staffing in terms of testing and, ideally, vaccinations.

Senator LANKFORD. Do others want to be able to comment on that?

Dr. KONETZKA. I will just add that the essential caregivers programs that were just mentioned, a handful of States at least implemented these even before the CDC opened up guidance about visits. And those may serve as a model, as a good model for how we should be moving as a country. Those are programs in which some family members could go in on a regular basis, and they took all the precautions that staff took, and I think those were generally very successful.

Senator LANKFORD. So would you recommend something like this in—let's skip past COVID. We are all looking forward to that day. We are past it. In whatever that looks like for us, we will still have tough choices in the days ahead. And obviously, a really difficult flu can have a catastrophic effect inside of a long-term care facility as well.

Would you recommend some of these same processes be carried over into a difficult flu season as well, for individuals in long-term care?

Dr. KONETZKA. Perhaps. But I think it is important to remember that reducing physical risk is not the only goal here. We need to find the right balance between quality of life and seeing family and friends, and reducing physical risk. I think the goal is probably not zero risk; the goal is to find the right balance.

Senator LANKFORD. I am glad to be able to hear you say that, because there does seem to be a concern about how we get to zero risk. And zero risk has a lot of emotional damage on a lot of families, and a lot of individuals in their isolation. And some of the individuals that I interact with will say things like, "I have been waiting for 10 months, and I've thought in my head over and over, once I get the vaccine this will be different." And they are experiencing right now nothing different for them, and they have had the vaccine.

So they are trying to find some hope in the middle of this as well. So thank all of you for the ongoing work that you have done.

The CHAIRMAN. Thank you, Senator Lankford.

Senator Casey—and, colleagues, Senator Casey has done three separate reports on this issue. He has put an enormous amount of effort into it, and we appreciate it. Senator Casey?

Senator CASEY. Mr. Chairman, thank you very much for having this hearing. I want to thank you and the ranking member. And, Mr. Chairman, I want to thank you for the work you have done to hold the prior administration accountable on these issues that relate to nursing homes and long-term care, and to work with me and with others to move this agenda forward, which we still have much work to do in connection with. I am just grateful for this opportunity. Senator Whitehouse earlier, in his introduction of Ms. Ramos, was highlighting some of the work that he has done with us as well, and we are grateful for that.

I want to start by offering at least, at a minimum, words of commendation to Ms. Ramos and other front-line workers. In your testimony very early on, you talked about, quote, "days filled with fear and sadness" in the work that you have done. And we want to commend that work.

I was especially moved by the reference you made to when you had contracted the virus and were not able to hug your son as you would want. And so many Americans have felt the same—that same sense of loss.

And the moment you talked about sitting with a long-term care resident and wanting to hold her hand, but being pulled away to the work that you had to do because of staffing issues—so we want to thank you and SEIU for standing up for workers like you.

We have to do more than offer words of commendation. We have to start voting with you—both parties, both Houses, both branches of government—to lift up the caregiving workforce. We are decades late in doing that. And so, I do not ask for your comment, I just want to let you know that we are thinking about you and realize that we have an obligation to you and those with whom you work.

My question will be preceded by a little bit of background. I want to direct my question to Dr. Konetzka. We know that, as many of us have referenced, now more than 178,000 residents and workers in long-term care have died from the COVID–19 virus.

This is a terrible, profound tragedy within the broader COVID– 19 tragedy. We know that, in Congress, we have an obligation to learn from the tragedy and to deliver a common-sense response.

I worked with Senator Toomey, my colleague from Pennsylvania, on work we did in connection with the Special Focus Facility program. We did some investigative work and made some changes, but now we have legislation that we have just recently reintroduced: the Nursing Home Reform Modernization Act.

It does basically three things. Number one, it expands the oversight of the Special Focus Facility program's Candidate Facility— that is a specific type of facility. Second, it increases the educational resources for the facilities that are underperforming. And third, it establishes an independent advisory council to inform Health and Human Services on how best to rank nursing home performance and foster quality improvements. I am grateful to be working with Senator Toomey, because some of this work can be and must be bipartisan.

Dr. Konetzka, do you think that there is merit in expanding the size of the Special Focus Facility program to more facilities and enhancing the oversight of underperforming nursing homes?

Dr. KONETZKA. Senator Casey, first of all, thank you for your persistent efforts on the issues of nursing homes and in the area of disparities. I am fully supportive of your efforts to expand the Special Focus Facility program. We all know that, even though there are many nursing homes that provide very good quality of care, there is a bottom tier of nursing homes that are chronically problematic. And that is the tier of nursing homes that the Special Focus Facility program is aimed at.

It has been a tiny program over the years, and I think you are absolutely right in wanting to expand that program and doing what we can to try to bring up that bottom tier.

Senator CASEY. Thanks very much, Doctor. And I know that we have about 30 seconds left, but just to ask quickly, Ms. Bottcher, with regard to transparency. I will just make it quick, without a prelude, to ask, what do you think we have to do to give families what they need to make informed decisions about nursing homes?

Ms. BOTTCHER. Well, of course knowledge is power. And so, having transparent data available for families, making it easy to read, being consumer-friendly, that will go a long way to helping families understand what is going on with their loved ones.

Senator CASEY. We look forward to working with you and the rest of the panel.

Thank you very much, Mr. Chairman.

The CHAIRMAN. Thank you for the good work, Senator Casey.

Senator Grassley?

Senator GRASSLEY. Thank you, Mr. Chairman.

Since we are talking about nursing homes, I think I ought to start by saying "thank you" to every American who has supported our seniors during this pandemic, because our nursing homes house the most vulnerable that we have in our society. And this has been a very challenging year for these seniors, but it has also been a very challenging year for our health-care workers.

Before I get to my first question for Mr. Dicken and Ms. Moten, let me lead in with this. Last year, the Department of Justice launched an investigation into four States' COVID–19 responses in nursing homes. These States were Michigan, New Jersey, New York, and Pennsylvania. They pressured nursing homes to admit residents who may have been infected with COVID–19. The CDC recommended that hospitals discharge patients with COVID–19 diagnosis only to nursing homes that are capable of implementing all recommended infection control procedures.

State officials who pressured nursing homes to admit untested or contagious COVID patients from hospitals likely increased the case rate and fatality risk for these residents. Meanwhile, State officials in other parts of the country—Florida is just one example—followed CDC's guidance, often with better results.

So to Mr. Dicken and Ms. Moten: how important is it for the Department of Justice to continue investigating these four States' violations of the civil rights of the nursing home residents and the failed duty to care?

Mr. DICKEN. Thank you, Senator Grassley, and I appreciate your long-term leadership on these issues. Certainly what we—we are aware that there are both Federal and State-level investigations ongoing. GAO continues to examine what the experience has been across all States, as this has affected all States. And there are two key points on that.

One, one reason why GAO has recommended that there needs to be more complete information that was only voluntarily reported at the Federal level on cases and deaths in nursing homes prior to May, is so that we can learn some of the lessons that we learned from the very uncertain and challenging times early in the pandemic.

And secondly, we have talked to—our ongoing work looks at a range of States across the country, and we are hearing common concerns about how best to get protective equipment, dealing with protecting hospitals. And these are challenges that have been faced throughout the country.

Ms. MOTEN. I want to echo the sentiments of Mr. Dicken. I think that it is important that we continue to investigate these four States in particular, and States across the country, as we are able to take those stumbling blocks and make them stepping stones.

You know, the reality is that we could have done a better job in a lot of these places. And while oftentimes our care community mirrors what was going on in other communities, our hospitals were able to handle infection control. And so I think we need to look into this so that we are able to figure out what system breakdowns we had in those different States and better understand them, so we do not repeat those same mistakes.

Senator GRASSLEY. Both Republican and Democrat Senators have warned President Biden that he should not terminate 56 U.S. attorneys, particularly those who have ongoing sensitive investigations.

One is Toni Bacon, the U.S. Attorney, Northern District, New York. Ms. Bacon previously served as the Justice Department's National Elder Justice Coordinator and currently has jurisdiction over Federal public correction crimes in the State. The State of New York under-counted nursing home deaths by as much as 50 percent, and State officials intentionally withheld data for months. Ms. Bacon is the obvious choice to continue a fair and unbiased investigation into possible violations of civil liberties of the elderly and public corruption.

So, to the same two people, Mr. Dicken and Ms. Moten, do you believe the U.S. Department of Justice must have a fair, unbiased, and experienced U.S. Attorney in the Northern District of New York, such as Ms. Bacon?

When you get done answering, I will have to say my time is up. But let's hear the answer.

Mr. DICKEN. Thank you, Senator Grassley. I cannot speak to the specifics there, but I certainly know that there are fair and complete investigations at the Federal and State levels. But I have not looked at that specific situation.

Senator GRASSLEY. Ms. Moten?

Ms. MOTEN. Again, I echo Mr. Dicken's position on that. I think that an unbiased party is definitely going to be needed to make the proper recommendations and to do a full investigation. But I cannot speak to the person you are asking about.

Senator GRASSLEY. Thank you, Mr. Chairman.

The CHAIRMAN. Thank you, Senator Grassley.

Just one fact, quickly, before we go to Senator Menendez. When you look at the top 10 States with the highest number of COVID deaths per occupied bed, they are evenly split between States led by Democratic and Republican Governors, which supports the proposition this was not a blue State/red State issue. It is a huge national tragedy for the country.

Senator Menendez?

Senator MENENDEZ. Thank you, Mr. Chairman.

Mr. Dicken, last June I led my House and Senate colleagues in a letter to then-Secretary Azar, and then-Administrator Verma, pleading for more resources, guidance, and support for nursing homes. At the time, New Jersey had already been on the front lines of the pandemic for over 2 months—2 months when we were fighting in the dark against an invisible enemy; 2 months when New Jerseyians suffered immeasurable losses and pain.

In that letter, I called for a comprehensive national testing plan. We did not get it. I asked for a strategy to ensure our nursing homes had sufficient PPE. I asked for a plan on staffing shortages, and how to care for COVID–19-positive residents. And I called for greater resources to improve reporting and communication.

We did not get all of those things. And when we did get something, it came slowly and, for many, too late. So that we can learn from the past, can you talk to us about the harm inflicted by the failure to put in place a national testing plan last spring?

Mr. DICKEN. Yes; thank you. And right, that is part of the broader work in the Federal response to the pandemic. GAO has also recommended that there be a national testing strategy, and that has not yet been implemented.

That is key for several reasons. The national testing strategy would help better target information on what resources and expertise can be used to try to control or prevent outbreaks. It also could ensure more consistency, so that State, Federal, and private entities work on common goals, and that there would be common information that could have more transparency.

Senator MENENDEZ. Thank you.

Dr. Gifford, I recently introduced the PREPARE Act and sent a letter with Congressman Pascrell to the administration requesting that infection control practices be improved in nursing homes to combat the future spread of COVID and other viruses.

Your plan also calls for a new focus on infection control by adding additional requirements to the infection preventionist position that is required in all facilities. Could you elaborate on your plan and how these changes would help provide a healthier environment for the residents you serve?

Dr. GIFFORD. Thank you, Senator Menendez, for all of your efforts on both PPE and infection control. We definitely have supported the infection preventionist program and requirements since the beginning. I think what we have learned is that you need to tailor that infection preventionist to the needs of the facility.

A large facility with 300 to 400 beds needs more than one person. A 20-bed facility in a rural community does not need the same amount. A facility that takes care of highly acute illness, and very sick individuals, may need more infection preventionists than those that have less acuity in there.

And so we would strongly support it being evidence-based. You also do not want to say it has to be one person, because if that person gets sick or is out on vacation or not working those days, you want to have good coverage on infection prevention throughout. So this should be covered by multiple people.

So we are asking for an evidence-based approach to addressing this infection preventionist in a nursing home.

Senator MENENDEZ. And one final question. Last week, the AHCA sent a letter to the administration asking for next steps for vaccinations at nursing homes. Now last week, we learned that in New Jersey only about half of our nursing home staff are vaccinated. Since the pharmacy partnership with retail pharmacies and nursing homes is drawing to a close, it seems to me we need to be sure we can still get people vaccinated in these facilities.

What are some of the more creative ways the Federal Government can partner with our nursing home partners to reach the stated goal of 75 percent of staff vaccinated by June 30th?

Dr. GIFFORD. Well, I think the initial plan they had, working with retail pharmacies and getting the vaccine out there, was a highly successful program. I think the challenge now is getting vaccine out. There just is not enough vaccine still coming out and being allocated into the program. And so, no matter how innovative a program you have, there is no vaccine being allocated out, other than for a handful of States.

We need to not let the gains that we have seen with vaccinations slip. It is also clear, I think as you heard from Ms. Ramos, that you need to have multiple people sitting down and listening and talking to staff and residents about what their concerns are with the vaccine, so that they can understand what is going on out there. And CDC is sort of working in that area, and we support that effort.

Senator MENENDEZ. Thank you, Mr. Chairman.

The CHAIRMAN. I thank my colleague. We are going to keep this going. Senator Crapo has been kind enough to say he will run the hearing while I run and vote. And I think I saw Senator Hassan. Perhaps she will be back soon.

Senator Crapo, if you will run it, I will be back very quickly.

Senator CRAPO [presiding]. I will do so. Thank you, Senator Wyden.

Do we have any Senators who are here at this time? Senator Thune?

[No response.]

Senator CRAPO. Senator Barrasso?

[No response.]

Senator CRAPO. Senator Warren?

[No response.]

Senator CRAPO. Senator Hassan?

[No response.]

Senator CRAPO. Well, if no Senator shows up, I will go back into some of my questions. Hold on a minute while I grab my stack of papers here.

All right; thank you. I am going to go next to you, Ms. Bottcher. You put in your testimony—you have outlined a five-point plan or a proposal that you are focusing on. I was interested—well, I was interested in all of those points. Your third point was basically to focus, if I understood it correctly, on safe access to in-person and virtual meetings between nursing home residents and their families.

Could you expand on that a little bit? Are you saying that we need to increase in-person, or just make sure that we focus both on in-person and virtual?

Ms. BOTTCHER. So, both in fact. And thank you for the question, Senator Crapo. AARP has advocated, when it is safe to do so, to allow for in-person visitation. And of course CMS updated those guidelines. But in-person visitation—we cannot lose sight of the fact that we still have to talk about infection control and follow those procedures.

There still has to be adequate staffing to be able to provide and support in-person visitation and all the other guidelines that CMS has put forward—and so all of that. It is a delicate balance, as we have talked about. In-person visitation would certainly help those who have had some mental decline without that social connectedness. And it would help with the mental health of the person, but we also have to do everything we can to provide for the safety of that person with regard to COVID.

Insofar as virtual visitation goes, we believe that Congress could do more to require that facilities facilitate virtual visitation when they cannot support in-person visitation. And of course we saw that throughout the pandemic with the use of cell phones, with the use of iPads. But this was not done consistently throughout nursing homes across the Nation.

Senator CRAPO. Thank you. I was just about ready to go to you, Dr. Konetzka, but I see that we may have Senator Thune with us. Do we? And if not, I do see Senator Daines.

Senator Daines, you may proceed.

Senator DAINES. Right. Thank you, Senator.

Well, I am glad to be part of this hearing today. This is something that has touched Montanans deeply. Over the past year, our Nation and my own State of Montana have experienced loss in so many ways. Our seniors have borne the brunt of this pandemic, in fact, so much so that States like New York have tried to cover up the true toll this pandemic has taken on nursing homes.

The reality is that more than one-third of all U.S. COVID–19 deaths are linked to long-term care facilities. We must do more to support our nursing home residents, many of whom have suffered with increased depression, anxiety, and worsening dementia due to COVID restrictions, and the isolation.

Throughout the pandemic, residents were deprived visits from sons, daughters, new grandbabies, staring through windows, listening to recordings of loved ones to try to keep those memories alive. And we know that extreme social isolation can have very serious health consequences and can even be deadly.

With nearly two-thirds of seniors having received their first shot, and millions of American being vaccinated every day, we are finally turning the corner. There is hope. Today, nursing home residents across the country can visit safely with their loved ones, and we have even seen examples of hugging their family members for the first time in a year.

We are making great strides. We are getting shots in arms across the country, currently at a pace of over 2 million per day, but there are folks who are reluctant to get the vaccine.

A February study by the CDC estimated low rates of vaccine uptake among nursing home staff at 38 percent, compared to nursing home residents at 78 percent. We need at least 75 percent of the population to be vaccinated for us to achieve herd immunity and get back to normal.

I decided to take part in the 5-year vaccine trial last year—it was offered in my home town of Bozeman, MT—because I want to do my part in helping to make Montanans feel confident about the vaccine.

My first question is to Mr. Dicken. Can you describe how well vaccine distribution in nursing homes is going and provide any analysis on the CDC's study on vaccine uptake?

Mr. DICKEN. Yes; thank you, Senator Daines. And you are right that as nursing homes have been prioritized for vaccine distribution, more than 99 percent of homes that participate in the Federal partnership have had at least one on-site clinic that could help offer vaccines to residents and staff.

That is more than 4.25 million vaccines that have been distributed to residents and staff in nursing homes as of early February. And that number continues to grow.

Senator, the CDC numbers you cited are correct that have had a larger share of residents who have taken the opportunity to get the vaccinations, and that during the first clinics that occurred under the partnership, a smaller share of staff had agreed to take the vaccinations.

There was hope that over time, as there continued to be more opportunity and clinics, that would increase. The comment that my fellow panelist, Ms. Ramos, her experience—as more staff see other colleagues who have been vaccinated and the decline in cases, we can only hope that that would increase their comfort with receiving vaccinations.

Senator DAINES. Thank you.

I have a question for Ms. Bottcher. Last year I teamed up with Senator Grassley on a bill that would allow for the creation of strike teams in States to help facilities that were being overwhelmed by COVID–19. This bill also supported tele-visitation programs so that nursing home residents would not be as isolated from family in the stresses of the pandemic.

Ms. Bottcher, can you speak to the benefits of virtual visits in lieu of in-person visits, and what barriers prevent residents from accessing tele-visit technology?

Ms. BOTTCHER. Certainly. Thank you so much for the question. AARP has long been supportive of virtual visits. And we have— when the pandemic unfolded and nursing homes were closed, families were shut off from their loved ones. And a lot of them did not already have that set up with their loved one.

And so it was incumbent upon nursing homes to facilitate that to the best extent, where they could. I think the shortcomings were the infection rates. As they rose in facilities with residents and staff, then you did not have enough staff to facilitate those virtual visits. You had some nursing homes that were concerned about passing around the technological devices to be able to facilitate that.

So there just was not a lot of support to be able to do that. So families were then troubled and became desperate. We heard from several families who were so desperate they would go to every single window around the nursing home and just start knocking until they found someone that they could talk to to wheel their loved one to the window. And they would call us just in frustration.

Some nursing facilities do not have strong broadband connection, or lack Internet access. That is also a problem that needs to be addressed.

And so, the extent to which we can require nursing homes to provide virtual visitation in lieu of in-person visitation when that cannot happen, that should be done.

Senator DAINES. Thank you. I see I am out of time.

Thank you, Senator.

Senator CRAPO. Thank you, Senator. Senator Warner?

Senator WARREN. Was that Senator Warren or Senator Warner?

Senator CRAPO. Warner.

Senator WARREN. Oh.

Senator CRAPO. I am sorry. Wait your turn. [Laughter.]

Senator WARREN. Sorry, Mark.

Senator WARNER. Thank you, Senator Crapo.

I want to—I have a couple of questions here. One, I want to start on the question of nursing home staffing. This is an issue I have been working on with Senator Tim Scott. We have to make sure— and obviously COVID has shown the ability of the facilities to recruit and retain quality staff is a challenge. It is oftentimes low pay. Part of that is due to the reimbursement rates, meaning the margins are quite thin for these facilities. And obviously post-COVID, I think this problem was only exacerbated.

I am going to start with Ms. Ramos. As a nursing home worker, could you talk a little bit about this issue and give any advice you might have on how we can better recruit and retain nursing home workers? And, Dr. Gifford, from the Association's standpoint, can you speak to this issue as well?

Ms. RAMOS. Hi; thank you for your question.

So like I said before, the quality of care and the short staffing had been issues before the pandemic. So the pandemic made things worse. For us health-care workers in the nursing home, it is a big challenge. Most of the time, we have 13 CNAs to 12 residents who are total care. So when you have that amount of residents per CNA, a lot of them stay in bed for long periods of time. And when the family members were coming in to visit, they were getting very upset, because they would come at 10:30 a.m. and their loved ones were in bed. So they would complain.

But as the pandemic hit, we were still working short, and as things got worse, we were lucky that we had a union that backed us up. And then we have complained for the ones who cannot speak for themselves, like our patients in the Alzheimer's unit. Our union supports us to speak up for them.

So with the pandemic, things got worse. And it is worse in the nursing home. We are still working short-staffed all the time, and our residents are not getting the quality care they deserve.

Senator WARNER. Dr. Gifford, did you have a comment?

Dr. GIFFORD. Yes. I think, as you heard from all the panelists today, the workforce needs to be improved. And we need better ways to recruit and retain. I think you have heard from us all today that, as you recognized, the tone of this is due to the underlying funding.

You know, the other challenge is, how do we recruit and retain beyond just the salaries? I think loan forgiveness programs are something we have been championing and we really need help with. That would go right to the workers. Tax credits for people who work in this sector. Subsidies to schools and technical schools to have their graduates working in long-term care.

What we have seen in many of those programs is students get sucked up by the hospitals and work elsewhere, and they do not come to work in long-term care. So we need to have specific programs that make us a priority. I mean, I think the one biggest lesson learned from this—and you heard it from everyone—is we were not a priority. So if we are going to make staffing a priority, we have to make loan forgiveness, tax credits, incentives to schools, a priority to get workers into long-term care. Otherwise, they will work in the other sectors. Thank you.

Senator WARNER. And let me just add, I stand with, I think, all our colleagues in a bipartisan way that we need to weed out the bad actors in this space. The star rating, I think, has had mixed success. But I also know from just a business perspective, the reimbursement rates are so low, and the margins are so thin, that those nursing homes that are trying to do the right thing—and I am particularly concerned now when we have seen nursing home populations, perhaps appropriately after COVID and people's concerns, fall 20, 25, 30 percent. I am not sure what the business model is going to look like, particularly in rural communities, so we can keep these facilities open with a level of quality where folks like Ms. Ramos can have adequate staffing.

Dr. Konetzka, could you—I know you have done a lot of research on this, including reimbursement rates. How can we make sure that the good operators are still able to operate, and how are we going to grapple with this issue of, in rural communities, 20-, 25-percent decrease in patient population? What is the model that is going to make this work?

Dr. KONETZKA. That is an excellent question, but it is a really hard one. This is the hard challenge to answer, right? Because it is almost definitely going to take resources. I think we generally underfund long-term care in this country. I agree with you that Medicaid rates in many States are very low, probably too low to take care of the level of need in a nursing home population.

I think, moving forward, we have to think about fundamental changes to the system. I think that there is an aging capital stock of nursing homes. There is financial fallout from the pandemic. And there are chronic problems such as under-staffing.

So I think we need to take a hard look at the underlying payment mechanism and the funding we inject into the system, and perhaps consider some bold changes.

Senator WARNER. Thank you, Mr. Chairman. I know Elizabeth is, I think, next——

Senator CRAPO. Unfortunately, Senator Thune came back. So it is going to be Senator Thune next. Elizabeth, we are getting there.

Senator Thune?

Senator WARNER. Famous last words there. [Laughter.]

Senator THUNE. Thank you, Mr. Chairman. Let me just say that the subject of today's hearing is one that I think we all wish we were not having to discuss, with the stories in our States——

[Loss of audio.]

Senator CRAPO. Senator Thune, have you been muted?

Senator THUNE. Am I on? Hello?

Senator CRAPO. Hello; we can hear you now.

Senator THUNE. Can you hear me now?

Senator CRAPO. Yes.

Senator THUNE. You have me? Okay. All right. Well, I will skip the preamble there——

[Loss of audio.]

Senator CRAPO. John, I think we are having trouble with your signal. We will give it about another 5 or 10 seconds, and then, Elizabeth, I think I am going to have to—oh, here he comes. Can you speak, John, and tell us if you can hear us?

[No response.]

Senator CRAPO. All right, Elizabeth, why don't you go?

Senator WARREN. All right; thank you, Mr. Chair. And I am sorry, Senator Thune, but I am sure we will get this straightened out.

When the coronavirus hit, nursing homes were ground zero. Today, at least 34,000 nursing home residents and 1,600 staff members have died of COVID–19. Responding to coronavirus is challenging for every health-care provider.

Genesis HealthCare, a nursing home chain with over 350 facilities across the country, was one provider that struggled.

Ms. Ramos, you work at Greenville Nursing Center, a Rhode Island nursing home owned by Genesis. From your testimony, it sounds like working at a facility last year was harrowing. Let me just ask: did you have the resources and the staff you needed to properly care for COVID–19 patients?

Ms. RAMOS. Thank you for your question. No, we did not have enough resources or the staff that we needed. But those, like I said before, are not new issues. Sometimes we have two residents with serious needs at the same time, but we have to choose who deserves our care. And every one of them deserves our care, 100 percent. But it is sad that we have been put in that situation all the time.

Senator WARREN. And you are right: it is sad to be put in that situation. But basically what you are saying is that you did not have the supplies, you did not have the staff you needed when the coronavirus hit. And I know that a lot of the nursing homes around the country were in the same boat, which is why Congress passed COVID–19 relief packages like the CARES Act earlier to get providers the resources they needed.

Now in January, I wrote to Genesis, which owns the nursing home where you work, and I received information that shows that they accepted $665 million in State and Federal grants and loans last year. And guess what Genesis did? It gave its then-CEO an approximately $2-million retention bonus just a few months before he left the company, which was and is in dire financial condition. In total, the CEO, George Hager, has received $8 million in compensation since January of 2020.

Ms. Ramos, you told us about how one of your co-workers died while trying to care for COVID–19 patients, while working at a facility with a $14 an hour starting wage. So let me just ask you your view on this. Should a top corporate executive have received a multi-million-dollar bonus while you were struggling to keep patients alive and keep yourself alive?

Or let me ask it another way. What could have been done to improve patient care with that $5.2-million retention bonus that the CEO received?

Ms. RAMOS. No, I do not think they should make millions of dollars in bonuses, because it is Medicare money. That money should be going to patient care.

So with that $5 million that he received, we could have paid a higher wage so we could attract more staff.

Senator WARNER. Right. More staff. More PPE. And that is exactly what Genesis should have done. It should have invested in workers like you.

So let me ask you, Dr. Gifford—you are here on behalf of the American Health Care Association, which represents nursing homes. Do you think it is right that nursing home CEOs received multi-million-dollar bonuses, while workers like Ms. Ramos fought for more PPE, more tests, and more resources?

[No response.]

Senator WARREN. Dr. Gifford?

Dr. GIFFORD. Senator, as a medical director, having worked in nursing homes in Rhode Island, I did not have the pleasure of working with Ms. Ramos there, but I saw firsthand—as you pointed out and Ms. Ramos has—how hard the CNAs work relative to everyone else. And they are really the lifeblood of an organization.

I think early on in this pandemic there was not PPE worldwide anywhere. And we were hearing from every type of facility out there about the need for getting PPE, and getting staffing. And we were calling for it. And what was available was not prioritized for nursing homes. It was going to hospitals and elsewhere. And I think the idea of how we prioritize and use that—the PRF funds that came to us were lifesaving. Many of the nursing homes out there are small family-run nursing homes, second and third generation——

Senator WARREN. So, I am sorry to interrupt, but that was not my question. My question was whether or not nursing home executives should be paid multi-million-dollar retention bonuses, or whether or not those millions of dollars should be invested in the resources that are needed to keep staff and residents safe and healthy.

Dr. GIFFORD. I think that is a good question, to think through how compensation is done at all levels and how are we going to be able to compete for retaining and recruiting staff at all levels throughout the health-care system. And that is something that we will need to look at. And I think we are fully supportive of transparency regarding how these funds were used going forward.

Senator WARNER. Well, I appreciate that you are going to look at it, but I just want to be clear on this. We cannot allow corporate greed to determine whether or not workers and seniors in this country live or die.

That is why I wrote to Genesis requesting information about their financial decisions. And today I am going to release their response, which comes in the wake of reports that Genesis will soon be under private-equity ownership.

I will be opening an investigation into for-profit nursing homes, including those run by private-equity firms. And the next time there is a pandemic, seniors should not be stuck in sub-par institutions run by greedy CEOs and vulture firms in order to make a quick buck.

Commerce needs to act now before tragedy strikes again. Thank you.

Thank you, Mr. Chairman.

Senator CRAPO. Thank you. And, Mr. Chairman, I see you are back. Senator Thune, I believe, is next.

The CHAIRMAN. I believe that is right.

Senator Thune?

Senator THUNE. Thank you, Mr. Chairman. Can you hear me this time?

The CHAIRMAN. Yes.

Senator THUNE. All right; we are back. Well, I appreciate the subject of today's hearing. Obviously it is a huge issue during the pandemic with a lot of nursing home residents isolated and unable to see their families, and with quality of care and staffing issues that this committee has looked at. This committee has, before the pandemic, and now more than ever, we need to address these issues to ensure that everyone's loved ones receive the care that they deserve.

Dr. Gifford, I understand at this time facilities are not required to report to CMS on staff and resident vaccination. Is there no CMS mandate or standard? How are your member facilities keeping track of vaccination records? And I am thinking about this in the context of future follow-up care once we know more about the longevity of COVID vaccines, or the need for boosters over time. So if you could address that.

And then, Mr. Dicken, is there anything GAO is recommending on reporting vaccinations in nursing facilities?

Dr. GIFFORD. Senator Thune, you are correct that currently there is no requirement. All the facilities are tracking vaccinations rates on their staff and residents internally.

There is a portal at the Centers for Disease Control called NHSN where you can report staff and resident vaccination rates. And we have been strongly urging our members to report that. We have been urging CMS and other entities to help sort of move that along. And we are fully open to transparency and having the information revealed out there, just for quality improvement purposes, as well as for family and residents.

We have also set a goal of getting 75 percent of the residents vaccinated. And we need that information to see how we have achieved that goal. So we are very supportive of that. Thank you.

Senator THUNE. Okay.

Mr. Dicken, is there anything GAO is recommending on reporting?

Mr. DICKEN. Yes; thank you, Senator Thune. And certainly GAO is continuing to track vaccine distribution, as well as efforts to assure that residents and staff and homes are offered vaccines, and to what extent that information is available and transparent.

I would note that there are other models in the nursing home setting. There is reporting now of vaccinations for flu or pneumococcal, and so certainly GAO has continued to track the experience in nursing homes in the current environment of COVID–19. GAO is continuing to track that and the efforts to make sure that there is data available, and that that can be made available, including at facility levels.

Senator THUNE. Okay; thank you.

Dr. Gifford, as we work to solve quality-of-care challenges, we also need to be mindful that access remains a priority as our population continues to age.

You testified the nursing home industry projects up to 1,600 closures in the aftermath of the pandemic. I expect census declines and COVID-related costs contributed to this. Could you shed further light on the causes of these closures, and if you can, project where in the Nation we might be at risk for closure? And of course, I am thinking particularly where I come from, like rural areas.

Dr. GIFFORD. Senator Thune, I think you are going to see the challenges, because the census in the facilities has dropped precipitously, from a little over 80 percent to under 70 percent. It has been about a 15-percent drop. That is not sustainable.

And so I think, particularly in the rural areas and their smaller facilities, they are more at risk. I think in States—which Dr. Konetzka has testified to—with poor Medicaid rates, particularly some of the inner city facilities where they have a large proportion of Medicaid, they are also at higher risk because they do not have the same resiliency to sort through this.

I think if we are going to make nursing homes a priority to avoid this and increase the staffing and make the PPE available that we need, it is going to have to come through, as Dr. Konetzka said, sort of a serious look at, what are the investments we are going to make? And how are we going to make this a priority going forward? Otherwise, I think in rural areas, like in your State, you will see closures. It is just not sustainable.

Senator THUNE. On the staffing issue, everybody on the panel has mentioned those challenges. I have heard that from facilities in South Dakota for years. Recognizing that Federal dollars are not unlimited, what solutions should policy-makers focus on to have the most immediate and positive impact when it comes to workforce staffing?

Anybody? And I know my time is expiring, so——

Ms. MOTEN. I think we need to be creative in terms of how we look at staffing, right? I will take the lead from both California and Florida, which have programs by which people graduating from social work, public health nursing, and one other program are required to participate in programs where they are going into these facilities.

So again, we should give them that infection control and universal health precaution education, and start looking at models with intergenerational aspects. And these are just very simple things logistically that we can do, especially as it pertains to our rural communities. Because we are going to start to see, as Dr. Gifford said, a lot of issues out in those rural communities where we have seen bed size compared to census drop drastically.

Senator THUNE. Thank you. Thank you, Mr. Chairman.

The CHAIRMAN. All right; thank you, Senator Thune.

Senator Hassan?

Senator HASSAN. Well, thank you so much, Chairman Wyden and Ranking Member Crapo, for the hearing. And I really appreciate all of the witnesses being here today. And I know it has been a long hearing, so thank you so much to you all for your testimony and your work.

Dr. Gifford, I want to start with a question for you. The COVID– 19 pandemic has killed more than 174,000 long-term care residents over the past year. More than 70 percent of all the COVID–19 deaths in my home State of New Hampshire have occurred in long-term care settings.

This pandemic exposed clear failures within these facilities, and in the oversight of these facilities. The failure to protect this vulnerable population during the pandemic is a national tragedy.

There are many reasons that this happened, and you have all discussed a number of them this morning, including the previous administration's failure to quickly and adequately respond, leaving nursing home workers and residents more vulnerable. But nursing homes themselves also need to take a hard look at their own role, and take responsibility for their failures.

So, Dr. Gifford, do you agree that nursing homes bear some of the blame for the tragic loss of life we have seen over the past year? And assuming that you do, what is the most important thing that went wrong? And what is happening now to correct it during this crisis and into the future?

Dr. GIFFORD. You know, I think you have heard from all of us that this pandemic exacerbated some underlying challenges that existed in the facilities, particularly around the staffing issues. But it also, I think, exposed the fact that we lacked a priority. We have seen in previous hurricanes and other disasters that the resources go to hospitals and other areas, and nursing homes are not a priority.

The other thing is, there was just a failure to learn over time what were the right things to do so we could get rapid lessons learned out there. So even, as Dr. Konetzka said, doing all the right things at the time would not have worked, because they were wrong for this virus.

I think how we learn from each other—we need to do that. We still do not know what the right frequency of testing is. We do not know whether opening up for family members to come in is going to be the right thing to do, and how to do it.

Those are critical things that we need to know going forward.

Senator HASSAN. But, Doctor—I am going to interrupt you, just because my time is limited. What have you learned that you can change? What could you do differently? Is it staffing that you need to really focus on?

Dr. GIFFORD. Well, I think we have taken a hard look at that, and I think we agree that we need to have 24-hour R.N. staffing, knowing R.N.s in a facility are really key to infection control. I have talked before about the infection preventions that are necessary. And we think you need to stockpile PPE for a 30-day supply. And we support that.

Senator HASSAN. Okay; so thank you.

I want to move to another issue, because I am sure that you saw the recent *New York Times* reporting on the failures of the Federal rating system for long-term care facilities, and its reliance on self-reported data.

There appears to be a widespread practice of inflating the number of reported staff responsible for patient care by including administrators, some who may not physically work in the facility. Staff shortages, as all the testimony has established today, have been a major issue during this pandemic. And not surprisingly, research suggests that better-staffed facilities lost fewer patients to COVID–19.

So, Dr. Gifford, given the disturbing record of some homes manipulating data and the importance of adequate staffing, does the Federal Government need to increase inspections and end the reliance on self-reporting?

Dr. GIFFORD. So, Senator, I think—a couple of things on the reporting system. There is this perception of self-reporting. I mean, it is composed of data from the surveyors, but that is not self-reported. The staffing data is from payroll data, which is auditable. And certainly we encourage people to follow the rules on that issue.

CMS has identified that there are many directors of nursing or nursing supervisors who have spent some time administratively and some time providing patient care. Some of that administrative time is calling families, so that is why they are counted in that program there.

So I want to make sure you understand what the process is there.

Senator HASSAN. I thank you for that. I am going to move on to a different issue. But as someone who has worked in a nursing home, I understand distinctly the difference between being on the phone to families and being at the bedside.

I want to turn quickly to Ms. Ramos before my time runs out, because even with vaccine supply increasing, reports suggest that about half of long-term care facility workers remain hesitant to take the vaccine.

And I am wondering, Ms. Ramos, how do you see access to paid sick leave impacting the willingness of front-line workers to take the vaccine?

Ms. RAMOS. Thank you for your question. I think that has a lot to do with it for workers, not only in health care, but in general. A lot of people are hesitant to take a vaccine because they know that there are side effects. And if they take a vaccine and they get sick, they are afraid that there will be consequences to pay, like they would use their sick time to pay them when they are going to need sick time when their family are sick. Or they will use education time, and when they want to spend time with their kids, they won't have it because they used that.

Or like for us health-care workers, we work every other weekend. So if we take a vaccine on a Friday, and on the weekend we get sick and we have to call out, we have to make it up the following weekend when we already have plans to spend it with our family. So I think it should be a system where you do not tell the companies to offer it, but it would be a law, like a mandate, so it would be better that way than just telling them to offer this and to offer that, because they will not follow up.

Senator HASSAN. Thank you very much. And thank you, Mr. Chair, for allowing me to go over time.

The CHAIRMAN. Thank you, Senator Hassan. And we are moving towards wrapping up, but there are a couple of areas I want to get into, because I think we may have missed them.

A question for you, Ms. Bottcher and Dr. Konetzka. My understanding is that CMS has not required that vaccination data be made available per facility. Now we are not talking about every single person's status; we are talking about the aggregate data on, say, this facility, X percentage have been vaccinated; this facility, Y percentage have been vaccinated.

That strikes me as important. What do you two think?

Ms. BOTTCHER. Senator, I think it is incredibly important. And in fact I spoke to one of our members yesterday, Mark Ferguson in Lake Charles, LA, and I posed the same question to him: how important is it that you know about the vaccination rate at your brother's facility? And he said it was extremely important. And in particular, although his brother has been vaccinated, it is important that we look to the future. And if they need a booster shot, or infection rates start climbing, he wants to know that information about his brother's facility.

The CHAIRMAN. All right.

Dr. Konetzka?

Dr. KONETZKA. I agree. I will just add that, yes, we certainly need that information to be public for consumers. They have a right to know the vaccination rates in our facilities they might be considering. It is also essential for researchers and for public health officials to have that data to track vaccination rates, to figure out what is working and what is not working, and whether vaccination is proceeding with equity.

So I think there is no excuse that those data are not made available publicly yet.

The CHAIRMAN. Good. And the last question I think on my end, and then I want to kind of sum up where we are: Dr. Konetzka, do you have any additional recommendations—I had to be on the floor voting for a bit—with respect to what can be done to deal with these yawning racial disparities, these enormous racial disparities? To some extent, they mirror society, as I touched on earlier, but to some extent they seem to be even more entrenched, and it is going to take more careful efforts to root them out. Do you have any final thoughts with respect to racial disparities in nursing homes?

Dr. KONETZKA. Yes, it is an incredibly important issue. So, as I said, I think we know that racial and ethnic disparities have been prominent in the pandemic, not only generally but also in nursing homes. At the same time, long before the pandemic, people of color tended to be in lower-quality nursing homes. And those nursing homes have a higher Medicaid census. Those nursing homes tend to have lower staffing ratios.

I think in the short run—and this goes back to your data question—in the short run, what we need is data on vaccinations to make sure that we are reaching their communities, the communities of color, but also the nursing homes within them, and that we are getting people vaccinated in those areas. We need to make sure that strike teams are also reaching those larger facilities in lower-income neighborhoods.

The long-run problem is harder, again because, as you said, it sort of reflects residential segregation and the problems that go along with the wider disparities in the health-care system. But in the short run, we can certainly target communities of color to try to reduce those disparities.

The CHAIRMAN. All of you have been a terrific panel, and as you can see, my colleagues kept coming back to these important points.

Dr. Konetzka, as you know, I think almost 3 hours ago I asked you about private equity, and the fact that they seemed to be bringing a "make money first, and patients somewhere later will be discussed" kind of philosophy, and colleagues kept talking about it all through the hearing.

So we thank you for that. And I could literally go person by person and mention your contributions. But I want to close——

Senator WHITEHOUSE. Mr. Chairman, I am back now—Senator Whitehouse.

The CHAIRMAN. Okay. Would you like to ask anything else? Or do you want to make——

Senator WHITEHOUSE. If I could drop in one question to Ms. Ramos——

The CHAIRMAN. Good. And then I will close it out. Go ahead.

Senator WHITEHOUSE. Ms. Ramos, when I introduced you, I described the amazing tragedy that you lived through with all of the fatalities at the Greenville Nursing Center, including a colleague, yourself getting the illness, the four of you having to try to manage—what was it?—two dozen COVID patients.

Could you just put as much of a personal experience before us of what this all felt like for you and your colleagues working in the Greenville Nursing Center, and what you have heard from other colleagues who have been doing the same work in our nursing homes?

Ms. RAMOS. Thank you for your question. So before COVID, we were going through those issues, and we had been fighting at the State level to pass the safe staffing, as you know, because it had been years and years that we had been working under-staffed, and the quality of care for our residents was getting worse and worse, and the pandemic made it even worse.

So in those times, I remember when our first unit got COVID. We were not allowed to visit our patients. We normally would take up a shift in those units because we had known them forever.

Senator WHITEHOUSE. You know them well. I mean, they are people in your life, right, the patients?

Ms. RAMOS. Yes. They are like a family to us. So a lot of—we kept texting our co-workers in that unit and encouraging them, and they kept telling us what was going on in that unit. If it was a normal day, we know that if somebody was dying, we could have stayed over after our shift and spent time with those residents, but because they were a COVID unit, we could not go there.

And we felt guilty when we heard such-and-such passed away and we could not be there. Their family could not be there for them. It was heartbreaking.

And then when it came to my unit, which is the Dementia unit, it was horrible. Like I said before in my opening statement, we were working short. There were 26 residents who were very ill, and the other CNA and I and a nurse and a housekeeper.

The nurse was overwhelmed. She have a lot to do. And she could not help us, and we could not help her. So we had to do the best we could. I remember my resident telling me she was scared. And I kept telling her, "It's okay." And then she was like, "No, can you stay with me?" And I couldn't stay with her to hold her hand. And I held her hand for a few seconds, and then I told her I had to go because somebody else needed me.

And she looked at me with a sad face, and she didn't want me to leave. And her family couldn't come in to hold her hand. And then I remember, that day a resident passed away. And then the funeral home couldn't come in to get the resident. They normally, on a regular day, before the pandemic, they came in and picked up the resident and we walked away once we put the resident in the bag, and we walked out the resident.

So our job was a resident passing away, and we had to—it was the hardest part—we had to put the resident in a bag, in a body bag. And those other residents, they are like a family, and we love them. So imagine if it's your own family who passed away at home and you have to put them in a body bag. And then we had to bring them outside.

So it was horrifying. We worked short all the time, and I am glad that we have a union that has our back. We made complaints, and the union did what they had to do. And then finally we got agency staff who came in to help us.

But the thing is, management were not there to help us. Like when we need help, we ask for help from management. If I am a CNA and a nurse, and another CNA is feeding a resident because that resident can't feed herself, then we call for help to come feed. They don't come to the floor. Another resident asked me, "I need to go to the bathroom."

So I have to make a choice right there and then. I have to leave that resident with the tray in front of them—that resident can't feed themselves—and take the other resident to the bathroom. Because with short staff, we don't have another staffer who would take over. And those are the choices that we had to make day to day before the pandemic, and with the pandemic, things got worse.

It is a sad situation, but I don't think it should just be a safe level that we're fighting for. Our union is fighting across the country to change the staffing of nursing homes. I think you guys have the power and that you can change it and have oversight in these nursing homes, and make it better for the quality of care for our residents and for our staff. Our staff are not leaving the nursing homes because they don't want to work in a nursing home; that is not the reason why they are leaving the nursing homes. They are leaving the nursing homes because the workload is a lot for the nurses and the CNAs. And they go work at the hospital where they will get less patients, and they pay them more than a nursing home.

They don't want to leave their residents, but they have to look at it with their health too at risk, and they don't want to go home exhausted after a long day at work, you know?

Senator WHITEHOUSE. Well, thank you so much, Ms. Ramos. People call you and your colleagues heroes for a reason. You are heroes of the heart, and I thank you for being here.

The CHAIRMAN. Ms. Ramos, you have another Senator who, I am sure, is very interested in your view as well, and we want to hear from her: Catherine Cortez Masto.

Senator CORTEZ MASTO. Thank you, Mr. Chairman and Ranking Member. This has been an incredible conversation.

Ms. Ramos, I am going to follow up because I truly agree with Senator Whitehouse. There are so many heroes on the front line right now, including you and so many at the SEIU and the work that you are doing.

My challenge has been—and I am hoping you can help with this—and I think the conversation you were having was, how do we attract more staff at the long-term care facilities?

Can you talk a little bit about the benefits and other things? What should we be doing? How do we attract them to make sure that we are not only getting them into the facilities because they are under-staffed, but taking care of them as well?

Ms. RAMOS. Thank you for your question. The way that we attract them is to put the starting rate higher than it is right now. Because nursing homes' starting rate is very low for

CNAs, and they can go to hospitals and make more, or they can work for agencies that are making double what we make.

So those are the challenges. And also, the staffing. They need to change the staffing in the nursing homes. Because if someone starts working in a nursing home and they end up having 12, 13 patients who are total care—they cannot do anything for themselves—within 3 months, they leave. And they get the experience that they need. They leave the nursing home, and they go to work somewhere else because, you know, they're like, "I can't do this job, because it's a lot and they don't pay enough."

So those are the main challenges that we face in the nursing homes. And I am grateful that I have a union that fights for better wages and better staffing in nursing homes, but when you're fighting for it State by State—we want this fight to go across the country.

Senator CORTEZ MASTO. Thank you. Thank you so much, and for your advocacy. It is so important.

Let me jump to, I believe it's Dr. Konetzka. I know there has been talk about private equity now being involved with long-term care, but can you opine on what sort of guard rails Congress should consider to ensure that additional resources that flow to long-term care facilities are invested in patient care and staff?

Dr. KONETZKA. Yes, it is an important question. And I think the first step is transparency. Right now, we just do not know where the money is flowing. So you know, we need to make reporting of those arrangements mandatory and assess where we are and whether current reimbursements are enough, or what else we need to invest into the system.

And then, I think the next step would be to consider some more oversight or regulation of these arrangements. When there is so much public money involved, I think some accountability is warranted. And we should be able to make sure, when we put Medicare and Medicaid money into nursing homes, that at least a certain proportion of it goes to patient care.

Senator CORTEZ MASTO. Thank you.

Again, this conversation today has been so helpful, I think to all of us. We so appreciate having this hearing today, Mr. Chairman, and I yield back to you.

The CHAIRMAN. I thank my colleague. And I know of her advocacy for seniors.

Here is my take on where things are. This has really been the area I have focused on in my time in public service. I was director of the Gray Panthers, ran the legal aid office for the elderly, and I have long known that, from sea to shining sea, there are persons who care deeply about the well-being of those patients in nursing homes.

And, Ms. Ramos, I can tell you—because I have visited with a couple of my colleagues when we were voting—you have left our members with a very clear call to action. You spelled it out: here are the problems, and the buck is not at the State level or the local level, or anywhere else; it is in the U.S. Congress. And the Senate Finance Committee has jurisdiction over this area.

I so appreciate what you have done. I appreciate all of you, and I think if I were to sum it up, despite all of the caring, good people who work in a number of nursing homes in America, we have still seen in the last year what I describe as a collision of mismanagement at every level. And Ms. Ramos started it off 3 hours ago when she talked about under-staffing and infection. And then she talked about the problems with PPE, not even being able to get basic protective equipment. And then she described, "Hey, by the way, we are also kind of in the dark. We have had difficulty getting information."

So I have had a number of opportunities over the years to hear about what needs to be done in terms of long-term care, and I think this has been a stellar panel. You have spelled it out.

Ms. Ramos has made it really clear. She is going to hold the Congress of the United States accountable. And that is exactly what we need. So I want you to know that I guess I am calling an end to the hearing for today, but let me tell you something. This hearing and the issues that we are going to be focused on, because of what you have said today and your call to action and accountability, is not something to be swept away. This is to be continued.

I thank you all. Terrific hearing, and I look forward to staying in touch.

Oh, I have one other matter. I would like to thank Ranking Member Crapo and all committee members for their participation. We thank our witnesses, of course, and for the information of all members, questions for the record should be submitted by 5 p.m. on Wednesday, March 24th. And with that, the hearing is adjourned.

Ms. RAMOS. Thank you.

[Whereupon, at 12:55 p.m., the hearing was concluded.]

Prepared Statement of Denise Bottcher, State Director, AARP Louisiana

Chairman Wyden, Ranking Member Crapo, and members of the committee, thank you for inviting AARP to testify today. My name is Denise Bottcher and I am the State director for AARP Louisiana. On behalf of our 38 million members, including over 425,000 in Louisiana, and all older Americans nationwide, AARP appreciates the opportunity to provide testimony at today's hearing. The situation in our nation's nursing homes and other long-term care facilities has been alarming since the beginning of the pandemic. Since then, AARP has consistently advocated for the health, safety and well-being of residents and staff.

These facilities have been ground zero in the fight against the coronavirus, representing a shockingly high share of COVID–19 deaths. Over 175,000 long-term care facility residents and staff have died—including almost 3,000 in Louisiana—due to COVID–19, representing about 35 percent of the deaths nationwide and over 30 percent of deaths in Louisiana, even though nursing home residents comprise less than one percent of the U.S. population.

These horrifying numbers are a tragedy and national disgrace. AARP has heard from thousands of people across the country whose loved ones—their mothers, fathers, grandparents, aunts, uncles, and dear friends—lost their lives, alone, in nursing homes. We recognize that even before the pandemic, many long-term care facilities struggled with basic infection control and adequate staffing. And we knew when the first COVID outbreak occurred at the Kirkwood facility, that the situation in these facilities was dire.

There were important steps taken, but too often the response was too slow and inadequate. Much more was and is needed now, and in the future, to protect residents, staff, their loved ones, and the surrounding communities from this disease. For the 4-week period ending February 14, the rates of COVID–19 cases and deaths in nursing homes were still higher than in late summer, according to AARP's Nursing Home Dashboard. That is unacceptable. While there may be a sense of relief with vaccines rolling out and cases and deaths in long-term care facilities finally declining, there are still too many deaths, and policy-makers and facilities are not relieved of their responsibility to protect nursing home residents. The consequences of not addressing the issues such as infection control, staffing, sufficient personal protective equipment and testing, oversight, accountability, and not following guidance is that someone's dad or mom dies. It is not a could act or should act situation, it is a must act situation. During the pandemic, AARP has urged action on a five-point plan to slow the spread and save lives:

1) Ensure facilities have adequate personal protective equipment for residents, staff, visitors, and others as needed, and prioritize regular and ongoing testing.
2) Improve transparency on COVID–19 and demographic data, vaccination rates of residents and staff by facility, and accountability for taxpayer dollars going to facilities.
3) Ensure access to in-person visitation following Federal and State guidelines for safety and require continued access to facilitated virtual visitation for all residents.
4) Ensure quality care for residents through adequate staffing, oversight, and in-person access to long-term care ombudsman.
5) Reject immunity and hold long-term care facilities accountable when they fail to provide proper care to residents.

Ensure Access to Personal Protective Equipment (PPE) and Testing

It is critical to provide PPE and ensure its consistent proper use by all staff caring for individuals in nursing homes, assisted living facilities, other residential care communities, home and community-based and other settings. PPE must be available for residents, staff, visitors, and surveyors.

Centers for Medicare and Medicaid Services (CMS) testing requirements for nursing home residents and staff have been an important step. We have strongly supported regular, prioritized testing of residents and staff as an important mechanism to prevent COVID–19 from entering nursing homes and other long-term care facilities, detect cases quickly, and stop transmission to additional residents and staff. Even with vaccines, we know that PPE and regular testing are still needed to stop the spread of coronavirus and other pathogens. AARP supports the funding in the American Rescue Plan Act for infection control and vaccine uptake support provided by quality improvement organizations to skilled nursing facilities. We also note that one of the best ways to keep people safe in nursing homes is to send fewer people to nursing homes who do not need that level of care.

Ensure Transparency on COVID–19, Demographic, and Vaccination Data, and Use of Funds by Providers

AARP has called for increased transparency of COVID–19 cases and deaths in long-term care facilities, including demographic data, such as race and ethnicity. We appreciated the CMS guidance and interim final rule with comment that took steps towards achieving greater transparency on COVID–19 cases and deaths and notification to residents, their representatives, and families about cases in the facility, as well as ensuring nursing homes are better prepared to respond to the public health emergency. While these reporting requirements are a necessary step, we believe care facilities should also report publicly daily whether they have confirmed COVID–19 cases and deaths, and that reporting should include demographic data.

The COVID–19 pandemic has shed light on the stark racial disparities affecting health outcomes for communities of color across the country. A recent national study found that nursing homes with a higher percentage of African American/Black or Hispanic residents had more than three times as many COVID–19 deaths as those that had a higher percentage of White residents. While there is a growing body of data that shows African Americans/Blacks, Hispanics, and American Indians and Alaska Natives are disproportionately impacted by the pandemic with higher rates of infection and death, more complete racial and ethnic data is still needed. Furthermore, there is insufficient data to fully demonstrate the impact of COVID–19 on Asian American and Pacific Islander (AAPI) communities, but some disaggregated data show mortality rates that are disproportionately high in some places.

To disrupt health disparities across the country, including those occurring within nursing homes and other long-term care facilities, we need better data. It is important that the Federal Government gather data and publicly report on COVID–19 cases, deaths, co-morbidities, and testing rates broken down into multiple demographic categories—while protecting patient privacy—including race, ethnicity, age, socioeconomic status, sexual orientation, gender identity, spoken/written language and disability. Data should also include venues such as hospitals, nursing homes, assisted living facilities, residential homes, and other locations. The information, disaggregated for all groups, should also be contrasted with 2019 numbers to truly understand the impact of COVID–19 on all communities. Collection, analysis, and regular public reporting of the detailed disaggregated information will help us effectively understand and respond to the crisis in a timely and focused way so that we can minimize the spread of the virus and improve health outcomes now and into the future. Indeed, given what we have learned in this crisis, improved data collection and reporting needs to be an ongoing practice for all long-term care facilities.

In addition, we believe vaccination data also needs to be broken down by age, race, and ethnicity for States, the Federal Government, and consumers to fully understand where the gaps are in vaccination administration. It is of utmost importance that this information be updated as quickly as possible, even daily. Furthermore, separate information about the number and percentage of residents and staff who have been vaccinated should be available by facility and State. While vaccines have given us all great hope of returning to normalcy, vaccines only work when they have been administered. We are deeply concerned about reports that there is a lack of vaccine confidence among long-term care staff. Policy-makers at the Federal and State level need to urgently focus their attention on this critical population to communicate clearly and credibly with these staff about the vaccines. Moreover, while the Long-Term Care Partnership with CVS and Walgreens was able to provide vaccines to residents and staff who wanted them, it is critical that vaccines remain available to new residents and staff, or those who initially opted out. We urge the Federal Government to work with States and long-term care facilities to ensure they can access and administer vaccines as needed.

We also need greater transparency on how the billions of dollars in taxpayer money from the Provider Relief Fund that have gone to facilities have been spent. Furthermore, if nursing homes or other long-term care facilities receive any additional dollars from the Provider Relief Fund or similar funds, AARP strongly urges that the administration and Congress ensure that such funding is used exclusively for the health, safety, and well-being of residents and staff, such as for PPE, testing, staffing, virtual visitation, infection control and other items that directly relate to resident care and well-being, prevention, and treatment. Facilities should be accountable for their use of taxpayer dollars, and funds should directly benefit residents.

Ensure Safe In-Person Visitation and Require Facilities to Provide and Facilitate Virtual Visitation

For many Americans living in nursing homes and other facilities, their friends and family provide not only a source of comfort, but also an important safety check. In-person visits, with some exceptions, have largely been halted over most of the past year.

We were pleased that CMS provided updated nursing home visitation guidance on March 10 that allows easier in-person visitation at nursing homes, while continuing to emphasize infection prevention and control practices for facilities, visitors, and others. This is very welcome news for nursing home residents and families.

In the year since the pandemic began, we have heard heartbreaking stories about the challenges families have had trying to see their relatives and the many important moments they missed. As we enter a new phase of this pandemic with the ongoing rollout of vaccines and growing knowledge about public health needs—including the safety, mental health, and social well-being of nursing home residents—it is vital that these vulnerable seniors can safely visit with their loved ones. Residents must be able to exercise their rights to visitation, and facilities should be held accountable for facilitating in-person visitation. AARP wrote to CMS on February 23 urging the agency to update its guidance, criteria, and support for safe in-person visitation.

While not a replacement for in-person visits, virtual visits can be an important lifeline for families, friends, and residents. We have urged Congress to require residential care facilities to make available and facilitate virtual visitation via video-conference or other technologies for residents and their loved ones. We also urge Congress to provide funding to support virtual visitation. AARP supports the bipartisan Advancing Connectivity during the Coronavirus to Ensure Support for Seniors Act (S. 57/H.R. 596), that would provide such funding, specifically grants to nursing homes to support virtual visits.

Ensure Adequate Staff, Oversight, and Access for Long-Term Care Ombudsmen

We are deeply concerned about staffing shortages at residential care facilities. AARP's Nursing Home Dashboard has consistently found over 25 percent of nursing homes nationally reporting a shortage of direct care workers since June 2020. It is essential that, at a minimum, staff/resident levels be maintained despite a potential reduction in workforce due to COVID–19 related circumstances. Many facilities had inadequate staff prior to the pandemic, and it is essential that staff be adequate to meet residents' many COVID- and non-COVID-related care needs, including infection control. Across the country, we have seen that higher staffing levels are associated with fewer deaths and COVID–19 cases in nursing homes. In addition, research shows that nursing homes with a registered nurse on staff help improve the quality of care. AARP supports funding in the American Rescue Plan Act for State strike teams in nursing homes with COVID–19 cases. AARP further urges Congress to take action to ensure that staffing levels in long-term care facilities are adequate, such as through pay and other compensation, paid leave, recruitment, training, and retention.

It also remains important for residents to have in-person access to long-term care ombudsmen, who play an important role in advocating for residents and their families.

More broadly, oversight from CMS and State survey agencies, including regular surveys, is vital now more than ever to ensure facilities are providing quality care and that resident health, safety, well-being, quality of life, and rights are protected. Strong enforcement action should be taken, when needed, to protect residents and ensure their rights. AARP also supports funding included in the American Rescue Plan Act for Elder Justice Act programs.

Reject Immunity for Nursing Homes and Other Long-Term Care Facilities and Hold Them Accountable

The pandemic has put residents' health, safety, and quality of care at unprecedented risk, as reflected by the horrific death tolls. We know that staff in many long-term care facilities are doing heroic work, putting their own health on the line to care for people in nursing homes. But sadly, AARP has heard from thousands of families across the country whose loved ones were not treated with the compassion or dignity that every American deserves. AARP strongly urges Congress to protect the safety of residents, including by maintaining the rights of residents and their families to seek legal redress to hold facilities accountable when residents are harmed, neglected, or abused.

Support Individuals to Remain in Their Homes and Communities

While we work to reform our Nation's long-term care facilities, we need to support the ability of people to remain in their homes and communities. Not only will this help people to live where they want to be, but also help to alleviate some of the challenges we are facing in our Nation's nursing homes. Furthermore, on average, for every one person residing in a nursing home, Medicaid can fund three individuals receiving community-based long-term care.

Congress must also look longer-term to give older adults and people with disabilities more options to live in their homes and communities, including more options to receive care at home, and more support for family caregivers who help make it possible. A family caregiver tax credit, as in the bipartisan, bicameral Credit for Caring Act, would help provide some financial relief to eligible family caregivers.

The pandemic has also highlighted the need to transform nursing homes, including by supporting or incentivizing small house nursing homes, such as Green Houses with private rooms and an empowered staff, making available private rooms, and creating a direct care ratio or medical loss ratio for nursing homes to ensure that public funds going to these facilities are used for resident care.

Families across the country are looking to Congress and the administration for swift action to protect the health and safety of their loved ones living in long-term care facilities now and in the future. We cannot wait any longer. Thank you again for your attention to this urgent challenge.

Questions Submitted for the Record to Denise Bottcher

Questions Submitted by Hon. Ron Wyden

Question. The Centers for Medicare and Medicaid Services (CMS) issued an interim final rule last year that required nursing homes to report COVID–19 data to the Centers for Disease Control and Prevention on a weekly basis beginning May 17, 2020. These data included COVID–19 infections, COVID–19 deaths, and the availability of key equipment and workers at individual nursing homes. The data have proved to be helpful for the public, policy-makers, and industry stakeholders to track the pandemic, and related issues, in these care settings. However, to date, CMS has *not* required nursing homes to provide such data prior to May 8, 2020, despite calls from Senate Democrats to do so. In September 2020, the Government Accountability Office (GAO) noted that "by not requiring nursing homes to submit data from the first 4 months of 2020, HHS is limiting the usefulness of the data in helping to understand the effects of COVID–19 in nursing homes." GAO went on to recommend that "HHS, in consultation with CMS and CDC, develop a strategy to capture more complete data on COVID–19 cases and deaths in nursing homes retroactively back to January 1, 2020."

Do you support GAO's recommendation? Why or why not? Please briefly explain.

Answer. Yes, AARP has supported the collection of data on COVID–19 cases and deaths in nursing homes retroactively prior to May 8th. Without this data, there is an incomplete State and national picture of COVID–19's impact on nursing home residents and staff. Given that nursing homes were not required to report COVID– 19 cases and deaths to the Centers for Medicare and Medicaid Services (CMS) until May, the numbers of COVID–19 cases and deaths reported by nursing homes are a significant undercount before June 2020 in this data source. Transparency is important and can help provide learnings to address issues and help make sure they do not happen again in the future.

Question. A recent paper published by the National Bureau of Economic Research noted that people who receive treatment in nursing homes owned by private equity firms have worse health outcomes than those living in facilities under other ownership structurers. This paper adds evidence to reports of worse outcomes associated with private equity's investment in the nursing home industry. Nursing homes have also become popular investments for real estate investment trusts (REITs), which often lease back properties to private equity firms or other related parties. The involvement of private equity in the nursing home industry has been of interest to the Finance Committee for more than a decade, and was a topic of interest for members during this hearing.

How would additional ownership transparency benefit families and patients as they consider nursing homes for themselves or their loved ones?

Answer. If consumers and their families have information about how a particular nursing home's ownership impacts or may impact the quality of care or quality of life residents receive in that nursing home, it could help them make more informed choices about whether that nursing home is appropriate for them and will meet their needs. It is important that information for consumers and their families is consumer-friendly and easily understandable.

Question. Section 6101 of the ACA sought to increase transparency of nursing home ownership structurers. To date, CMS has not fully implemented or enforced this section of the ACA, although the agency does have existing reporting mechanisms for nursing home ownership that provide a certain amount of information to the public. As the committee considers the changing ownership landscape in the nursing home industry, would implementing section 6101 provide sufficient transparency? Would you suggest additional measures the committee should consider?

Answer. Fully implementing current law is an important step. We suggest that the committee seek technical assistance from the Centers for Medicare and Medicaid Services and consult with researchers and others who have more closely examined private equity ownership to see what gaps may remain, and what additional measures may be needed to capture relevant data and information that may be important to families and the general public.

Question. COVID–19's toll on nursing homes has not been limited to viral infections. Residents have suffered mentally and physically, and had less access to family members and patient advocates. On March 10, 2021, the Centers for Medicare and Medicaid Services issued new guidance that allows for residents to more easily receive visitors. On the same day, the Centers for Disease Control and Prevention issued Updated Healthcare Infection Prevention and Control Recommendations in Response to COVID–19, which stated "quarantine is no longer recommended for residents who are being admitted to a post-acute care facility if they are fully vaccinated and have not had prolonged close contact with someone with SARS–coV–2 infection in the prior 14 days." The committee has received written testimony for this hearing from medical experts raising concerns that the new guidance may be overly permissive, and could put nursing home residents in danger, particularly if COVID–19 variants breakthrough vaccine protections. On the other hand, some advocates have called for more permissive visitation guidelines.

Do you view the guidance as properly balanced? Do you think there needs to be adjustments to protect the safety of residents and workers?

Answer. Throughout the pandemic, scientists across the globe have worked hard to better understand this virus and the disease it causes. We appreciate that as the science has progressed, the Centers for Medicare and Medicaid Services (CMS) and the Centers for Disease Control and Prevention (CDC) have adapted their ongoing guidance related to nursing homes. Informed learnings about public health needs— including the physical safety, mental health, and social well-being of nursing home residents—and ongoing vigilance to ensure these things is vital, especially given the impact of COVID–19 on nursing home residents and staff. Continued learnings, assessment, and information based on science, should inform guidance from CMS and CDC, which is important on these issues and will continue to be going forward.

Question. Preliminary research conducted by Columbia University researchers suggests that the Pfizer and Moderna vaccines were up to 12 times less effective at neutralizing the B.1.351 COVID–19 variant ("South African variant") than earlier strains of the coronavirus.[1]

---

[1] https://www.nature.com/articles/s41586-021-03398-2_reference.pdf?utm_medium=affiliate&utm_source=commission_junction&utm_campaign=3_nsn6445_deeplink_PID100024933&utm_content=deeplink.

The researchers also found that convalescent plasma was 9 times less effective against the South African variants, leading them to write "[t]aken together, the overall findings are worrisome, particularly in light of recent reports that both Novavax and Johnson & Johnson vaccines showed a substantial drop in efficacy in South Africa."[2] The researchers went on to write, "mutationally, this virus is traveling in a direction that could ultimately lead to escape from our current therapeutic and prophylactic interventions directed to the viral spike. If the rampant spread of the virus continues and more critical mutations accumulate, then we may be condemned to chasing after the evolving SARS–CoV–2 continually, as we have long done for influenza virus."[3] The Centers for Disease Control and Prevention (CDC) has previously found suspected cases of reinfection among nursing home residents who previously tested positive for COVID–19.[4] Similarly, a paper published earlier this year in *The Lancet* suggested that a resurgence in COVID–19 cases in the Brazilian city of Manaus may have been due to a new variant (known as P1 or "Brazilian variant") "may evade immunity generated in response to previous infections."[5]

The South African and Brazilian variants continue to circulate in the United States.[6] What is your level of concern about the danger that these and other COVID–19 variants may pose to nursing homes, particularly residents who have been most vulnerable to the disease?

Answer. While vaccines give us all great hope of returning to normalcy and we have seen declines in facility cases and deaths, given the impact of COVID–19 on residents and staff, continued vigilance is needed to ensure their health, safety, and well-being, including access to sufficient personal protective equipment (PPE) and testing. More than 182,000 residents and staff of nursing homes and other long-term care facilities have died due to COVID–19, representing about one-third of all COVID–19 deaths nationwide to date. These horrifying numbers are a tragedy and national disgrace, and we must take every precaution to prevent any further outbreaks.

Throughout the pandemic, scientists across the globe have worked hard to better understand this virus and the disease it causes. We appreciate that as the science has progressed, the Centers for Medicare and Medicaid Services (CMS) and the Centers for Disease Control and Prevention (CDC) have adapted their ongoing guidance related to nursing homes. Continued learnings and guidance from CMS and CDC will be important going forward.

Question. Is additional surveillance necessary to detect the spread of viral variants? What types of surveillance, if any, should be implemented in regards to the nursing home industry specifically?

Answer. Ongoing and improved public health surveillance related to COVID–19 and variants is important to understand how they are impacting individuals and the population overall. The Centers for Disease Control and Prevention (CDC) and Centers for Medicare and

---

[2] https://www.nature.com/articles/s41586-021-03398-2_reference.pdf?utm_medium=affiliate&utm_source=commission_junction&utm_campaign=3_nsn6445_deeplink_PID100024933&utm_ content=deeplink.
[3] https://www.nature.com/articles/s41586-021-03398-2_reference.pdf?utm_medium=affiliate&utm_source=commission_junction&utm_campaign=3_nsn6445_deep-link_PID100024933&utm_ content=deeplink.
[4] https://www.cdc.gov/mmwr/volumes/70/wr/mm7008a3.htm.
[5] https://www.thelancet.com/article/S0140-6736(21)00183-5/fulltext.
[6] https://www.cdc.gov/coronavirus/2019-ncov/transmission/variant-cases.html.

Medicaid Services (CMS) should work together to determine what types of additional surveillance, if any, should be implemented in relation to the nursing home industry. AARP has urged greater transparency around COVID– 19 and nursing homes, including on COVID–19 cases and deaths, demographic data, and vaccination rates of residents and staff by facility. If there is additional surveillance, timely information should be shared with the public, residents, families, and staff.

Question. In the event that additional vaccinations and/or booster shots are needed to protect against variants, do you have a view on what would be the best model to accomplish such a rollout, and what would be a reasonable amount of time?

Answer. We would encourage looking at the successes, experiences, and lessons learned from the Pharmacy Partnership for Long-Term Care Program and other State experiences with vaccinations in long-term care facilities. Using a model informed by those experiences, and perhaps similar to the Partnership, would be a good place to start. Timing should be informed by that previous experience and the protocol for additional vaccinations and/or booster shots, but once such vaccinations or booster shots are available they should be administered as effectively, efficiently, and quickly as possible. Given the risk to older populations, nursing home and other long-term care facility residents and older Americans should be prioritized. There should also be a clear plan from the beginning to ensure ongoing access to additional vaccinations and/or booster shots for residents and staff after the initial roll-out.

Question. What lessons can be drawn from the experience of the CVS-Walgreen Long-Term Care Partnership in regards to additional vaccination campaigns?

Answer. It is important to learn from what worked well in terms of the successful vaccination of residents and staff, as well as other lessons including the importance of educating residents, staff, and families about the vaccine and building vaccine confidence, especially among staff; having multiple ways to get consent for vaccination; ensuring sufficient vaccine supply and addressing initial distribution problems; improved allocation of the number of needed doses; and having a clear plan from the beginning to ensure ongoing access to additional vaccinations and/or booster shots for residents and staff after the initial rollout.

Question Submitted by Hon. Patrick J. Toomey

Question. Prior to the COVID–19 pandemic, I worked alongside my Pennsylvania colleague Senator Casey to address the quality of care for nursing homes residents. We were successful in pressing the Centers for Medicare and Medicaid Services (CMS) to publicize both participants and candidates affiliated with the Special Focus Facility (SFF) program, which provides more frequent oversight of facilities that consistently fail to meet Federal safety and care requirements.

Specific to this issue, Senator Casey and I reintroduced the Nursing Home Reform Modernization Act (S. 782) on March 16, 2021, which would expand the SFF program to ensure that all facilities nominated as candidates for the program receive additional oversight. Our legislation would also increase educational resources for underperforming facilities and create an independent advisory panel to inform CMS on how best to rank nursing home performance.

AARP has been instrumental in crafting our legislation and has endorsed the bill. Can you discuss the impact this legislation will have on nursing home residents?

Answer. AARP appreciates the bipartisan work that you and Senator Casey put into the Nursing Home Reform Modernization Act. Importantly, as you note, your bill would expand the number of nursing homes in the Special Focus Facility (SFF) Program to identify and increase transparency around those facilities with a history of serious quality issues and ensure they receive more frequent inspections. Inspections can help identify important quality of care issues or problems that must be addressed by a facility to ensure resident health and safety.

The legislation also includes vital consumer protections to help ensure appropriate oversight and accountability for nursing homes and requires consumer participation in an Advisory Council examining processes for ranking nursing homes prior to the establishment of such a ranking system. It is important for consumers to have representation on this Advisory Council, so that their voices and experiences help inform the Council's work.

Question Submitted by Hon. John Barrasso

Question. A top concern of Wyoming nursing facilities is making sure there are enough staff to care for residents.

Many Wyoming nursing homes provide professional development and other educational opportunities to attract and maintain their staff.

Can you discuss solutions related to workforce development you believe will improve the ability of nursing facilities to attract and maintain direct care staff?

Answer. COVID–19 exacerbated existing direct care staff shortages that pre-dated the pandemic. It is essential that, at a minimum, staff/resident levels be maintained despite a potential reduction in workforce due to COVID–19 related circumstances. Across the country, we have seen that higher staffing levels are associated with fewer deaths and COVID–19 cases in nursing homes. In addition, research shows that nursing homes with a registered nurse on staff help improve the quality of care. AARP supported funding in recently enacted legislation for State strike teams in nursing homes with COVID–19 cases. This would help provide additional support to facilities when they need it most. AARP has further urged Congress to act to ensure that staffing levels in long-term care facilities are adequate, such as through pay and other compensation, paid leave, recruitment, training, and retention.

Questions Submitted by Hon. Todd Young

Question. As outlined in many of your testimonies, the visiting restrictions and isolation necessitated by the COVID–19 pandemic took a heavy toll on the emotional and mental health of many nursing home residents separated from their family members and other loved ones. Fortunately, with increased vaccination and declining COVID–19 deaths, many of these restrictions have been lifted.

While we hope that restrictions of this scale will not be necessary again, it is worth examining ways to alleviate the negative emotional and mental health effects that isolation may have on nursing home residents. The use of technology, for one, has allowed residents to interact virtually with family and other loved ones from whom they are otherwise separated. Expanded use of telehealth has also helped residents access routine health-care services while limiting spread of the coronavirus.

What are some lessons learned from the public health emergency in terms of the integration of technology in nursing homes—both in helping residents visit virtually with loved ones and in accessing health-care services?

Answer. The COVID–19 pandemic increased the use of technology in nursing homes for virtual visits with loved ones and accessing health-care services through telehealth. While not a replacement for in-person visits, virtual visits can be an important lifeline for families, friends, and residents both as a source of comfort and an important safety check. Access to these visits is important. Among the lessons learned are the importance of access to the necessary technology, including video-conference or similar technology to enable residents to see their family and friends, and funding for it; designated staff to facilitate virtual visits with residents (including assisting with the use of the technology and scheduling visits); regular cleaning and disinfecting of devices; and the availability of broadband access to use the technology. It is also important for facilities to communicate clearly with residents and families about how to access virtual visits.

The use of telehealth in nursing homes during the pandemic has helped ensure more efficient and effective access to health care. Telehealth is an effective way to deliver care while preserving physical distancing and minimizing risk of COVID–19 exposure. In addition, telehealth may enable the participation of family caregivers in the visit with the consent of the resident. This could help with care coordination, care continuity, a smooth discharge from a skilled nursing facility, and care at home post-discharge. AARP has supported greater access to telehealth for Medicare beneficiaries, and CMS has made many temporary changes to increase telehealth access during the public health emergency. Data from these temporary administrative policy changes should be examined before they are made permanent by congressional action. Specifically, individual telehealth services should be reviewed for their impact on quality of care and disparities. We would also encourage policymakers to fully update and enforce the Health Insurance Portability and Accountability Act (HIPAA)—to reflect changes in technology and utilization—alongside making permanent policy changes. We also note that the use of telehealth is a tool meant to supplement, not replace, necessary in-person care.

Question. How do you anticipate this type of technology continuing to be used beyond the pandemic?

Answer. Beyond the pandemic, virtual visits can enable residents to visit with loved ones who may be unable to visit in person for a variety of reasons, including but not limited to distance or illness. Virtual visits can also be helpful and important if a resident is sick or not feeling well, to enable a larger group of individuals to visit with a resident, and to enable family and friends to check in on their loved ones. Technology can also help enable the participation of family caregivers—with the consent of the resident—to assist with care coordination, care continuity, a smooth discharge from a skilled nursing facility, and care at home post-discharge.

Submitted by Hon. Sherrod Brown, a U.S. Senator from Ohio

Congress of the United States
Washington, DC 20510
November 15, 2019

Kewsong Lee
Co-Chief Executive Officer
The Carlyle Group
1001 Pennsylvania Avenue, NW
Washington, DC 20004–2505

Glenn A. Youngkin
Co-Chief Executive Officer
The Carlyle Group
1001 Pennsylvania Avenue, NW
Washington, DC 20004-2505

Dear Messrs. Lee and Yonugkin:

We are writing to request information regarding the Carlyle Group's (Carlyle) investment in companies providing nursing home care and other long-term care services and to request information about your firm's structure and finances as it relates to these companies.

Private equity funds often operate under a model where they purchase controlling interests in companies for a short time, load them up with debt, strip them of their assets, extract exorbitant fees, and sell them at a profit—implementing drastic cost-cutting measures at the expense of consumers, workers, communities, and taxpayers. For that reason, we have concerns about the rapid spread and effect of private equity investment in many sectors of the economy, especially industries that affect vulnerable populations and rely primarily on taxpayer-funded programs such as Medicare and Medicaid, like the nursing home industry. We are particularly concerned about your firm's investment in large for-profit nursing home chains, which research has shown often provide worse care than not-for-profit faci1ities.[48] In light of these concerns, we request information about your firm, the portfolio companies in which it has invested, and the performance of those investments.

Nursing homes provide a wide range of important medical and personal care services to a growing and vulnerable elderly population, with 1.3 million residents in the United States currently receiving care in more than 15,000 facilities.[49] For decades, reports and data have highlighted the shocking living conditions found in many nursing home and other long-term

---

[48] *International Journal of Health Services,* "Ownership, Financing, and Management Strategies of the 10 largest for-profit nursing home chains in the United States," Charlene Harrington et al., 2011, *https://www.ncbi.nlm.nih.gov/pubmed/22053531;* Kaiser Family Foundation, "Reading the Stars: Nursing Home Quality Star Ratings, Nationally and by State," May 2015, *http://files.kff.org/attachment/issue-brief-reading-the-stars-nursing-home-quality-star-ratings-nationally-and-by-state.*

[49] National Center for Health Statistics, "Long-term Care Providers and Services Users in the United States, 2015–2016," February 2019, *https://www.cdc.gov/nchs/data/series/sr_03/sr03_43-508.pdf.*

care facilities across the country.[50] Twelve years ago, for example, journalists uncovered how a group of private investment firms acquired 49 nursing homes, including a facility in Florida where managers slashed the number of registered nurses by half and cut supply and activity budgets. Residents, meanwhile, suffered from preventable infections and injuries.[51] Last year, news reports similarly detailed how a for-profit nursing home employed drastic cost cutting measures, "exposed its roughly 25,000 patients to increasing health risk,' and ultimately filed for bankruptcy—all after a private equity firm acquired the company.[52]

This is particularly concerning given the fact that two-thirds of nursing home residents rely on government-sponsored health insurance coverage, meaning both not-for-profit and for-profit nursing homes benefit from government funding.[53] Medicaid is the primary payer[54] for nursing home care, with Medicare and Medicaid combined covering approximately 75 percent of nursing home residents.[55] In 2015, taxpayers sent more than $55 billion to the nursing home industry to cover the costs of long-term care. These reports and corresponding research raise serious questions about the role of private equity firms in the nursing home care industry, and the extent to which these firms' emphasis on profits and short-term return is responsible for declines in quality of care. They also raise concerns over the stewardship of taxpayer dollars, when—in many cases—these facilities continue to receive Medicare and Medicaid funding despite their decline in quality.

The majority of nursing facilities—almost 70%—are for-profit, and over half are chain-affiliated.[56] The overwhelming majority of research conducted over the last 2 decades shows that for-profit and chain affiliated[57] companies provide a lower quality of care and experience more serious health and safety deficiencies when compared to non-profit facilities.[58]

---

[50] *New York Times,* "At Many Homes, More Profit and Less Nursing," Charles Duhigg, September 23, 2017, *https://www.nytimes.com/2007/09/23/business/23nursing.html; Reveal,* "The rats sensed she was going to pass away," Jennifer Gollan, September 18, 2019, *https://www.revealnews.org/article/elderly-often-face-neglect-in-california-care-homes-that-exploit-work-ers/.*

[51] *New York Times,* "At Many Homes, More Profit and Less Nursing," Charles Duhigg, September 23, 2017, *https://www.nytimes.com/2007/09/23/business/23nursing.html.*

[52] *Washington Post,* "Overdoses, bedsores, broken bones: What happened when a private-equity firm sought to care for society's most vulnerable," Peter Whoriskey and Dan Keating, November 25, 2018, *https://www.washingtonpost.com/business/economy/opioid-overdoses-bedsores-and-broken-bones-what-happened-when-a-private-equity-firm-sought-profits-in-caring-for-societys-most-vulnerable/2018/11/25/09089a4a-ed14-11e8-baac-2a674e91502b_story.html.*

[53] Kaiser Family Foundation, "Distribution of Certified Nursing Facility Residents by Primary Payer Source," accessed on Nov. 14, 2019, *https://www.kff.org/other/state-indicator/distribution-of-certified-nursing-facilities-by-primary-payer-source/?currentTimeframe=0&sortModel=%7B%22colId%22:%22Location%22,%22sort%22:%22asc%22%7D.*

[54] Kaiser Family Foundation, "Medicaid's Role in Nursing Home Care," June 20, 2017, *https://www.kff.org/infographic/medicaids-role-in-nursing-home-care/.*

[55] Kaiser Family Foundation, "Distribution of Certified Nursing Facility Residents by Primary Payer Source," accessed on Nov. 14, 2019, *https://www.kff.org/other/state-indicator/distribution-of-certified-nursing-facilities-by-primary-payer-source/?currentTimeframe=0&sortModel=%7B%22colId%22:%22Location%22,%22sort%22:%22asc%22%7D.*

[56] National Center for Health Statistics, "Long-term Care Providers and Services Users in the United States, 2015–2016," February 2019, *https://www.cdc.gov/nchs/data/series/sr_03/sr03_43-508.pdf.*

[57] Facilities owned or leased by "an organization that owns two or more long-term care facilities."

[58] *International Journal of Health Services,* "Ownership, Financing, and Management Strategies of the 10 largest for-profit nursing home chains in the United States," Charlene Harrington et al., 2011; *Medical Care Research and Review,* "Nursing home profit status and quality of care: Is there any evidence of an association?", Michael P. Hillmer et al., April 2005, *https://www.ncbi.nlm.nih.gov/pubmed/15750174.*

Additionally, for-profit facilities receive the lowest scores in the Centers for Medicare and Medicaid Services' (CMS) nursing home rating system that takes into account, state health inspections, staffing ratios and quality measures.[59]

Private equity investment appears to exacerbate the problems faced at chain-affiliated for-profit nursing homes. Studies show that private equity-owned facilities generally "deliver poorer quality of care" than other chain-affiliated for-profit facilities; are likely to try to reduce cost by "substituting expensive but skilled RNs with cheaper and less skilled nurses;" and "report significantly higher number of deficiencies" that climb with more years of private equity ownership. As a result, private equity-owned nursing homes have 21% higher deficiencies, 25% lower nursing staff skill mix, and "worse results on pressure sore prevention . . . and [higher] pressure ulcer [] risk prevalence."[60] That was reportedly the case at HCR ManorCare—the second largest for-profit nursing home chain in the United States. In the years following its acquisition by your firm, "the number of citations increased for, among other things, neither preventing nor treating bed sores; medication errors; not providing proper care for people who need special services such as injections, colostomies and prostheses; and not assisting patients with eating and personal hygiene."[61]

Moreover, while the quality of service declines, the complicated ownership and operating structure of these investments "limit legal remedies available to aggrieved residents."[62] For example, after a resident died at the private-equity-owned Habana Health Care Center (as a result of "a wound [that] should have been detected much earlier"), a family member tried to sue the owners of the facility, only to discover that the facility's complicated ownership structure "meant that even if she prevailed in court, the investors' wallets would likely be out of reach."[63] Shifting funds to other affiliated entities, or to the private equity firm itself, to immunize itself from liability for judgments against a target company is a widespread practice in the private equity industry.

Private equity investment in this sector has increased over the last few decades. The Government Accountability Office found that over the span of 10 years ending in 2008, private investment firms acquired approximately 1,900 unique nursing homes.[64] Today, private equity firms own or operate several large for-profit chains that control hundreds of facilities and provide nursing home care among other long-term care services.[65] Carlyle reportedly owns or has had investments in companies providing nursing home care. In order to help us understand

[59] Kaiser Family Foundation, "Reading the Stars: Nursing Home Quality Star Ratings, Nationally and by State," May 2015, *http://files.kff.org/attachment/issue-brief-reading-the-stars-nursing-home-quality-star-ratings-nationally-and-by-state.*

[60] *Journal of Health Care Finance,* "Private Equity Ownership of Nursing Homes: Implications for Quality," Rohit Pradhan et al., June–July 2014, *http://healthfinancejournal.com/index.php/johcf/article/view/12.*

[61] *Washington Post,* "Overdoses, bedsores, broken bones: What happened when a private-equity firm sought to care for society's most vulnerable," Peter Whoriskey and Dan Keating, November 25, 2018, *https://www.washingtonpost.com/business/economy/opioid-overdoses-bed-sores-and-broken-bones-what-happened-when-a-private-equity-firm-sought-profits-in-caring-for-societys-most-vulnerable/2018/11/25/09089a4a-ed14-11e8-baac-2a674e91502b_story.html.*

[62] *Journal of Health Care Finance,* "Private Equity Ownership of Nursing Homes: Implications for Quality," Rohit Pradhan et al., June–July 2014, *http://healthfinancejournal.com/index.php/johcf/article/view/12.*

[63] *New York Times,* "At Many Homes, More Profit and Less Nursing," Charles Duhigg, September 23, 2007, *https://www.nytimes.com/2007/09/23/business/23nursing.html.*

[64] Government Accountability Office, "Nursing Homes: Complexity of Private Investment Purchases Demonstrates Need for CMS to Improve the Usability and Completeness of Ownership Data," September 2010, *https://www.gao.gov/assets/320/310562.pdf.*

[65] IQVIA, "U.S. Elder Care Market Summary," September 2019, *https://www.skainfo.com/reports/u.s.-elder-care-market-summary.*

your firm' s role in the nursing home sector, we ask that you provide answers to the following questions no later than November 29, 2019.

1. Please provide the disclosure documents and information enumerated in Sections 501 and 503 of the Stop Wall Street Looting Act.[66]
2. Which nursing home or other long-term care service companies, including all affiliates or related entities, does Carlyle have a stake in or own? Please provide the name of and a brief description of the services each company provides—including the number of facilities that it owns or operates.
    a. Which nursing home or other long-term care companies, including all affiliates or related entities, has Carlyle had a stake in or owned in the past 20 years? Please provide the name of and a brief description of the services each company provides or provided—including the number of nursing home and other long-term care facilities that it owned or operated.
    b. For each nursing home or other long-term care service company Carlyle had a stake in or owned in the past 20 years, including all affiliates or related entities, please provide the following information for each year that the firm have had a stake in or owned this company and the 5 years preceding the firm's investment.
        I. The name of the company
        II. Total number of facilities, by type of facility
        III. Ownership stake
        IV. Total revenue, and the total revenue from Medicare, and from Medicaid
        V. Total transaction, advisory, or other fees collected after the acquisition of the company
        VI. Net income
        VII. Total number of employees for each facility
        VIII. Total number of patients for each facility, and the total number whose care is paid for by Medicare, and by Medicaid
        IX. Other private-equity firms that own a stake in the company
3. Private-equity firms reportedly employ sale-leaseback arrangements in order to quickly recover investments. For each company listed in questions 2(a) and 2(b), please list the number of nursing home or other long-term care facilities for which you acquired real estate assets, and whether a sale-lease-back agreement has been executed for any of those companies or facilities.
4. Has any nursing home or other long-term care company, including all affiliates or related entities, in which Carlyle has an ownership stake or has had an ownership stake in the last 20 years received Section 232 Department of Housing and Urban Development (HUD)-insured mortgages? If so, please provide the name of each facility and the total value of each loan insured by HUD.
5. Has any nursing home or other long-term care company, including all affiliates or related entities, in which Carlyle has an ownership stake or has had an ownership stake in the last 20 years, been placed in receivership? Please provide the name of each facility.

---

[66] Stop Wall Street Looting Act, S. 2155, *https://www.congress.gov/bill/116th-congress/senate-bill/2155.*

6. Has any nursing home or other long-term care company, including all affiliates or related entities, in which Carlyle has an ownership stake or has had an ownership stake in the last 20 years, been found to have violated any federal or state laws or regulations? If so, please provide a complete list, including the date and description, of all such violations. Please also include a list of all deficiencies identified in state or federal surveys of the facilities owned by the company for each year.
7. Has any nursing home or other long-term care company, including all affiliates or related entities, in which Carlyle has an ownership stake or has had an ownership stake in the last 20 years, reached a settlement with any federal or state law enforcement entity related to a potential violation of any federal or state laws or regulations or deficiencies in providing care? If so, please provide a complete list, including the date and description, of all such settlements.
8. Has any nursing home or other long-term care company, including all affiliates or related entities, in which Carlyle has an ownership stake or has had an ownership stake in the past 20 years, reached a settlement with any individual who was provided services by the company related to a potential violation of any federal or state laws or regulations or deficiencies in providing care? If so, please provide a complete list, including the date and description, of all such settlements.

Thank you for your attention to this matter.
Sincerely,
Elizabeth Warren
United States Senator
Sherrod Brown United States Senator

Mark Pocan
Member of Congress

* * *

Congress of the United States
Washington, DC 20510
November 15, 2019

Arnold Whitman
Chairman
Formation Capital
3500 Lenox Road, Suite 510
Atlanta, Georgia 30326

Brian Beckwith
Formation Capital
3500 Lenox Road, Suite 510
Atlanta, Georgia 30326

Dear Messrs. Whitman and Beckwith:

We are writing to request information regarding Formation Capital's (Formation) investment in companies providing nursing home care and other long-term care services and to request information about your firm' s structure and finances as it relates to these companies.

Private equity funds often operate under a model where they purchase controlling interests in companies for a short time, load them up with debt, strip them of their assets, extract exorbitant fees, and sell them at a profit—implementing drastic cost-cutting measures at the expense of consumers, workers, communities, and taxpayers. For that reason, we have concerns about the rapid spread and effect of private equity investment in many sectors of the economy, especially industries that affect vulnerable populations and rely primarily on taxpayer-funded programs such as Medicare and Medicaid, like the nursing home industry. We are particularly concerned about your firm's investment in large for-profit nursing home chains, which research has shown often provide worse care than not-for-profit facilities.[67] In light of these concerns, we request information about your firm, the portfolio companies in which it has invested, and the performance of those investments.

Nursing homes provide a wide range of important medical and personal care services to a growing and vulnerable elderly population, with 1.3 million residents in the United States currently receiving care in more than 15,000 facilities.[68] For decades, reports and data have highlighted the shocking living conditions found in many nursing home and other long-term care facilities across the country.[69] Twelve years ago, for example, journalists uncovered how a group of private investment firms acquired 49 nursing homes, including a facility in Florida where managers slashed the number of registered nurses by half and cut supply and activity budgets. Residents, meanwhile, suffered from preventable infections and injuries.[70] Last year, news reports similarly detailed how a for-profit nursing home employed drastic cost cutting measures, "exposed its roughly 25,000 patients to increasing health risk," and ultimately filed for bankruptcy—all after a private equity firm acquired the company.[71]

This is particularly concerning given the fact that two-thirds of nursing home residents rely on government-sponsored health insurance coverage, meaning both not-for-profit and for-profit

[67] *International Journal of Health Services,* "Ownership, Financing, and Management Strategies of the 10 largest for-profit nursing home chains in the United States," Charlene Harrington et al., 2011, *https://www.ncbi.nlm.nih.gov/pubmed/22053531;* Kaiser Family Foundation, "Reading the Stars: Nursing Home Quality Star Ratings, Nationally and by State," May 2015, *http://files.kff.org/attachment/issue-brief-reading-the-stars-nursing-home-quality-star-ratings-nationally-and-by-state.*

[68] National Center for Health Statistics, "Long-term Care Providers and Services Users in the United States, 2015–2016," February 2019, *https://www.cdc.gov/nchs/data/series/sr_03/sr03_43-508.pdf.*

[69] *New York Times,* "At Many Homes, More Profit and Less Nursing," Charles Duhigg, September 23, 2017, *https://www.nytimes.com/2007/09/23/business/23nursing.html; Reveal,* "The rats sensed she was going to pass away," Jennifer Gollan, September 18, 2019, *https://www.revealnews.org/article/elderly-often-face-neglect-in-california-care-homes-that-exploit-workers/.*

[70] *New York Times,* "At Many Homes, More Profit and Less Nursing," Charles Duhigg, September 23, 2017, *https://www.nytimes.com/2007/09/23/business/23nursing.html.*

[71] *Washington Post,* "Overdoses, bedsores, broken bones: What happened when a private-equity firm sought to care for society's most vulnerable," Peter Whoriskey and Dan Keating, November 25, 2018, *https://www.washingtonpost.com/business/economy/opioid-overdoses-bedsores-and-broken-bones-what-happened-when-a-private-equity-firm-sought-profits-in-caring-for-societys-most-vulnerable/2018/11/25/09089a4a-ed14-11e8-baac-2a674e91502b_story.html.*

nursing homes benefit from government funding.[72] Medicaid is the primary payer[73] for nursing home care, with Medicare and Medicaid combined covering approximately 75 percent of nursing home residents.[74] In 2015, taxpayers sent more than $55 billion to the nursing home industry to cover the costs of long-term care. These reports and corresponding research raise serious questions about the role of private equity firms in the nursing home care industry, and the extent to which these firms' emphasis on profits and short-term return is responsible for declines in quality of care. They also raise concerns over the stewardship of taxpayer dollars, when—in many cases—these facilities continue to receive Medicare and Medicaid funding despite their decline in quality.

The majority of nursing facilities—almost 70%—are for-profit, and over half are chain-affiliated.[75] The overwhelming majority of research conducted over the last 2 decades shows that for-profit and chain affiliated[76] companies provide a lower quality of care and experience more serious health and safety deficiencies when compared to non-profit facilities.[77]

Additionally, for-profit facilities receive the lowest scores in the Centers for Medicare and Medicaid Services' (CMS) nursing home rating system that takes into account, state health inspections, staffing ratios and quality measures.[78]

Private equity investment appears to exacerbate the problems faced at chain-affiliated for-profit nursing homes. Studies show that private equity-owned facilities generally "deliver poorer quality of care" than other chain-affiliated for-profit facilities; are likely to try to reduce cost by "substituting expensive but skilled RNs with cheaper and less skilled nurses;" and "report significantly higher number of deficiencies" that climb with more years of private equity ownership. As a result, private equity-owned nursing homes have 21% higher deficiencies, 25% lower nursing staff skill mix, and "worse results on pressure sore prevention . . . and [higher] pressure ulcer [] risk prevalence."[79] That was reportedly the case at HCR ManorCare—the second largest for-profit nursing home chain in the United States. In the years following its acquisition by a private equity firm, "the number of citations increased for, among other things, neither preventing nor treating bed sores; medication errors; not providing proper

---

[72] Kaiser Family Foundation, "Distribution of Certified Nursing Facility Residents by Primary Payer Source," accessed on Nov. 14, 2019, *https://www.kff.org/other/state-indicator/distribution-of-certified-nursing-facilities-by-primary-payer-source/?currentTimeframe=O&sortModel=%7B%22colId%22:%22Location%22.%22sort%22:%22asc%22%7D.*

[73] Kaiser Family Foundation, "Medicaid's Role in Nursing Home Care," June 20, 2017, *https://www.kff.org/infographic/medicaids-role-in-nursing-home-care/.*

[74] Kaiser Family Foundation, "Distribution of Certified Nursing Facility Residents by Primary Payer Source," accessed on Nov. 14, 2019, *https://www.kff.org/other/state-indicator/distribution-of-certified-nursing-facilities-by-primary-payer-source/?currentTimeframe=O&sortModel=%7B%22colId%22:%22Location%22,%22sort%22:%22asc%22%7D.*

[75] National Center for Health Statistics, "Long-term Care Providers and Services Users in the United States, 2015–2016," February 2019, *https://www.cdc.gov/nchs/data/series/sr_03/sr03_43-508.pdf.*

[76] Facilities owned or leased by "an organization that owns two or more long-term care facilities."

[77] *International Journal of Health Services,* "Ownership, Financing, and Management Strategies of the ten largest for-profit nursing home chains in the United States," Charlene Harrington et al., 2011; *Medical Care Research and Review,* "Nursing home profit status and quality of care: Is there any evidence of an association?", Michael P. Hillmer et al., April 2005, *https://www.ncbi.nlm.nih.gov/pubmed/15750174.*

[78] Kaiser Family Foundation, "Reading the Stars: Nursing Home Quality Star Ratings, Nationally and by State," May 2015, *http://files.kff.org/attachment/issue-brief-reading-the-stars-nursing-home-quality-star-ratings-nationallyand-by-state.*

[79] *Journal of Health Care Finance,* "Private Equity Ownership of Nursing Homes: Implications for Quality," Rohit Pradhan et al., June–July 2014, *http://healthfinancejournal.com/index.php/johcf/article/view/12.*

care for people who need special services such as injections, colostomies and prostheses; and not assisting patients with eating and personal hygiene."[80]

Moreover, while the quality of service declines, the complicated ownership and operating structure of these investments "limit legal remedies available to aggrieved residents."[81] For example, after a resident died at the private-equity-owned Habana Health Care Center (as a result of "a wound [that] should have been detected much earlier"), a family member tried to sue the owners of the facility, only to discover that the facility's complicated ownership structure "meant that even if she prevailed in court, the investors' wallets would likely be out of reach."[82] Shifting funds to other affiliated entities, or to the private equity firm itself, to immunize itself from liability for judgments against a target company is a widespread practice in the private equity industry.

Private equity investment in this sector has increased over the last few decades. The Government Accountability Office found that over the span of 10 years ending in 2008, private investment firms acquired approximately 1,900 unique nursing homes.[83] Today, private equity firms own or operate several large for-profit chains that control hundreds of facilities and provide nursing home care among other longterm care services.[84] Formation reportedly owns or has had investments in companies providing nursing home care. In order to help us understand your firm's role in the nursing home sector, we ask that you provide answers to the following questions no later than November 29, 2019.

1. Please provide the disclosure documents and information enumerated in Sections 501 and 503 of the Stop Wall Street Looting Act.[85]
2. Which nursing home or other long-term care service companies, including all affiliates or related entities, does Formation have a stake in or own? Please provide the name of and a brief description of the services each company provides—including the number of facilities that it owns or operates.
    a. Which nursing home or other long-term care companies, including all affiliates or related entities, has Formation had a stake in or owned in the past 20 years? Please provide the name of and a brief description of the services each company provides or provided-including the number of nursing home and other long-term care facilities that it owned or operated.
    b. For each nursing home or other long-term care service company Formation had a stake in or owned in the past 20 years, including all affiliates or related entities,

---

80 *Washington Post,* "Overdoses, bedsores, broken bones: What happened when a private-equity firm sought to care for society's most vulnerable," Peter Whoriskey and Dan Keating, November 25, 2018, *https://www.washingtonpost.com/business/economy/opioid-overdoses-bed-sores-and-broken-bones-what-happened-when-a-private-equity-firm-sought-profits-in-caring-for-societys-most-vulnerable/2018/11/25/09089a4a-ed14-11e8-baac-2a674e91502b_story.html.*

81 *Journal of Health Care Finance,* "Private Equity Ownership of Nursing Homes: Implications for Quality," Rohit Pradhan et al., June–July 2014, *http://healthfinancejournal.com/index.php/johcf/article/view/12.*

82 *New York Times,* "At Many Homes, More Profit and Less Nursing," Charles Duhigg, September 23, 2007, *https://www.nytimes.com/2007/09/23/business/23nursing.html.*

83 Government Accountability Office, "Nursing Homes: Complexity of Private Investment Purchases Demonstrates Need for CMS to Improve the Usability and Completeness of Ownership Data," September 2010, *https://www.gao.gov/assets/320/310562.pdf.*

84 IQVIA, "U.S. Elder Care Market Summary," September 2019, *https://www.skainfo.com/reports/u.s.-elder-care-market-summary.*

85 Stop Wall Street Looting Act, S. 2155, *https://www.congress.gov/bill/116th-congress/senate-bill/2155.*

please provide the following information for each year that the firm have had a stake in or owned this company and the 5 years preceding the firm's investment.

I. The name of the company
II. Total number of facilities, by type of facility
III. Ownership stake
IV. Total revenue, and the total revenue from Medicare, and from Medicaid
V. Total transaction, advisory, or other fees collected after the acquisition of the company
VI. Net income
VII. Total number of employees for each facility
VIII. Total number of patients for each facility, and the total number whose care is paid for by Medicare, and by Medicaid
IX. Other private-equity firms that own a stake in the company

3. Private-equity firms reportedly employ sale-leaseback arrangements in order to quickly recover investments. For each company listed in questions 2(a) and 2(b), please list the number of nursing home or other long-term care facilities for which you acquired real estate assets, and whether a sale-lease-back agreement has been executed for any of those companies or facilities.
4. Has any nursing home or other long-term care company, including all affiliates or related entities, in which Formation has an ownership stake or has had an ownership stake in the last 20 years received Section 232 Department of Housing and Urban Development (HUD)-insured mortgages? If so, please provide the name of each facility and the total value of each loan insured by HUD.
5. Has any nursing home or other long-term care company, including all affiliates or related entities, in which Formation has an ownership stake or has had an ownership stake in the last 20 years, been placed in receivership? Please provide the name of each facility.
6. Has any nursing home or other long-term care company, including all affiliates or related entities, in which Formation has an ownership stake or has had an ownership stake in the last 20 years, been found to have violated any federal or state laws or regulations? If so, please provide a complete list, including the date and description, of all such violations. Please also include a list of all deficiencies identified in state or federal surveys of the facilities owned by the company for each year.
7. Has any nursing home or other long-term care company, including all affiliates or related entities, in which Formation has an ownership stake or has had an ownership stake in the last 20 years, reached a settlement with any federal or state law enforcement entity related to a potential violation of any federal or state laws or regulations or deficiencies in providing care? If so, please provide a complete list, including the date and description, of all such settlements.
8. Has any nursing home or other long-term care company, including all affiliates or related entities, in which Formation has an ownership stake or has had an ownership stake in the past 20 years, reached a settlement with any individual who was provided services by the company related to a potential violation of any federal or state laws or regulations or deficiencies in providing care? If so, please provide a complete list, including the date and description, of all such settlements.

Thank you for your attention to this matter.
Sincerely,
Elizabeth Warren
United States Senator
Mark Pocan
United States Congress
Sherrod Brown
United States Senator

* * *

Congress of the United States
Washington, DC 20510
November 15, 2019
Ronald E. Silva
President and Chief Executive Officer
Fillmore Capital Partners
Four Embarcadero Center, Suite 710
San Francisco, CA 94111

Dear Mr. Silva:

We are writing to request information regarding Fillmore Capital Partners' (Fillmore) investment in companies providing nursing home care and other long-term care services and to request information about your firm's structure and finances as it relates to these companies.

Private equity funds often operate under a model where they purchase controlling interests in companies for a short time, load them up with debt, strip them of their assets, extract exorbitant fees, and sell them at a profit—implementing drastic cost-cutting measures at the expense of consumers, workers, communities, and taxpayers. For that reason, we have concerns about the rapid spread and effect of private equity investment in many sectors of the economy, especially industries that affect vulnerable populations and rely primarily on taxpayer-funded programs such as Medicare and Medicaid, like the nursing home industry. We are particularly concerned about your firm's investment in large for-profit nursing home chains, which research has shown often provide worse care than not-for-profit facilities.[86] In light of these concerns, we request information about your firm, the portfolio companies in which it has invested, and the performance of those investments.

Nursing homes provide a wide range of important medical and personal care services to a growing and vulnerable elderly population, with 1.3 million residents in the United States currently receiving care in more than 15,000 facilities.[87] For decades, reports and data have highlighted the shocking living conditions found in many nursing home and other long-term

[86] *International Journal of Health Services,* "Ownership, Financing, and Management Strategies of the 10 largest for-profit nursing home chains in the United States," Charlene Harrington et al., 2011, *https://www.ncbi.nlm.nih.gov/pubmed/22053531;* Kaiser Family Foundation, "Reading the Stars: Nursing Home Quality Star Ratings, Nationally and by State," May 2015, *http://files.kff.org/attachment/issue-brief-reading-the-stars-nursing-home-quality-star-ratings-nationally-and-by-state.*

[87] National Center for Health Statistics, "Long-term Care Providers and Services Users in the United States, 2015–2016," February 2019, *https://www.cdc.gov/nchs/data/series/sr_03/sr03_43-508.pdf.*

care facilities across the country.[88] Twelve years ago, for example, journalists uncovered how a group of private investment firms acquired 49 nursing homes, including a facility in Florida where managers slashed the number of registered nurses by half and cut supply and activity budgets. Residents, meanwhile, suffered from preventable infections and injuries.[89] Last year, news reports similarly detailed how a for-profit nursing home employed drastic cost cutting measures, "exposed its roughly 25,000 patients to increasing health risk," and ultimately filed for bankruptcy—all after a private equity firm acquired the company.[90]

This is particularly concerning given the fact that two-thirds of nursing home residents rely on government-sponsored health insurance coverage, meaning both not-for-profit and for-profit nursing homes benefit from government funding.[91] Medicaid is the primary payer[92] for nursing home care, with Medicare and Medicaid combined covering approximately 75 percent of nursing home residents.[93] In 2015, taxpayers sent more than $55 billion to the nursing home industry to cover the costs of long-term care. These reports and corresponding research raise serious questions about the role of private equity firms in the nursing home care industry, and the extent to which these firms' emphasis on profits and short-term return is responsible for declines in quality of care. They also raise concerns over the stewardship of taxpayer dollars, when—in many cases—these facilities continue to receive Medicare and Medicaid funding despite their decline in quality.

The majority of nursing facilities—almost 70%—are for-profit, and over half are chain-affiliated.[94] The overwhelming majority of research conducted over the last 2 decades shows that for-profit and chain affiliated[95] companies provide a lower quality of care and experience more serious health and safety deficiencies when compared to non-profit facilities.[96]

---

[88] *New York Times,* "At Many Homes, More Profit and Less Nursing," Charles Duhigg, September 23, 2017, *https://www.nytimes.com/2007/09/23/business/23nursing.html; Reveal,* "The rats sensed she was going to pass away," Jennifer Gollan, September 18, 2019, *https://www.revealnews.org/article/elderly-often-face-neglect-in-california-care-homes-that-exploit-workers/.*

[89] *New York Times,* "At Many Homes, More Profit and Less Nursing," Charles Duhigg, September 23, 2017, *https://www.nytimes.com/2007/09/23/business/23nursing.html.*

[90] *Washington Post,* "Overdoses, bedsores, broken bones: What happened when a private-equity firm sought to care for society's most vulnerable," Peter Whoriskey and Dan Keating, November 25, 2018, *https://www.washingtonpost.com/business/economy/opioid-overdoses-bedsores-and-broken-bones-what-happened-when-a-private-equity-firm-sought-profits-in-caring-for-societys-most-vulnerable/2018/11/25/09089a4a-ed14-11e8-baac-2a674e91502b*_story.html.

[91] Kaiser Family Foundation. "Distribution of Certified Nursing Facility Residents by Primary Payer Source," accessed on Nov. 14, 2019, *https://www.kff.org/other/state-indicator/distribution-of-certified-nursing-facilities-by-primary-payer-source/?currentTimeframe=O&sortModel=%7B%22colId%22:%22Location%22.%22sort%22:%22asc%22%7D.*

[92] Kaiser Family Foundation, "Medicaid's Role in Nursing Home Care," June 20, 2017, *https://www.kff.org/infographic/medicaids-role-in-nursing-home-care/.*

[93] Kaiser Family Foundation, "Distribution of Certified Nursing Facility Residents by Primary Payer Source," accessed on Nov. 14, 2019, *https://www.kff.org/other/state-indicator/distribution-of-certified-nursing-facilities-by-primary-payer-source/?currentTimeframe=O&sortModel=%7B%22colId%22:%22Location%22,%22sort%22:%22asc%22%7D.*

[94] National Center for Health Statistics, "Long-term Care Providers and Services Users in the United States, 2015–2016," February 2019, *https://www.cdc.gov/nchs/data/series/sr_03/sr03_43-508.pdf.*

[95] Facilities owned or leased by "an organization that owns two or more long-term care facilities."

[96] *International Journal of Health Services,* "Ownership, Financing, and Management Strategies of the 10 largest for-profit nursing home chains in the United States," Charlene Harrington et al., 2011; *Medical Care Research and Review,* "Nursing home profit status and quality of care: Is there any evidence of an association?", Michael P. Hillmer et al., April 2005, *https://www.ncbi.nlm.nih.gov/pubmed/15750174.*

Additionally, for-profit facilities receive the lowest scores in the Centers for Medicare and Medicaid Services' (CMS) nursing home rating system that takes into account, state health inspections, staffing ratios and quality measures.[97]

Private equity investment appears to exacerbate the problems faced at chain-affiliated for-profit nursing homes. Studies show that private equity-owned facilities generally "deliver poorer quality of care" than other chain-affiliated for-profit facilities; are likely to try to reduce cost by "substituting expensive but skilled RNs with cheaper and less skilled nurses;" and "report significantly higher number of deficiencies" that climb with more years of private equity ownership. As a result, private equity-owned nursing homes have 21% higher deficiencies, 25% lower nursing staff skill mix, and "worse results on pressure sore prevention . . . and [higher] pressure ulcer [] risk prevalence."[98] That was reportedly the case at HCR ManorCare—the second largest for-profit nursing home chain in the United States. In the years following its acquisition by a private equity firm, "the number of citations increased for, among other things, neither preventing nor treating bed sores; medication errors; not providing proper care for people who need special services such as injections, colostomies and prostheses; and not assisting patients with eating and personal hygiene."[99]

Moreover, while the quality of service declines, the complicated ownership and operating structure of these investments "limit legal remedies available to aggrieved residents."[100] For example, after a resident died at the private-equity-owned Habana Health Care Center (as a result of "a wound [that] should have been detected much earlier"), a family member tried to sue the owners of the facility, only to discover that the facility's complicated ownership structure "meant that even if she prevailed in court, the investors' wallets would likely be out of reach."[101] Shifting funds to other affiliated entities, or to the private equity firm itself, to immunize itself from liability for judgments against a target company is a widespread practice in the private equity industry.

Private equity investment in this sector has increased over the last few decades. The Government Accountability Office found that over the span of 10 years ending in 2008, private investment firms acquired approximately 1,900 unique nursing homes.[102] Today, private equity firms own or operate several large for-profit chains that control hundreds of facilities and provide nursing home care among other long-term care services.[103] Fillmore reportedly owns or has had investments in companies providing nursing home care. In order to help us

---

[97] Kaiser Family Foundation, "Reading the Stars: Nursing Home Quality Star Ratings, Nationally and by State," May 2015, *http://files.kff.org/attachment/issue-brief-reading-the-stars-nursing-home-quality-star-ratings-nationally-and-by-state.*

[98] *Journal of Health Care Finance,* "Private Equity Ownership of Nursing Homes: Implications for Quality," Rohit Pradhan et al., June–July 2014, *http://healthfinancejournal.com/index.php/johcf/article/view/12.*

[99] *Washington Post,* "Overdoses, bedsores, broken bones: What happened when a private-equity firm sought to care for society's most vulnerable," Peter Whoriskey and Dan Keating, November 25, 2018, *https://www.washingtonpost.com/business/economy/opioid-overdoses-bed-sores-and-broken-bones-what-happened-when-a-private-equity-firm-sought-profits-in-caring-for-societys-most-vulnerable/2018/11/25/09089a4a-ed14-11e8-baac-2a674e91502b_story.html.*

[100] *Journal of Health Care Finance,* "Private Equity Ownership of Nursing Homes: Implications for Quality," Rohit Pradban et al., June–July 2014, *http://healthfinancejournal.com/index.php/johcf/article/view/12.*

[101] *New York Times,* "At Many Homes, More Profit and Less Nursing," Charles Duhigg, September 23, 2007, *https://www.nytimes.com/2007/09/23/business/23nursing.html.*

[102] Government Accountability Office, "Nursing Homes: Complexity of Private Investment Purchases Demonstrates Need for CMS to Improve the Usability and Completeness of Ownership Data," September 2010, *https://www.gao.gov/assets/320/310562.pdf.*

[103] IQVIA, "U.S. Elder Care Market Summary," September 2019, *https://www.skainfo.com/reports/u.s.-elder-care-market-summary.*

understand your firm's role in the nursing home sector, we ask that you provide answers to the following questions no later than November 29, 2019.

1. Please provide the disclosure documents and information enumerated in Sections 501 and 503 of the Stop Wall Street Looting Act.[104]
2. Which nursing home or other long-term care service companies, including all affiliates or related entities, does Fillmore have a stake in or own? Please provide the name of and a brief description of the services each company provides—including the number of facilities that it owns or operates.
   a. Which nursing home or other long-term care companies, including all affiliates or related entities, has Fillmore had a stake in or owned in the past 20 years? Please provide the name of and a brief description of the services each company provides or provided—including the number of nursing home and other long-term care facilities that it owned or operated.
   b. For each nursing home or other long-term care service company Fillmore had a stake in or owned in the past 20 years, including all affiliates or related entities, please provide the following information for each year that the firm have had a stake in or owned this company and the 5 years preceding the firm's investment.
      I. The name of the company
      II. Total number of facilities, by type of facility
      III. Ownership stake
      IV. Total revenue, and the total revenue from Medicare, and from Medicaid
      V. Total transaction, advisory, or other fees collected after the acquisition of the company
      VI. Net income
      VII. Total number of employees for each facility
      VIII. Total number of patients for each facility, and the total number whose care is paid for by Medicare, and by Medicaid
      IX. Other private-equity firms that own a stake in the company
3. Private-equity firms reportedly employ sale-leaseback arrangements in order to quickly recover investments. For each company listed in questions 2(a) and 2(b), please list the number of nursing home or other long-term care facilities for which you acquired real estate assets, and whether a sale-lease-back agreement has been executed for any of those companies or facilities.
4. Has any nursing home or other long-term care company, including all affiliates or related entities, in which Fillmore has an ownership stake or has had an ownership stake in the last 20 years received Section 232 Department and Urban Development (HUD)-insured mortgages? If so, please provide the name of each facility and the total value of each loan insured by HUD.
5. Has any nursing home or other long-term care company, including all affiliates or related entities, in which Fillmore has an ownership stake or has had an ownership stake in the last 20 years, been placed in receivership? Please provide the name of each facility.

[104] Stop Wall Street Looting Act, S. 2155, *https://www.congress.gov/bill/116th-congress/senate-bill/2155.*

6. Has any nursing home or other long-term care company, including all affiliates or related entities, in which Fillmore has an ownership stake or has had an ownership stake in the last 20 years, been found to have violated any federal or state laws or regulations? If so, please provide a complete list, including the date and description, of all such violations. Please also include a list of all deficiencies identified in state or federal surveys of the facilities owned by the company for each year.
7. Has any nursing home or other long-term care company, including all affiliates or related entities, in which Fillmore has an ownership stake or has had an ownership stake in the last 20 years, reached a settlement with any federal or state law enforcement entity related to a potential violation of any federal or state laws or regulations or deficiencies in providing care? If so, please provide a complete list, including the date and description, of all such settlements.
8. Has any nursing home or other long-term care company, including all affiliates or related entities, in which Fillmore has an ownership stake or has had an ownership stake in the past 20 years, reached a settlement with any individual who was provided services by the company related to a potential violation of any federal or state laws or regulations or deficiencies in providing care? If so, please provide a complete list, including the date and description, of all such settlements.

Thank you for your attention to this matter.
Sincerely, Elizabeth Warren
United States Senator

Sherrod Brown
United States Senator

Mark Pocan
United States Congress

* * *

Congress of the United States
Washington, DC 20510
November 15, 2019

Charles R. Kaye
Co-Chief Executive Officer
Warburg Pincus LLC
450 Lexington Ave. New York, NY 10017

Joseph P. Landy
Co-Chief Executive Officer
Warburg Pincus LLC
450 Lexington Ave. New York, NY 10017

Dear Messrs. Kaye and Landy:

We are writing to request information regarding Warburg Pincus LLC's (Warburg Pincus) investment in companies providing nursing home care and other long-term care services and to request information about your firm's structure and finances as it relates to these companies.

Private equity funds often operate under a model where they purchase controlling interests in companies for a short time, load them up with debt, strip them of their assets, extract exorbitant fees, and sell them at a profit -implementing drastic cost-cutting measures at the expense of consumers, workers, communities, and taxpayers. For that reason, we have concerns about the rapid spread and effect of private equity investment in many sectors of the economy, especially industries that affect vulnerable populations and rely primarily on taxpayer-funded programs such as Medicare and Medicaid, like the nursing home industry. We are particularly concerned about your firm's investment in large for-profit nursing home chains, which research has shown often provide worse care than not-for-profit facilities.[105] In light of these concerns, we request information about your firm, the portfolio companies in which it has invested, and the performance of those investments.

Nursing homes provide a wide range of important medical and personal care services to a growing and vulnerable elderly population, with 1.3 million residents in the United States currently receiving care in more than 15,000 facilities.[106] For decades, reports and data have highlighted the shocking living conditions found in many nursing home and other long-term care facilities across the country.[107] Twelve years ago, for example, journalists uncovered how a group of private investment firms acquired 49 nursing homes, including a facility in Florida where managers slashed the number of registered nurses by half and cut supply and activity budgets. Residents, meanwhile, suffered from preventable infections and injuries.[108] Last year, news reports similarly detailed how a for-profit nursing home employed drastic cost cutting measures, "exposed its roughly 25,000 patients to increasing health risk," and ultimately filed for bankruptcy—all after a private equity firm acquired the company.[109]

This is particularly concerning given the fact that two-thirds of nursing home residents rely on government-sponsored health insurance coverage, meaning both not-for-profit and for-profit

---

[105] *International Journal of Health Services,* "Ownership, Financing, and Management Strategies of the 10 largest for-profit nursing home chains in the United States," Charlene Harrington et al., 2011, *https://www.ncbi.nlm.nih.gov/pubmed/22053531;* Kaiser Family Foundation, "Reading the Stars: Nursing Home Quality Star Ratings, Nationally and by State," May 2015, *http://files.kff.org/attachment/issue-brief-reading-the-stars-nursing-home-quality-star-ratings-nationally-and-by-state.*

[106] National Center for Health Statistics, "Long-term Care Providers and Services Users in the United States, 2015–2016," February 2019, *https://www.cdc.gov/nchs/data/series/sr_03/sr03_43-508.pdf.*

[107] *New York Times,* "At Many Homes, More Profit and Less Nursing," Charles Duhigg, September 23, 2017, *https://www.nytimes.com/2007/09/23/business/23nursing.html; Reveal,* "The rats sensed she was going to pass away," Jennifer Gollan, September 18, 2019, *https://www.revealnews.org/article/elderly-often-face-neglect-in-california-care-homes-that-exploit-workers/.*

[108] *New York Times,* "At Many Homes, More Profit and Less Nursing," Charles Duhigg, September 23, 2017, *https://www.nytimes.com/2007/09/23/business/23nursing.html.*

[109] *Washington Post,* "Overdoses, bedsores, broken bones: What happened when a private-equity firm sought to care for society's most vulnerable," Peter Whoriskey and Dan Keating, November 25, 2018, *https://www.washingtonpost.com/business/economy/opioid-overdoses-bedsores-and-broken-bones-what-happened-when-a-private-equity-firm-sought-profits-in-caring-for-societys-most-vulnerable/2018/11/25/09089a4a-ed14-11e8-baac-2a674e91502b_story.html.*

nursing homes benefit from government funding.[110] Medicaid is the primary payer[111] for nursing home care, with Medicare and Medicaid combined covering approximately 75 percent of nursing home residents.[112] In 2015, taxpayers sent more than $55 billion to the nursing home industry to cover the costs of long-term care. These reports and corresponding research raise serious questions about the role of private equity firms in the nursing home care industry, and the extent to which these firms' emphasis on profits and short-term return is responsible for declines in quality of care. They also raise concerns over the stewardship of taxpayer dollars, when—in many cases—these facilities continue to receive Medicare and Medicaid funding despite their decline in quality.

The majority of nursing facilities—almost 70%—are for-profit, and over half are chain-affiliated.[113] The overwhelming majority of research conducted over the last 2 decades shows that for-profit and chain affiliated[114] companies provide a lower quality of care and experience more serious health and safety deficiencies when compared to non-profit facilities.[115]

Additionally, for-profit facilities receive the lowest scores in the Centers for Medicare and Medicaid Services' (CMS) nursing home rating system that takes into account, state health inspections, staffing ratios and quality measures.[116]

Private equity investment appears to exacerbate the problems faced at chain-affiliated for-profit nursing homes. Studies show that private equity-owned facilities generally "deliver poorer quality of care" than other chain-affiliated for-profit facilities; are likely to try to reduce cost by "substituting expensive but skilled RNs with cheaper and less skilled nurses;" and "report significantly higher number of deficiencies" that climb with more years of private equity ownership. As a result, private equity-owned nursing homes have 21% higher deficiencies, 25% lower nursing staff skill mix, and "worse results on pressure sore prevention . . . and [higher] pressure ulcer [] risk prevalence."[117] That was reportedly the case at HCR ManorCare—the second largest for-profit nursing home chain in the United States. In the years following its acquisition by a private equity firm, "the number of citations increased for, among other things, neither preventing nor treating bed sores; medication errors; not providing proper

---

[110] Kaiser Family Foundation, "Distribution of Certified Nursing Facility Residents by Primary Payer Source," accessed on Nov. 14, 2019, *https://www.kff.org/other/state-indicator/distribution-of-certified-nursing-facilities-by-primary-payer-source/?currentTimeframe=0&sortModel=%7B%22colId%22:%22Location%22.%22sort%22:%22asc%22%7D.*

[111] Kaiser Family Foundation, "Medicaid's Role in Nursing Home Care," June 20, 2017, *https://www.kff.org/infographic/medicaids-role-in-nursing-home-care/.*

[112] Kaiser Family Foundation, "Distribution of Certified Nursing Facility Residents by Primary Payer Source," accessed on Nov. 14, 2019, *https://www.kff.org/other/state-indicator/distribution-of-certified-nursing-facilities-by-primary-payer-source/?currentTimeframe=0&sortModel=%7B%22colId%22:%22Location%22.%22sort%22:%22asc%22%7D.*

[113] National Center for Health Statistics, "Long-term Care Providers and Services Users in the United States, 2015–2016," February 2019, *https://www.cdc.gov/nchs/data/series/sr_03/sr03_43-508.pdf.*

[114] Facilities owned or leased by "an organization that owns two or more long-term care facilities."

[115] *International Journal of Health Services,* "Ownership, Financing, and Management Strategies of the 10 largest for-profit nursing home chains in the United States," Charlene Harrington et al., 2011; *Medical Care Research and Review,* "Nursing home profit status and quality of care: Is there any evidence of an association?", Michael P. Hillmer et al., April 2005, *https://www.ncbi.nlm.nih.gov/pubmed/15750174.*

[116] Kaiser Family Foundation, "Reading the Stars: Nursing Home Quality Star Ratings, Nationally and by State," May 2015, *http://files.kff.org/attachment/issue-brief-reading-the-stars-nursing-home-quality-star-ratings-nationally-and-by-state.*

[117] *Journal of Health Care Finance,* "Private Equity Ownership of Nursing Homes: Implications for Quality," Rohit Pradhan et al., June–July 2014, *http://healthfinancejournal.com/index.php/johcf/article/view/12.*

care for people who need special services such as injections, colostomies and prostheses; and not assisting patients with eating and personal hygiene."[118]

Moreover, while the quality of service declines, the complicated ownership and operating structure of these investments "limit legal remedies available to aggrieved residents."[119] For example, after a resident died at the private-equity-owned Habana Health Care Center (as a result of "a wound [that] should have been detected much earlier"), a family member tried to sue the owners of the facility, only to discover that the facility's complicated ownership structure "meant that even if she prevailed in court, the investors' wallets would likely be out of reach."[120] Shifting funds to other affiliated entities, or to the private equity firm itself, to immunize itself from liability for judgments against a target company is a widespread practice in the private equity industry.

Private equity investment in this sector has increased over the last few decades. The Government Accountability Office found that over the span of 10 years ending in 2008, private investment firms acquired approximately 1,900 unique nursing homes.[121] Today, private equity firms own or operate several large for-profit chains that control hundreds of facilities and provide nursing home care among other long-term care services.[122] Warburg Pincus reportedly owns or has had investments in companies providing nursing home care. In order to help us understand your firm's role in the nursing home sector, we ask that you provide answers to the following questions no later than November 29, 2019.

1. Please provide the disclosure documents and information enumerated in Sections 501 and 503 of the Stop Wall Street Looting Act.[123]
2. Which nursing home or other long-term care service companies, including all affiliates or related entities, does Warburg Pincus have a stake in or own? Please provide the name of and a brief description of the services each company provides—including the number of facilities that it owns or operates.
    a. Which nursing home or other long-term care companies, including all affiliates or related entities, has Warburg Pincus had a stake in or owned in the past 20 years? Please provide the name of and a brief description of the services each company provides or provided—including the number of nursing home and other long-term care facilities that it owned or operated.
    b. For each nursing home or other long-term care service company Warburg Pincus had a stake in or owned in the past 20 years, including all affiliates or related entities, please provide the following information for each year that the firm have

[118] *Washington Post,* "Overdoses, bedsores, broken bones: What happened when a private-equity firm sought to care for society's most vulnerable," Peter Whoriskey and Dan Keating, November 25, 2018, *https://www.washingtonpost.com/business/economy/opioid-overdoses-bed-sores-and-broken-bones-what-happened-when-a-private-equity-firm-sought-profits-in-caring-for-societys-most-vulnerable/2018/11/25/09089a4a-ed14-11e8-baac-2a674e91502b*_story.html.

[119] *Journal of Health Care Finance,* "Private Equity Ownership of Nursing Homes: Implications for Quality," Rohit Pradhan et al., June–July 2014, *http://healthfinancejournal.com/index.php/johcf/article/view/12.*

[120] *New York Times,* "At Many Homes, More Profit and Less Nursing," Charles Duhigg, September 23, 2007, *https://www.nytimes.com/2007/09/23/business/23nursing.html.*

[121] Government Accountability Office, "Nursing Homes: Complexity of Private Investment Purchases Demonstrates Need for CMS to Improve the Usability and Completeness of Ownership Data," September 2010, *https://www.gao.gov/assets/320/310562.pdf.*

[122] IQVIA, "U.S. Elder Care Market Summary," September 2019, *https://www.skainfo.com/reports/u.s.-elder-care-market-summary.*

[123] Stop Wall Street Looting Act, S. 2155, *https://www.congress.gov/bill/116th-congress/senate-bill/2155.*

had a stake in or owned this company and the 5 years preceding the firm's investment.

I. The name of the company
II. Total number of facilities, by type of facility
III. Ownership stake
IV. Total revenue, and the total revenue from Medicare, and from Medicaid
V. Total transaction, advisory, or other fees collected after the acquisition of the company
VI. Net income
VII. Total number of employees for each facility
VIII. Total number of patients for each facility, and the total number whose care is paid for by Medicare, and by Medicaid
IX. Other private-equity firms that own a stake in the company

3. Private-equity firms reportedly employ sale-leaseback arrangements in order to quickly recover investments. For each company listed in questions 2(a) and 2(b), please list the number of nursing home or other long-term care facilities for which you acquired real estate assets, and whether a sale-lease-back agreement has been executed for any of those companies or facilities.
4. Has any nursing home or other long-term care company, including all affiliates or related entities, in which Warburg Pincus has an ownership stake or has had an ownership stake in the last 20 years received Section 232 Department of Housing and Urban Development (HUD)-insured mortgages? If so, please provide the name of each facility and the total value of each loan insured by HUD.
5. Has any nursing home or other long-term care company, including all affiliates or related entities, in which Warburg Pincus has an ownership stake or has had an ownership stake in the last 20 years, been placed in receivership? Please provide the name of each facility.
6. Has any nursing home or other long-term care company, including all affiliates or related entities, in which Warburg Pincus has an ownership stake or has had an ownership stake in the last 20 years, been found to have violated any federal or state laws or regulations? If so, please provide a complete list, including the date and description, of all such violations. Please also include a list of all deficiencies identified in state or federal surveys of the facilities owned by the company for each year.
7. Has any nursing home or other long-term care company, including all affiliates or related entities, in which Warburg Pincus has an ownership stake or has had an ownership stake in the last 20 years, reached a settlement with any federal or state law enforcement entity related to a potential violation of any federal or state laws or regulations or deficiencies in providing care? If so, please provide a complete list, including the date and description, of all such settlements.
8. Has any nursing home or other long-term care company, including all affiliates or related entities, in which Warburg Pincus has an ownership stake or has had an ownership stake in the past 20 years, reached a settlement with any individual who was provided services by the company related to a potential violation of any federal or state laws or regulations or deficiencies in providing care? If so, please provide a complete list, including the date and description, of all such settlements.

Thank you for your attention to this matter.
Sincerely, Elizabeth Warren
United States Senator

Sherrod Brown
United States Senator

Mark Pocan
United States Congress

* * *

Fillmore Capital Partners LLC
Four Embarcadero Center, Suite 710
San Francisco CA 94111

December 18, 2019
The Honorable Elizabeth Warren
The Honorable Sherrod Brown
Mark Pocan, Member of Congress
Congress of the United States
Washington DC 20510
RE: United States Congress—Letter of November 15, 2019

Dear Senator Warren, Senator Brown and Congressman Pocan:

This will confirm receipt of an electronic copy of your above-referenced letter directed to Fillmore Capital Partners in which you make certain representations about private equity companies and request information about Fillmore Capital Partners and affiliates. In preparing for response, we explored the basis for your written request for detailed proprietary information. I note that in your role as Democratic members of the House and Senate you have proposed a bill entitled the "Stop Wall Street Looting Act of 2019" with the goal of enhancing government scrutiny of the private equity sector. Your letter to Fillmore Capital Partners advocates for the points you believe support passage of the Act and requests information that would presumably be used as part of the effort to pass this Act. Please find below my response to your letter, which is tailored to your request and the circumstances, based on information readily available at this time.

First, I would like to share a high level review of my observations of the nursing home industry as a whole so that we have the proper context here. In my opinion it is counterproductive to paint any sector with a broad-brush, be it the investment or nursing home sector. I have personal experience with the healthcare industry as a caregiver to my mom and dad, both veterans of WWII, as well as countless other family members and friends. To hold the hand of the dying is both difficult and life changing. In addition to my role with Fillmore, I have served as a board chairperson for several ownership companies, some of which had affiliations with the long-term care industry and the operation of nursing homes. These are my general observations as an individual, caregiver, trustee of an IDD individual and as a board chair-person.

It should come as no surprise to you that I disagree with the portrayal of individuals and businesses affiliated with the private equity sector and nursing home industry as "uncaring" and "profit-seeking." The nursing home industry and healthcare providers in general in this Country employ some of the most hardworking and caring citizens in the U.S. Every day 24/7/365, healthcare providers touch the lives of tens of millions of individuals and families, many of which are your constituents, in an attempt to provide care, comfort and solutions. With respect to nursing or long-term care, in most cases these are patients whose family could not care for them or would not care for them. They are patients who were ready to discharge from hospitals with no place to go. They are patients with mental and physical conditions in need of the services that only a nursing home is willing to provide. They are for the most part, our elderly population who have little to no income, living on the edge of life with no alternatives. For profit and non-profit nursing home operators serve our communities whether they be urban, suburban or in rural parts of the U.S. Many providers do so with 50 plus year-old facilities, limited financial resources, outdated regulations, labor and skill challenges, enduring general disdain from the uninformed. As my Marine Corps mother said at 87, "getting old ain't for the faint of heart." Nursing home operators have provided services in States with Medicaid reimbursement rates that do not even cover the actual costs of the care provided to citizens of their State, yet operators have often continued to provide the resources needed to support those locations. In some communities the nursing facility is the only healthcare resource, the largest employer, and even provides coffee for local first responders. Nursing homes, and the caregivers in them, have served and continue to serve as a critical resource for the elderly and infirm U.S. population.

As you are aware, effective in 2012 Congress reduced planned Medicare reimbursement rates for nursing homes in by 11.1%. At the time the then President of the Alliance for Quality Nursing Home Care stated that lawmakers would as a result be "faced with an increased threat to local seniors' access to care." Recent closure of nursing facilities in rural areas in multiple States has in fact threatened seniors' access to care. Without question rural communities will continue to struggle with access to healthcare, long-term care, medication management and hospice care. Industry leaders with whom I have spoken, have grave concerns regarding how the future needs of the baby boomer elderly will be met given the current lack of Federal and State support for the nursing home industry in the U.S. Adequate funding is needed to help your constituents who have to rely on government funding to receive care. Much like the aging infrastructure issue this Country faces with regard to housing for those with low income, the physical plant locations for many nursing homes are reaching the end of their useful life. Industry leaders have cautioned that given the current economic realities, even with State, Federal and private sector support, it is doubtful that providers will be able to develop new or replace old facilities. It cannot be disputed that the industry is already one of the most heavily regulated, scrutinized and targeted for litigation in the Country. Without changes in reimbursement to offset escalating costs overall, many facilities that are needed by the senior population simply will not survive.

With regard to your specific requests for information, the first requests information that could be required in the event the Act were passed. Because the Act has not passed we are not educated about the requirements of the Act and are not in a position to respond to this request. The response to request #2(a) is simple and is already known to CMS and most State SNF licensure authorities. The response to requests #2(b) through #8 involves asking affiliates of Fillmore Capital to gather a significant amount of information, much of which has already been provided to government agencies and is otherwise publicly available. As of this date the Fillmore and Golden Living affiliated Golden Living Center operators no longer operate nursing homes. Therefore, those affiliates have limited personnel to locate and retrieve the information requested. I can, however, provide some basic information that I have obtained, such as for #4 I am not aware of any HUD financing related to Golden Living Centers; for #5, no Golden Living Center licensed operator was placed in receivership at any time; for #6, very few, if any, operators could answer 'no' as the nursing home industry is very heavily regulated and frequently assessed fines for alleged violations. CMS has public data readily available to you from which you can identify nursing facility surveys. #7 and #8 request information subject to confidentiality obligations which our affiliates with very limited resources would have to research.

I have noticed that numerous references cited in your letter are sources that have for many years criticized and opposed both nursing home operators and their affiliated holding companies/owners. They have pure disdain for what caregivers do, many in aging facilities with few modern amenities. Of course, nursing home providers care for your Medicaid constituents, generally frail and declining with numerous health challenges 24/7/365 for less than $140 per day and, as my mother would once again say, that ain't for the faint of heart! I hope you will find this response beneficial. I am willing to make time to further discuss this and attempt to create understanding in order to replace disdain. It is also my understanding that there are many nursing home operator representatives who are willing to work closely with Congress to share information and pursue solutions that are in the overall best interest of your constituents.

Finally, as an example of the positive impact investors can have on the healthcare industry, please review the websites of two Fillmore affiliated healthcare organizations which are defying the odds to successfully provide needed state-of-the-art services, *www.Salude.com* and *www.alixarx.com.* Salude is a specially constructed skilled nursing facility which is ranked by CMS as the #1 skilled nursing care facility in the U.S., out of 15,000 nationally. AlixaRx is a unique remote automated pharmacy solution developed for nursing care, to make needed medications more readily available in rural communities by providing on-demand medication and patient medication management. Unfortunately, these concepts are not likely to come to your communities soon as they require financial resources beyond what are currently available in most States and communities in order to succeed.

With Respect, Ronald E. Silva
President and CEO

* * *

Akin Gump
Strauss Hauer and Feld LLP

Raphael A. Prober
Confidential Treatment Requested
November 29, 2019

VIA E–MAIL
The Honorable Elizabeth Warren
United States Senate
9 Hart Senate Office Building
Washington, DC 20510

The Honorable Sherrod Brown
United States Senate
503 Hart Senate Office Building
Washington, DC 20510

The Honorable Mark Pocan
United States House of Representatives
1421 Longworth House Office Building
Washington, DC 20510

Re: November 15, 2019 Letter to Warburg Pincus, LLC

Dear Senator Warren, Senator Brown, and Congressman Pocan:

On behalf of Warburg Pincus, LLC ("Warburg Pincus"), we write in response to your letter dated November 15, 2019 (the "Letter") in which you requested information regarding investments made by funds managed by Warburg Pincus in skilled nursing facilities.

Funds managed by Warburg Pincus, since its founding in 1966, have made over 150 healthcare investments. In the last 20 years, only two investments made by funds managed by Warburg Pincus were in the skilled nursing home care industry; the first of which was exited in 2002 and the second of which was exited in 2011. Since 2011, no fund managed by Warburg Pincus has made or held any investments in skilled nursing facilities. Below, please find information on the investments exited in 2002 and 2011, which constitute the only investments covered by your Letter.[124]

Since its founding in 1966, Warburg Pincus has predominantly pursued a strategy of growth investing at scale, with the vast majority of the investments made in growth stage or early stage companies. Over the years, funds managed by Warburg Pincus have successfully invested in growth companies as well as companies at other stages of development, from building early-stage and start-up companies, to providing capital to meet the needs of existing businesses and, to a lesser extent, to investing in later-stage transactions and special situations, typically in circumstances in which growth is a key aspect of the investment thesis. The firm's early-stage and growth investing approach is thesis-driven, pursuing extensively researched themes and ideas. The firm also prefers to invest with accomplished management teams who are investing in the transactions alongside the firm. As evidence of the firm's successful focus on growth investing, the firm's portfolio investments have completed over 170 initial public offerings.

[124] Funds managed by Warburg Pincus also invested in two companies focused on the assisted living industry, Brandywine Senior Care (invested in 2006, exited in 2010) and The Covenant Group (invested in 2007, exited in 2011).

Warburg Pincus aims to build lasting companies that will perform well in growing industries—the goal in every investment is to create a larger, thriving business by making long-term investments and creating value. Warburg Pincus believes that this approach positions the investors in the funds it manages, which include pension funds that benefit multiple categories of public and private employees, to receive attractive risk-adjusted long-term returns over the course of economic and capital markets cycles.

In 2000, funds managed by Warburg Pincus invested in Centennial Healthcare Corporation ("Centennial"). At the time, Centennial was a publicly traded operator of approximately 100 skilled nursing facilities, of which 6 were owned, 64 were leased, and 30 were managed, and had operations in 22 states. During that period, the skilled nursing home care industry was severely challenged due to, among other things, reduced reimbursement rates, high leverage, high labor costs due to a labor shortage, and high litigation expenses due to industry-wide regulatory issues and increasing patient liability tort claims. Four of the seven largest home chains had filed for bankruptcy, with a fifth imminent (which subsequently also filed for bankruptcy). Centennial itself faced these challenges. Warburg Pincus's investment thesis was that the industry was poised to recover due to, among other things, an increasing demand for long-term nursing care because of an aging population. In light of that investment thesis, funds managed by Warburg Pincus acquired approximately 52% of Centennial in 2000, with management and other investors (Welsh Carson and South Atlantic Capital) owning the rest. Despite management's efforts to turn Centennial around in this challenging environment, the company filed for bankruptcy in 2002. No dividends were paid to any fund managed by Warburg Pincus during the period of ownership, nor did Warburg Pincus itself charge or collect any transaction, advisory or other fees, consistent with the firm's long-standing practice not to charge such fees for any services provided by Warburg Pincus employees to portfolio companies.

Based on the same investment thesis for Centennial, funds managed by Warburg Pincus co-founded Florida Healthcare Properties ("Florida Healthcare") in 2001, owning approximately 75% of the company during much of its ownership tenure, with other health care executives and management owning the rest. Over time, Florida Healthcare came to operate approximately 127 skilled nursing facilities in 17 states and the District of Columbia. Sale-leasebacks were not part of the company's business model—the company leased almost all of its facilities from third parties. The funds managed by Warburg Pincus exited their investment in Florida Healthcare in 2011. (The company's name had since been changed to Lavie Care Centers.) Once again, Warburg Pincus did not charge or collect any transaction, advisory or other fees.

Warburg Pincus's involvement in the operations of its portfolio companies, like Centennial and Florida Healthcare, is that of an investor. While Warburg Pincus nominees often sit on the boards of directors of its portfolio companies (and held seats on the boards of directors of both Centennial and Florida Healthcare during the periods of ownership), the role and responsibility of such board representatives is one of oversight of the company's executive management team and assistance in the strategic direction of the company. The executive management teams of portfolio companies are responsible for the day-to-day operations of the portfolio companies. As a general matter, the information provided to board members is designed to assist them in discharging their oversight duties.

We hope the information that Warburg Pincus has provided herein with respect to the two investments exited nearly a decade ago is helpful to your review.

* * *

The information and data included in this response contains sensitive information—including confidential and proprietary information—and we request that such information be treated accordingly and that it not be released to any third parties. Production of this information and data is not intended to constitute a waiver of the attorney-client, attorney work product, or any other applicable rights or privileges in this or any other forum, and Warburg Pincus expressly reserves its rights in this regard.

Sincerely, Raphael A. Prober
Counsel for Warburg Pincus

* * *

The Carlyle Group
1001 Pennsylvania Avenue, NW, Suite 220
Washington, DC 20004–2505

November 29, 2019
Senator Elizabeth Warren
309 Hart Senate Office Building
Washington, DC 20510–4543

Senator Sherrod Brown
503 Hart Senate Office Building
Washington, DC 20510–4543

Congressman Mark Pocan
1421 Longworth House Office Building
Washington, DC 20510–4543

Dear Senators Warren, Brown and Congressman Pocan:

We received your inquiry dated November 15, 2019 regarding The Carlyle Group's investments in companies providing nursing home care and other long-term care services. We appreciate your interest in the subject.

The Carlyle Group ("Carlyle") is a global investment firm with deep industry expertise that deploys private capital across four business segments: Corporate Private Equity, Real Assets, Global Credit, and Investment Solutions. With $222 billion of assets under management, Carlyle's purpose is to invest wisely and create value on behalf of its investors, many of whom are public pensions. Carlyle has expertise in various industries, including aerospace, defense and government services, consumer and retail, energy and power, financial services, healthcare, industrial, real estate, technology and business services, telecommunications and media, and transportation. The portfolio companies owned by Carlyle investment funds employ 900,000 people globally and more than 100,000 in the United States. Since its founding in 1987, the firm has invested $103 billion in 643 Corporate Private Equity transactions. More than 2,600 investors from 94 countries entrust Carlyle with their capital.

The healthcare sector has been a core focus area for Carlyle for over 25 years. Carlyle's investments in healthcare companies have spanned geographies—including North America, Europe, South America, and Asia—and subsectors within healthcare—including leading providers of clinical care, preeminent research organizations, reliable manufacturers of medical devices and pharmaceutical products, and reputable service providers that facilitate access to timely and high-quality care. Our portfolio of investments, within healthcare and across other industries, also spans investment strategies, including investing in growth-oriented companies to support their expansions. Regardless of the geography, subsector, or investment strategy, we seek to invest behind healthcare companies that can capitalize on growth opportunities, drive better health outcomes for patients, and bring improvements to the healthcare system. As part of our investment process, we also evaluate the environmental, social, and governance aspects of a company, which takes into consideration key stakeholders, including patients, payors, customers, and employees.

Today, neither Carlyle nor any nor its investment funds owns any equity interest in any company that operates nursing facilities[125] in the United States.[126] In 2007, an investment fund managed by Carlyle acquired a majority equity investment in HCR ManorCare, Inc. ("the Company" or "HCR"), which operated skilled nursing, assisted living and home healthcare facilities. Carlyle never managed the operations of the company. However, employees of Carlyle served as members of the Board of Directors of HCR, and the Board of Directors ensured that the Company had appropriate policies and procedures in place to assess and address clinical quality at HCR's facilities. For example, under Carlyle's ownership, HCR ManorCare established an Independent Advisory Committee on Quality, which provided advice and recommendations to the Company's Board of Directors on ways to measure, maintain and improve quality care for HCR ManorCare patients and residents.

During Carlyle's ownership, quality and care delivery remained a key priority for the Company.[127] From 2007–2017, HCR's total staffing, hands on caregiving staff and nursing staff all increased. The Centers for Medicare and Medicaid Services ("CMS") rated HCR ManorCare's regulatory compliance above industry average. At the time of Carlyle's exit, HCR ManorCare's CMS Five Star Rating[128] Data show that the facilities were at or above industry average for overall, quality measures, staffing and registered nurse staffing. In fact, most of the centers received four or five stars. From 2013–2017, HCR ManorCare's serious safety incident rate was better than the national average in each and every year. During the same period, the average CMS quality measure star rating was considered outstanding by CMS, with 88% of centers receiving four or five stars.

---

[125] See the Nursing Home Compare site of *medicare.gov*: "Nursing home is a term that includes both skilled nursing facilities and nursing facilities. Skilled nursing facilities (SNF) are those that participate in both Medicare and Medicaid. Nursing facilities (NF) arc those that participate in Medicaid only. Nursing homes primarily engage in providing residents skilled nursing care and related services for residents who require medical or nursing care and rehabilitation services for the rehabilitation of injured, disabled, or sick individuals." *(https://www.medicare.gov/NursingHomeCompare/Resources/Glossary.html).*

[126] Carlyle Real Estate funds do hold investments in real estate on which private pay senior living communities, independent communities and assisted living communities are operated. However, the companies in which Carlyle's Real Estate funds hold investments do not operate these facilities.

[127] All data referenced in this letter provided to Carlyle by HCR ManorCare.

[128] The Centers for Medicare and Medicaid Services created the Five-Star Rating System to allow consumers to assess nursing homes on health inspections, staffing and quality measures.

Management of real estate assets is a necessary part of operating in the nursing facility industry, and, during Carlyle's ownership, HCR, like other companies in the industry, engaged in a number of transactions involving its real estate holdings. Those transactions included a 2011 sale-lease-back transaction in which HCP, Inc. acquired a portion of HCR's real estate assets and leased those facilities back to HCR. HCP, Inc. subsequently transferred those assets to Quality Care Properties, Inc.

Following our initial investment, several legislative events and CMS actions created reimbursement headwinds that negatively impacted the company's financial performance. These measures reduced the company's reimbursement and/or increased its costs by hundreds of millions of dollars. As an example, Medicare rates for the industry and HCR for 2019 are lower than they were in 2011 due to rate cuts and changes in rate methodology. The entire skilled nursing facility industry has been negatively affected by these changes. In fact, The Medicare Payment Advisory Committee (MedPAC), the agency that provides the U.S. Congress with analysis and policy advice, estimated the margin for the entire skilled nursing facility industry was less than 1.0% in 2017.[129] Numerous other companies in the industry have filed for bankruptcy, exited long-term care or were financially distressed during this time, including Genesis, Signature, Extendicare, Skyline, Kindred, Golden Living and Consulate.

Given these changes in reimbursement, HCR ManorCare had been working on a plan to recapitalize its balance sheet in a manner designed to promote the long-term financial health of the Company and maintain quality of care. For legal reasons, the company filed for pre-packaged bankruptcy in 2018. Patient care was not compromised. All creditors and employees continued to be paid during the bankruptcy proceedings and not a single creditor (other than the Company's landlord, Quality Care Properties) lost capital as a result of the bankruptcy filing. As a result of this restructuring, HCR ManorCare became a wholly owned subsidiary of ProMedica Health System in 2018. Carlyle owns no interest in either HCR ManorCare or ProMedcia. ProMedica, an acute care health system, bought HCR ManorCare because it is a high-quality provider. ProMedica would not have acquired HCR if it did not believe that HCR provides high quality patient care.

Carlyle takes pride in its approach to responsible investing. We thank you for your inquiry in this subject.

Sincerely, Stacey Dion

Managing Director, Global Government Affairs

Prepared Statement of Hon. Mike Crapo, a U.S. Senator from Idaho

At the national, State and local levels, the pandemic has challenged our sense of normalcy. It has tested every institution of daily life we know, threatening the physical and economic health of our Nation. Americans from all walks of life have experienced a year full of tremendous hardship and tragedy. It is the people living and working in our Nation's nursing homes, however, who bore an outsized burden.

[129] Per MedPAC March 2019 Report to Congress.

More than 174,000 people died as COVID–19 ravaged our long-term care facilities. That number represents almost one-third of all U.S. deaths that have occurred during the pandemic.

Both long-stay nursing homes and short-stay post-acute skilled nursing facilities rely on direct care workers—such as licensed practical nurses, certified nursing assistants, and personal care aides—to provide most hands-on care. These workers are in close physical contact with residents, assisting with bathing, dressing, and eating. Current data shows that long-term care workers are typically female, and a disproportionate share are women of color.

Many of these direct care workers live paycheck to paycheck. Over the past year, they have put their lives on the line. We owe them a debt of gratitude. Thank you to the dedicated nursing home workers like Adelina Ramos, one of our witnesses.

These workers hear Americans calling them heroes, but they are often underappreciated when on the job. To these front-line workers, please know that the sacrifices you are making every day do not go unnoticed or unappreciated.

Today, we will hear from a number of expert witnesses who will provide key insights into nursing home conditions over the past year. This testimony will help us better understand exactly what happened, when it happened, and why it happened. It will give us insight into policies that produced results, as well as areas that need improvement.

Hearings are just one oversight tool this committee uses to hold government agencies, the health-care industry, and individual providers accountable. Another key part of oversight is securing reliable and accurate data. Transparent data reporting brings accountability and helps drive decision-making. As we look to the future, it is vital that all States report accurate COVID–19 data. That is the only way for economists, researchers, advocacy organizations, and policy-makers to tackle the challenges facing the nursing home sector head-on.

This is not a job for the Federal Government alone. Multiple Federal, State, and local programs and partnerships work to support the health-care needs of our Nation's most vulnerable populations. We must work together—in an honest and transparent manner—to safeguard our nursing home residents and the workers who care for them.

Over the weekend, *The New York Times* published the results of an investigation into the Centers for Medicare and Medicaid Services (CMS) nursing home five-star rating system. The investigation questions the objectivity and accuracy of the CMS star ratings system. This rating system, which was first implemented during the Obama administration, is designed to help beneficiaries, their families, and caregivers compare nursing home quality more easily.

Care Compare is another online tool available to help seniors, the disabled, and their families find out if a particular nursing home facility meets Federal health and safety standards, staffing levels, and quality performance metrics.

After several bipartisan hearings held by the Finance Committee during 2019, CMS implemented changes to Nursing Home Compare that specifically denote nursing homes that have been cited for incidents of abuse, neglect, or exploitation. That may have been a start, but clearly there is a lot more work that needs to be done.

I am grateful to each of our witnesses for the work that they are doing and for taking the time to join us today. Their expertise will help us advance public policies that slow the spread of COVID–19 and lessen its devastating impacts on our Nation's elderly and the disabled.

Prepared Statement of John E. Dicken, Director, Health Care, Government Accountability Office

COVID-19 in Nursing Homes: HHS Has Taken Steps in Response to Pandemic, But Several GAO Recommendations Have Not Been Implemented

Why GAO Did This Study

The COVID-19 pandemic has had a disproportionate impact on the 1.4 million elderly or disabled residents in the nation's more than 15,000 Medicare- and Medicaid-certified nursing homes, who are often in frail health and living in close proximity to one another. HHS, primarily through CMS and CDC, has led the pandemic response in nursing homes.

The CARES Act includes a provision for GAO to conduct monitoring and oversight of the federal government's efforts to prepare for, respond to, and recover from the COVID-19 pandemic. GAO has examined the government's response to COVID-19 in nursing homes through its CARES Act reporting (GAO-21-265, GAO-21-191, GAO-20-701, and GAO-20-625).

This testimony will summarize the findings from these reports. Specifically, it describes COVID-19 trends in nursing homes and their experiences responding to the pandemic, and HHS's response to the pandemic in nursing homes.

To conduct this previously reported work, GAO reviewed CDC data, agency guidance, and other relevant information on HHS's response to the COVID-19 pandemic. GAO interviewed agency officials and other knowledgeable stakeholders. In addition, GAO supplemented this information with updated data from CDC on COVID-19 cases and deaths reported by nursing homes as of February 2021.

What GAO Found

GAO's review of data from the Centers for Disease Control and Prevention (CDC) found that winter 2020 was marked by a significant surge in the number of COVID-19 cases and deaths in nursing homes. However, CDC data as of February 2021, show that both cases and deaths have declined by more than 80 percent since their peaks in December 2020. With the introduction of vaccines, observers are hopeful that nursing homes may be beginning to see a reprieve. Nevertheless, the emergence of more highly transmissible virus variants warrants the need for continued vigilance, according to public health officials.

GAO's prior work has found that nursing homes have faced many difficult challenges battling COVID-19. While challenges related to staffing shortages have persisted through the pandemic, challenges related to obtaining Personal Protective Equipment (PPE) and conducting COVID-19 tests—although still notable—have generally shown signs of improvement since summer 2020. Further, with the decline in nursing homes cases, the Centers for Medicare and Medicaid Services (CMS) updated its guidance in March 2021 to expand resident visitation, an issue that has been an ongoing challenge during the pandemic. Some new challenges have also emerged as vaccinations began in nursing homes, such as reluctance among some staff to receive a COVID-19 vaccine.

The Department of Health and Human Services (HHS), primarily through CMS and the CDC, has taken steps to address COVID-19 in nursing homes. However, HHS has not implemented several relevant GAO recommendations, including:

- HHS has not implemented GAO's recommendation related to the Nursing Home Commission report, which assessed the response to COVID-19 in nursing homes. CMS released the Nursing Home Commission's report and recommendations in September 2020. When the report was released, CMS broadly outlined the actions the agency had taken, but the agency did not provide a plan that would allow it to track its progress. GAO recommended in November 2020 that HHS develop an implementation plan. As of February 2021, this recommendation had not been implemented.
- HHS has not implemented GAO's recommendation to fill COVID-19 data voids. CMS required nursing homes to begin reporting the number of cases and deaths to the agency effective May 8, 2020. However, CMS made the reporting of the data prior to this date optional. GAO recommended in September 2020 that HHS develop a strategy to capture more complete COVID-19 data in nursing homes retroactively back to January 1, 2020. As of February 2021, this recommendation had not been implemented.

Implementing GAO's recommendations could help address some of the challenges nursing homes continue to face and fill important gaps in the federal government's understanding of, and transparency around, data on COVID-19 in nursing homes. In addition to monitoring HHS's implementation of past recommendations, GAO has ongoing work related to COVID-19 outbreaks in nursing homes and CMS's oversight of infection control and emergency preparedness.

Chairman Wyden, Ranking Member Crapo, and Members of the Committee:

I am pleased to be here today to discuss our work on Coronavirus Disease 2019 (COVID-19) in nursing homes. Just over a year ago, a Washington State nursing home was battling one of the first major COVID-19 outbreaks in the United States. Today, the COVID-19 pandemic has reached nearly all of the more than 15,000 Medicare- and Medicaid-certified nursing homes in the country, resulting in a disproportionately high number of COVID-19 deaths among residents.

While the nation's 1.4 million nursing home residents are a small share of the total U.S. population (less than 1 percent), they comprise nearly 30 percent of COVID-19 deaths reported by the Centers for Disease Control and Prevention (CDC). Nursing home residents are at a high risk for COVID-19 infection and death because the virus has a high mortality rate among elderly adults and those with underlying health conditions.

In addition, the congregate nature of nursing homes, with staff caring for multiple residents and shared communal spaces, as well as high incidence rates in the surrounding community, can increase the risk that COVID-19 will enter the home and easily spread. Further, efforts to reduce the spread of COVID-19 in nursing homes have required changes in typical nursing home practices—such as restricting visitors and isolating residents exposed to COVID-19—raising concerns for vulnerable residents, who may have less social interaction and third party oversight of their care.

The Centers for Medicare & Medicaid Services (CMS), an agency within the Department of Health and Human Services (HHS), is responsible for ensuring that nursing homes meet federal quality standards to participate in the Medicare and Medicaid programs.[130] In response to the pandemic, HHS, primarily through CMS and CDC, has taken a series of actions with nursing homes, such as providing guidance, developing targeted inspections to improve infection control practices, and distributing testing devices to homes.[131] In addition, in May 2020, CDC began collecting weekly COVID-19 data from nursing homes through its National Healthcare Safety Network system.

The CARES Act includes a provision for us to conduct monitoring and oversight of the federal government's efforts to prepare for, respond to, and recover from the COVID-19 pandemic.[132] In response to the CARES Act, we have examined the response to COVID-19 in nursing homes in four reports since June 2020. To help inform today's discussion, my testimony will summarize our findings on nursing home issues from these reports.[133] In particular, my statement will address:

1. COVID-19 trends in nursing homes and their experiences responding to the COVID-19 pandemic, and
2. HHS's response to the COVID-19 pandemic in nursing homes.

In addition, I will highlight key actions that we recommended HHS take and the current status of those recommendations. While my comments today focus on the findings of our CARES Act reports, they are also informed by our longer-term body of work examining nursing home oversight and quality prior to the pandemic.

To conduct the work for the previously issued reports on which my comments are based, we reviewed CDC data, agency guidance, and other relevant information on HHS's response to the COVID-19 pandemic. We interviewed agency officials, as well as researchers with experience in infection control, advocates for individuals residing in nursing homes and their families, national associations representing nursing homes, and representatives from associations representing state and local officials.

---

[130] To monitor compliance with these standards, CMS enters into agreements with state survey agencies in each state government to conduct inspections, including recurring comprehensive standard surveys and as-needed investigations. CMS's Center for Clinical Standards and Quality has responsibility for overseeing state survey agencies' survey and certification activities, among others.

[131] In our May 2020 report, we found that infection control deficiencies were widespread and persistent in nursing homes in the years prior to the COVID-19 pandemic. See GAO, *Infection Control Deficiencies Were Widespread and Persistent in Nursing Homes Prior to COVID-19 Pandemic*, GAO-20-576R, (Washington, D.C.: May 20, 2020).

[132] Pub. L. No. 116-139, § 19010(b), 134 Stat. 281, 579 (2020).

[133] See GAO, *COVID-19: Critical Vaccine Distribution, Supply Chain, Program Integrity, and Other Challenges Require Focused Federal Attention*, GAO-21-265, (Washington, D.C.: Jan. 28, 2021); *COVID-19: Urgent Actions Needed to Better Ensure an Effective Federal Response*, GAO-21-191, (Washington, D.C.: Nov. 30, 2020);*COVID-19: Federal Efforts Could Be Strengthened by Timely and Concerted Actions*, GAO-20-701, (Washington, D.C.: Sept. 21, 2020); and *COVID-19: Opportunities to Improve Federal Response and Recovery Efforts*, GAO-20-625, (Washington, D.C.: June 25, 2020).

More detailed information on our methodology can be found in the issued reports.[134]

In addition, we supplemented this information with updated data from CDC on COVID-19 reported by nursing homes for the week ending February 7, 2021.[135] We analyzed the CDC data as they were reported by nursing homes to CDC and publicly posted by CMS. We did not otherwise independently verify the accuracy of the information with these nursing homes. We assessed the reliability of the data sets used in our analyses by checking for missing values and obvious errors and reviewing relevant CMS and CDC documents. We determined the data were sufficiently reliable for the purposes of our reporting objective.

We conducted the work on which this statement is based in accordance with generally accepted government auditing standards. Those standards require that we plan and perform the audit to obtain sufficient, appropriate evidence to provide a reasonable basis for our findings and conclusions based on our audit objectives. We believe that the evidence obtained provides a reasonable basis for our findings and conclusions based on our audit objectives.

Nursing Home COVID-19 Cases and Deaths Are Declining after Winter Surge; Persistent Challenges Remain in Pandemic Response

After a Winter Surge, CDC Data Show a Decline in COVID-19 Cases and Deaths among Nursing Home Residents and Staff to Levels Closer to Those of Fall 2020

Our analysis of CDC data shows that winter 2020 was marked by a significant surge in the number of COVID-19 cases and deaths for nursing home residents and staff. Specifically, during mid-December 2020, there were more than 33,600 new resident cases and 28,600 new staff cases, which was more than twice as high as the prior case number peaks in summer 2020. CDC data show that cases and deaths in nursing homes are on the decline. Specifically, as of the week ending February 7, 2021, resident and staff cases have both declined by more than 80 percent since their peaks in December 2020.

The changing weekly COVID-19 death counts in nursing homes generally moved in the same direction as changes in the country as a whole. With the introduction of vaccines, observers are hopeful that nursing homes may be beginning to see a reprieve; however, the emergence of more highly transmissible virus variants warrants the need for continued vigilance, according to public health officials.[136] (See Figure 1).

---

[134] For example, see GAO-21-265.

[135] We analyzed the most recent data available on February 18, 2021. The CDC data on COVID-19 in nursing homes were accessed on February 18, 2021, for the week ending February 7, 2021, from https://data.cms.gov/Covid19-nursing-home-data. For the data on COVID-19 in nursing homes, we analyzed and reported data that had been determined by CDC and CMS to pass quality assurance checks for data entry errors. According to CDC, data used in this analysis are part of a live data set, meaning that facilities can make corrections to the data at any time.

[136] These numbers are likely underreported because they do not include data for the 998 nursing homes (6.5 percent) that did not report COVID-19 data to CDC for the week ending February 7, 2021, or that submitted data that failed data quality assurance checks. The week ending May 31, 2020, is the first single week of data reported to CDC. The week ending May 24 is the only earlier week of data, and could potentially include cases and deaths for multiple weeks dating back to January 1, 2020, for those homes which voluntarily reported such data. It is therefore not comparable with data for other weeks, and we excluded it. According to CDC, data used in this analysis are part of a live data set, meaning that facilities can make corrections to the data at any time.

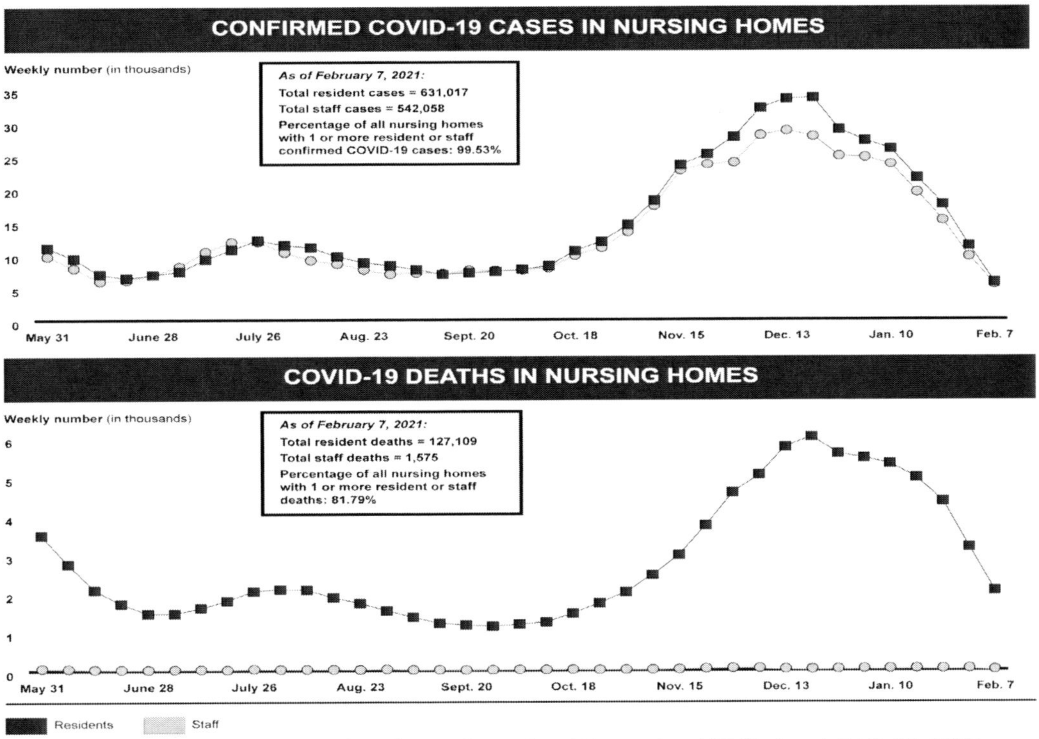

Source: GAO analysis of Centers for Disease Control and Prevention (CDC) data. | GAO-21-402T.

Notes: Dates refer to the end of a week (e.g., May 31 refers to the entire week from May 25 through May 31).

According to CDC, data used in this analysis are part of a live data set, meaning that facilities can make corrections to the data at any time. Data presented reflect the data downloaded as of February 18, 2021, which includes data through the week ending February 7, 2021. We excluded data for the week ending May 24, 2020, because it is the first week for which data are available from the CDC and could include cases and deaths from multiple weeks dating back to January 1, 2020.

Weekly and cumulative case and death counts are likely underreported because they do not include data for the nursing homes that did not report COVID-19 data to CDC for that week or from nursing homes that submitted data that failed data quality assurance checks. Additionally, as we previously reported, the Centers for Medicare & Medicaid Services (CMS) does not require nursing homes to *(cont.)* report data prior to May 2020, although nursing homes may do so voluntarily. We recommended that the Secretary of Health and Human Services—in consultation with CMS and CDC—develop a strategy to capture more complete data on confirmed COVID-19 cases and deaths in nursing homes retroactively to January 1, 2020. See GAO, *COVID-19: Federal Efforts Could Be Strengthened by Timely and Concerted Actions*, GAO-20-701, (Washington, D.C.: Sept. 21, 2020).

Weekly staff deaths reported for the weeks ending May 31 through February 7 ranged from 13 (week ending September 20, 2020) to 61 (week ending May 31, 2020).

Figure 1. New weekly confirmed COVID-19 cases and deaths among U.S. nursing home residents and staff, as reported by Medicare and Medicaid-certified nursing homes, May 31, 2020, through Feb 7, 2021.

Some Challenges Nursing Homes Faced Persisted While Other New Challenges Have Emerged

In our prior CARES Act reports, we found that nursing homes have faced many difficult challenges battling COVID-19.[137] While challenges related to staffing shortages have persisted through the pandemic, challenges related to obtaining Personal Protective Equipment (PPE) and conducting COVID-19 tests—although still notable—have generally shown signs of improvement since summer 2020. Further, with the decline in nursing home cases, CMS updated its guidance in March 2021 to expand resident visitation, an issue that has been an ongoing and persistent challenge during the pandemic. Some new challenges have also emerged as vaccinations started for nursing home residents and staff. (See Table 1). Some of these challenges, such as staffing shortages, obtaining PPE, and conducting testing, are critically important for infection control.

Table 1. Key pandemic challenges experienced by nursing homes

Challenge	Description	Status
Visitation	Through interviews with researchers, advocacy organizations, and national association officials from July 2020 to February 2021, we consistently heard that nursing homes have faced an ongoing tension between providing residents with important visitation and minimizing the potential for a COVID-19 outbreak: • The restriction of visitors has negatively affected residents' mental and physical health. Researchers and advocacy organizations have noted that the isolation resulting from decreased visitation can cause loneliness, anxiety, and depression among residents. • The restriction of visitors has created limited oversight of facilities through the exclusion of resident advocates, such as family members and ombudsmen	Challenge has persisted throughout pandemic
Staffing	In our reviews of data from the Centers for Disease Control and Prevention (CDC) and interviews with advocacy organization and national association officials from July 2020 through January 2021, we consistently found that nursing home staffing challenges were difficult and ongoing throughout the pandemic: • CDC data from July through December 2020 consistently show that about one in five nursing homes were reporting to CDC that they had a shortage of nurse aides or other support staff.[a] • From nursing home associations we interviewed, we heard that many alternative staffing sources have been used to fill critical gaps, such as seeking help from staffing agencies, sharing staff between other local providers, and using emergency waivers to hire nurse aides who had yet to complete their certification. As of January 2021, we continued to hear that staff are exhausted, face burn-out from emotional trauma, need to quarantine due to exposure to or illness from the virus, or stay home to take care of family members—all of which further strains staffing resources.	Challenge has persisted throughout pandemic
Personal Protective Equipment (PPE)	According to our reviews of data from the CDC and interviews with advocacy organization and national association officials from July 2020 to January 2021, shortages of PPE in nursing homes have improved since the beginning of the COVID-19 pandemic but remain an issue: • CDC data show that, as recently as December 2020, about 10 percent of nursing homes did not have a one-week supply of at	Challenge has generally shown improvement

[137] See GAO-20-701; GAO-21-265; GAO-21-191; and GAO-20-625.

Challenge	Description	Status
	• least one of the following: N95 respirators, surgical masks, gloves, eye protection, or gowns (a decrease from about 22 percent of nursing homes in July 2020). • In interviews with advocacy organizations and national association officials from July 2020 to January 2021, we heard that, while challenges maintaining PPE supplies in reserve is an ongoing concern, supply shortages have become less severe over time.	
Testing	According to our reviews of CDC data and interviews with a researcher and with nursing home association officials in November 2020 and January 2021, nursing homes' ability to use testing to identify infected residents and staff through testing protocols has improved over the course of the pandemic, but at a high cost to nursing homes: • Nursing homes have reported to CDC improved testing capacity. Specifically, the number of nursing homes testing for COVID-19 in both staff and residents has increased by 48 percentage points—from 35 to 83 percent—between August 16, 2020, and November 22, 2020, the last week complete data for overall testing were available. • Although data reported in December 2020 by nursing homes found that less than 2 percent of nursing homes would be unable to test all staff or residents within the week if needed, nursing home association officials note that the high cost of continuous testing is not sustainable indefinitely.	Challenge has generally shown improvement
Vaccinations	According to our reviews of a CDC analysis of vaccination data and interviews with nursing home and state and local government officials, nursing homes face some emerging challenges related to vaccinations: • A February 2021 CDC study estimated low rates of vaccine uptake among nursing home staff (38 percent) compared to nursing home residents (78 percent) participating in the Pharmacy Partnership for Long-Term Care Program.[b] • In interviews with nursing home and state and local government association officials since the vaccines were first administered in December 2020, we heard about reluctance among some nursing home staff to receive the COVID-19 vaccine, in addition to hearing about uncertainty around certain aspects of vaccination distribution and requirements earlier in the year.	Emerging challenge

Source: GAO review of CDC data and interviews. | GAO-21-402T.

[a]According to CDC's data documentation, other support staff may include certified nursing assistants, medication aides, and medication technicians as reported to CDC by the provider.

[b]R. Gharpure, et al., "Early COVID-19 First-Dose Vaccination Coverage Among Residents and Staff Members of Skilled Nursing Facilities Participating in the Pharmacy Partnership for Long-Term Care Program—United States, December 2020-January 2021," Centers for Disease Control and Prevention Morbidity and Mortality Weekly Report, vol. 70, no. 5 (2021): 178-182.

HHS Has Taken Steps in Response to COVID-19, but Several Relevant GAO Recommendations Have Not Been Implemented

Our prior CARES Act reports have described how HHS, primarily through CMS and CDC, has taken a series of actions to address COVID-19 in nursing homes, such as providing guidance to nursing homes on infection control practices and issuing waivers and regulatory flexibilities.[138]

[138] For example, in March 2020 CMS waived the requirement that a nursing home not employ nurse aides for more than 4 months unless they meet certain training and certification requirements. This was done to address potential staffing shortages in nursing homes due to the COVID-19 pandemic.

Examples of other actions include:

- Temporarily suspending state survey agencies' standard surveys and many complaint investigations, instead shifting to targeted infection prevention and control surveys and high-priority complaint investigations.[139]
- Creating a new reporting requirement for nursing homes to report weekly COVID-19 cases and deaths for residents and staff as of May 8, 2020.
- Distributing antigen diagnostic tests and associated point-of-care testing instruments to nursing homes.
- Distributing billions of dollars in payments from the Provider Relief Fund, established with funds provided under the CARES Act and other COVID-19 relief laws, as direct payments to assist nursing homes with responding to COVID-19.[140]
- Convening the Coronavirus Commission on Safety and Quality in Nursing Homes (the Nursing Home Commission) in June 2020, which was tasked with assessing the response to the COVID-19 pandemic in nursing homes and made recommendations for additional actions CMS could take.
- Establishing the Pharmacy Partnership for Long-Term Care Program in October 2020, an agreement with CVS, Walgreens, and Managed Health Care Associates Inc. to provide and administer COVID-19 vaccines to residents of long-term care facilities, including nursing homes.
- Directing nursing homes to expand resident visitation beginning in March 2021, after previously restricting visitors and non-essential health care personnel in nursing homes, except in certain compassionate care situations, to reduce the transmission of COVID-19.[141]

However, HHS has not implemented several of our recommendations that could help the agency address some of the challenges nursing homes have faced and fill important voids in the federal government's understanding of, and transparency around, data on COVID-19 in nursing homes. (See app. I for a description of related GAO reports and the status of their recommendations.)

---

[139] On June 1, CMS issued survey re-prioritization guidance as part of its nursing home reopening strategy. Specifically, once a state enters phase 3—a threshold based on factors including case status in the community and the nursing home, as well as access to testing, PPE, and adequate staffing—state survey agencies were authorized to expand beyond conducting targeted infection control surveys and high-priority complaint investigations to include lower-priority complaint investigations. See Centers for Medicare & Medicaid Services, "COVID-19 Survey Activities, CARES Act Funding, Enhanced Enforcement for Infection Control Deficiencies, and Quality Improvement Activities in Nursing Homes," QSO-20-31-ALL, (Baltimore, Md.: June 1, 2020). On August 17, CMS revised this guidance to authorize traditional, comprehensive, standard surveys and lower-priority complaint investigations as soon as state survey agencies have the resources, such as staff and PPE. See Centers for Medicare & Medicaid Services, "Enforcement Cases Held During the Prioritization Period and Revised Survey Prioritization," QSO-20-35-ALL, (Baltimore, Md.: Aug. 17, 2020).

[140] As of January 15, 2021, $5 billion in Provider Relief Funds had been allocated for nursing homes and $4.764 billion had been disbursed.

[141] CMS restricted visitors and non-essential health care personnel in nursing homes from March through September 2020. In September 2020, CMS issued guidance that allowed for nursing homes to resume visitations depending on certain factors.

- *HHS has not implemented our recommendation related to the Nursing Home Commission report.* CMS released the Nursing Home Commission's final report in September 2020, which includes 27 recommendations organized under 10 themes—such as Testing and Screening, Equipment and PPE, Workforce (staffing), and Visitation—that are paired with over 100 specific action steps for CMS.[142] CMS released a response to the report broadly outlining the actions the agency has taken to date as part of its response to the COVID-19 pandemic, but the agency did not provide an implementation plan that would allow it to track and report progress toward the Commission's recommendations.

  We recommended in November 2020 that the Administrator of CMS quickly develop a plan that further details how the agency intends to respond to and implement, as appropriate, the 27 recommendations in the final report of the Coronavirus Commission on Safety and Quality in Nursing Homes. HHS neither agreed nor disagreed with our recommendation; instead, it highlighted actions CMS has taken related to Commission recommendations and indicated that it would refer to and act upon the Nursing Home Commission's recommendations as appropriate. CMS reiterated this position in February 2021.
- *HHS has not implemented our recommendation to fill COVID-19 data voids.* HHS, through CMS, implemented a COVID-19 reporting requirement for nursing homes effective May 8, 2020 (noted briefly above).[143] CMS made the reporting of the data prior to May 8, 2020, optional. As a result, CMS's data do not capture the early months of the pandemic.[144]

  We recommended in September 2020 that the Secretary of HHS, in consultation with CMS and CDC, develop a strategy to capture more complete data on confirmed COVID-19 cases and deaths in nursing homes retroactively back to January 1, 2020, and clarify the extent to which nursing homes had reported data before May 8, 2020.[145] Although HHS partially agreed with this recommendation and indicated that it continues to consider how to implement this recommendation, the agency had taken no specific actions, as of February 2021.

We maintain the importance of our recommendations. Specifically, we maintain that developing a plan for whether CMS will proceed with the Nursing Home Commission's recommendations and, if so, how it will do so would improve the agency's ability to systematically consider the Nursing Home Commission's recommendations going forward. We also maintain that collecting data on COVID-19 cases and deaths from nursing homes retroactively would better inform the government's continued response to, and recovery from,

---

[142] MITRE, *Coronavirus Commission on Safety and Quality in Nursing Homes: Commission Final Report*, PRS Release Number 20-2382, September 2020.

[143] 85 Fed. Reg. 27,550, 27,627 (May 8, 2020) (to be codified at 42 C.F.R. § 483.80(g)). CMS is responsible for ensuring that nursing homes meet federal quality standards to participate in the Medicare and Medicaid programs.

[144] Nursing homes are required to self-report data regarding COVID-19 cases and deaths among residents and staff, PPE supplies, and staffing shortages, among other things, at least weekly through CDC's National Healthcare Safety Network.

[145] Also in September 2020, GAO identified gaps in COVID-19 data for racial and ethnic minority groups, and, among other things, recommended that CDC take steps to help ensure its ability to comprehensively assess the long-term health outcomes of persons with COVID-19, including by race and ethnicity. HHS agreed with the recommendation and as of February 2021, CDC is reviewing the quality of the demographic data and assessing potential opportunities to enhance the collection of race and ethnicity data.

the COVID-19 pandemic, and we maintain that HHS could ease the burden by incorporating data previously reported to CDC or to state or local public health offices.

We also have recommendations from work completed prior to the pandemic that have yet to be fully implemented by CMS. Implementation of these recommendations could improve HHS's oversight of nursing homes both generally and during a pandemic. For example, in our 2019 report on abuse in nursing homes, we made six recommendations, including recommending that CMS require state survey agencies to immediately notify law enforcement of any reasonable suspicion of a crime against a resident, and that CMS provide more guidance to state survey agencies on the information nursing homes should include on facility-reported incidents. CMS agreed with our recommendations.[146] These recommendations have relevance prior to, during, and after the COVID-19 pandemic, because with reduced visitors or ombudsmen presence in nursing homes, and with the decrease or elimination of surveyor presence, there may be a higher risk of residents being abused and of that abuse going unreported.[147] This risk is higher than it needs to be because CMS has not yet implemented our relevant recommendations.

In addition to monitoring HHS's implementation of past recommendations, we have ongoing work examining COVID-19 outbreaks in nursing homes, as well as CMS's oversight of infection prevention and control protocols and the adequacy of emergency preparedness standards for emerging infectious diseases in nursing homes.

In summary, the COVID-19 pandemic has underscored the importance of issues we have previously raised about nursing home quality and oversight while pointing to new vulnerabilities unique to the pandemic. Effective federal oversight and support for nursing homes are especially critical during times of widespread disease outbreak, as the pandemic has demonstrated. As nursing homes are prioritized for vaccination, there is hope that COVID-19 cases and deaths in these homes will continue to decline. Going forward, our work on COVID-19 in nursing homes remains important for informing future pandemic responses, as well as for addressing longer-standing challenges that have put residents' health and safety at risk, as indicated by our prior recommendations.

Chairman Wyden, Ranking Member Crapo, and Members of the Committee, this concludes my prepared statement. I would be pleased to respond to any questions that you may have at this time.

Appendix I: Description of Selected GAO Reports on Nursing Homes with Recommendations

The following table summarizes the status of relevant recommendations from GAO's prior reports on nursing home oversight with the status as of the most recent detailed update. According to the Centers for Medicare & Medicaid Services (CMS), as of March 2021, there are no additional updates on the status of these recommendations, as the agency's focus has been on responding to the pandemic.

---

[146] See GAO, *Nursing Homes: Improved Oversight Needed to Better Protect Residents from Abuse.* GAO-19-433. (Washington, D.C.: June 13, 2019).

[147] State surveyors evaluate nursing homes' compliance with federal quality standards.

Table 1. Description of selected GAO reports on nursing homes with recommendations, April 2011 through November 2020

Date	Title	Summary of recommendations
November 2020	*COVID-19: Urgent Actions Needed to Better Ensure an Effective Federal Response* (GAO-21-191)	GAO made one recommendation related to nursing homes that the Centers for Medicare & Medicaid Services (CMS) should quickly develop a plan that further details how the agency intends to respond to and implement, as appropriate, the 27 recommendations in the final report of the Coronavirus Commission on Safety and Quality in Nursing Homes, which CMS released on September 16, 2020. The Department of Health and Human Services (HHS) neither agreed nor disagreed with our recommendation and, as of February 2021, HHS/CMS had not implemented this recommendation.
September 2020	*COVID-19: Federal Efforts Could Be Strengthened by Timely and Concerted Actions* (GAO-20-701)	GAO made one recommendation related to nursing homes that HHS, in consultation with CMS and the Centers for Disease Control and Prevention (CDC), develop a strategy to capture more complete data on confirmed COVID-19 cases and deaths in nursing homes retroactively to January 1, 2020, in order to address gaps in the new reporting requirements on COVID-19 cases and deaths in nursing homes. HHS partially agreed with this recommendation and, as of February 2021, HHS had not implemented this recommendation.
June 2019	*Nursing Homes: Improved Oversight Needed to Better Protect Residents from Abuse* (GAO-19-433)	GAO made six recommendations, including that CMS require state survey agencies to immediately notify law enforcement of any reasonable suspicion of a crime against a resident, and that CMS provide more guidance to state survey agencies on the information nursing homes should include on facility-reported incidents. HHS agreed with the recommendations and, as of February 2020, HHS had not implemented these recommendations.
April 2019	*Management Report: CMS Needs to Address Gaps in Federal Oversight of Nursing Home Abuse Investigations That Persisted in Oregon for at Least 15 Years* (GAO-19-313R)	GAO made three recommendations, including that CMS ensure all state survey agencies are meeting federal requirements for investigating alleged abuse, and that the results are shared with CMS. HHS agreed with the recommendations and, as of November 2019, HHS had implemented one of the three recommendations.
November 2016	*Nursing Homes: Consumers Could Benefit from Improvements to the Nursing Home Compare Website and Five-Star Quality Rating System* (GAO-17-61)	GAO made four recommendations, including that CMS should add information to the Five-Star System that allows consumers to compare nursing homes nationally. HHS agreed with three of the four recommendations and, as of July 2019, HHS had implemented three of the four recommendations.
October 2015	*Nursing Home Quality: CMS Should Continue to Improve Data and Oversight* (GAO-16-33)	GAO made three recommendations, including that CMS implement a clear plan for ongoing auditing of self-reported data and establish a process for monitoring oversight modifications to better assess their effects. HHS agreed with GAO's recommendations. As of 2020, HHS had implemented these three recommendations.
April 2011	*Nursing Homes: More Reliable Data and Consistent Guidance Would Improve CMS Oversight of State Complaint Investigations* (GAO-11-280)	GAO made seven recommendations aimed at ensuring CMS's complaints database is reliable, strengthening CMS's assessment of state survey agencies' performance in managing complaints, and increasing accountability for managing the complaints process. HHS generally agreed with our recommendations. As of October 2019, HHS had implemented two of these seven recommendations and indicated it would not be taking action on a third (GAO closed this as not implemented).

Source: GAO. | GAO-21-402T.

Note: The hyperlinks to these reports provide additional details about the recommendations and their statuses.

Appendix II: Related GAO Reports

CARES Act Reports

COVID-19: Critical Vaccine Distribution, Supply Chain, Program Integrity, and Other Challenges Require Focused Federal Attention. GAO-21-265. Washington, D.C.: January 28, 2021.

COVID-19: Urgent Actions Needed to Better Ensure an Effective Federal Response. GAO-21-191. Washington, D.C.: November 30, 2020.

COVID-19: Federal Efforts Could Be Strengthened by Timely and Concerted Actions. GAO-20-701. Washington, D.C.: September 21, 2020.

COVID-19: Opportunities to Improve Federal Response and Recovery Efforts. GAO-20-625. Washington, D.C.: June 25, 2020.

Other GAO Reports

Infection Control Deficiencies Were Widespread and Persistent in Nursing Homes Prior to COVID-19 Pandemic. GAO-20-576R. Washington, D.C.: May 20, 2020.

Elder Abuse: Federal Requirements for Oversight in Nursing Homes and Assisted Living Facilities Differ. GAO-19-599. Washington, D.C.: August 19, 2019.

Nursing Homes: Improved Oversight Needed to Better Protect Residents from Abuse. GAO-19-433. Washington, D.C.: June 13, 2019.

Management Report: CMS Needs to Address Gaps in Federal Oversight of Nursing Home Abuse Investigations That Persisted in Oregon for at Least 15 Years. GAO-19-313R. Washington, D.C.: April 15, 2019.

Nursing Homes: Consumers Could Benefit from Improvements to the Nursing Home Compare Website and Five-Star Quality Rating System. GAO-17-61. Washington, D.C.: November 18, 2016.

Nursing Home Quality: CMS Should Continue to Improve Data and Oversight. GAO-16-33. Washington, D.C.: October 30, 2015.

Antipsychotic Drug Use: HHS Has Initiatives to Reduce Use among Older Adults in Nursing Homes, but Should Expand Efforts to Other Settings.
GAO-15-211. Washington, D.C.: January 30, 2015.

Nursing Homes: More Reliable Data and Consistent Guidance Would Improve CMS Oversight of State Complaint Investigations. GAO-11-280. Washington, D.C.: April 7, 2011.

Questions Submitted for the Record to John E. Dicken

Questions Submitted by Hon. Ron Wyden

Question. What changes do you recommend to the Five-Star system so it will better reflect patients' outcomes of care and inform residents and loved ones about the quality and safety of nursing homes?

Answer. We last reported on the Five-Star Quality Rating System (Five-Star System) in November 2016 (see GAO–17–61). We made four recommendations in that report, three of which have been implemented by the Centers for Medicare and Medicaid Services (CMS) and one of which remains unimplemented.

With regard to the unimplemented recommendation, we recommended that, to help improve the Five-Star System's ability to enable consumers to understand nursing home quality and make distinctions between high- and low-performing homes, the Administrator of CMS should add information to the Five-Star System that allows consumers to compare nursing homes nationally. The Department of Health and Human Services (HHS) did not concur with this recommendation. In July 2019, CMS officials told us they do not plan to implement this recommendation, and as of March 2021 CMS had not informed us of steps taken to address the recommendation. However, we maintain that adding national comparison information is important, especially for those consumers who live near State borders or have multi-State options.

We also recommended in that report that CMS evaluate the feasibility of adding consumer satisfaction information to the Five-Star System. HHS concurred with this recommendation and provided us with such a study dated October 2017, leading us to close the recommendation as implemented. However, the study described "wide-spread consensus that measuring satisfaction of nursing home residents and families is crucial to understanding resident experience and to informing consumers on choosing a nursing home." This suggests that CMS could better inform residents and their loved ones about the quality and safety of nursing homes by taking the next step of adding consumer satisfaction information to the Five-Star System.

As GAO continues to evaluate the federal response to COVID–19 in nursing homes and the effects of the pandemic on the safety and welfare of nursing home residents, we will also monitor challenges the pandemic will pose for CMS's Five-Star System going forward. For example, nursing home inspection results are one key element of the Five-Star System's ratings, but many standard inspections have not occurred or have been delayed during this national emergency, consistent with CMS's guidelines. Thus, the information consumers receive from the Five-Star System will be a less timely and accurate representation of care provided during the pandemic.

Question. The involvement of private equity in the nursing home industry has been of interest to the Finance Committee for more than a decade, and the role of private equity and for profit ownership in the nursing home industry was raised in testimony and questions at the hearing. The Government Accountability Office (GAO) considered this issue in a 2010 report, "Nursing Homes: Complexity of Private Investment Purchases Demonstrates Need for CMS to

Improve the Usability and Completeness of Ownership Data." Please provide an update on the status of the recommendations made in this report.

Answer. The 11 recommendations from that report, GAO–10–710, are closed. Five were closed as implemented, and six were closed as not implemented. The recommendations not implemented are summarized in the following paragraphs, but full details are available in the report and on the GAO website.

Three of the recommendations not implemented relate to the Patient Protection and Affordable Care Act (PPACA), which expanded the ownership and control reporting requirements for Medicare and Medicaid nursing homes. At the time we reported, these PPACA requirements had not yet been implemented, and we recommended that HHS consider requiring certain types of reporting as it developed the regulations to implement these requirements. For each of these recommendations, CMS told GAO that it had taken steps to obtain the recommended information by making changes to its provider enrollment application form. However, in each case GAO assessed that the changes did not specifically or sufficiently address the information targeted by our recommendations. Because CMS had not indicated any plans to take further actions at the time these recommendations were closed, GAO considered them to be closed and not implemented.

The other three recommendations not implemented related to information HHS should require nursing homes to report or to actions HHS should take to ensure the usability, accuracy, and completeness of nursing home ownership information. In the case of our recommending an additional reporting requirement, CMS told GAO that, upon further review, it had determined that taking action would represent an undue burden on providers, given the existing functionality of its provider enrollment system, and that the agency considered the matter closed. In the other two cases, CMS told GAO about actions it had taken related to the recommendations and said that the agency had no further updates and considered the matters closed.

GAO currently has ongoing work related to the quality of nursing homes with chain ownership, including private equity owners, which should provide more up-to-date information on this topic.

Question. During the hearing, several Senators and witnesses raised the importance of the Federal Government collecting and publishing information from individual nursing homes that show the rate of vaccinations for residents and staff. Since that time, a bipartisan group of senators have sent a letter to the U.S. Department of Health and Human Services calling on it to take steps to begin this data collection. Has GAO issued any recommendations in relation to this issue?

Answer. The Federal Government's collection and reporting of nursing home vaccination data is important for providing insight into nursing home quality of care and protecting the vulnerable nursing home population. We made two recommendations related to this issue in our March 2021 CARES Act report (see GAO–21–387).

First, we recommended that the Secretary of HHS should ensure that the Director of the CDC collects data specific to the COVID–19 vaccination rates in nursing homes and makes these data publicly available to better ensure transparency and that the necessary information is available to improve ongoing and future vaccination efforts for nursing home residents and staff. HHS neither agreed nor disagreed with this recommendation.

In response to our recommendation, HHS said it is working towards better data transparency and noted that nursing homes have an opportunity to voluntarily report data through the National Healthcare Safety Network (NHSN) tracking system. However, according to CDC, as of February 17, 2021, around 14 percent of nursing homes are voluntarily reporting staff vaccination data through NHSN and around 18 percent are voluntarily reporting resident vaccination data. We maintain that more complete data on COVID–19 vaccinations in nursing homes will be important for CMS's ongoing efforts to monitor nursing home quality and that making these data transparent through public reporting provides consumers with insight into how well nursing homes are caring for their residents.

Second, we recommended that the Secretary of HHS should ensure that the Administrator of CMS, in consultation with CDC, requires nursing homes to offer COVID–19 vaccinations to residents and staff and design and implement associated quality measures. HHS neither agreed nor disagreed with this recommendation.

In response to our recommendation, HHS indicated that CMS is "actively evaluating" whether changes need to be made to its infection control requirements regarding the COVID–19 vaccine and that CMS and CDC "have made progress in developing quality measures related to COVID–19 vaccination." We note that CMS already requires nursing homes to offer influenza and pneumococcal vaccinations to nursing home residents; given the significant threat COVID–19 poses to nursing home residents, with a mortality rate far exceeding that of influenza, we maintain the importance of this recommendation for protecting the vulnerable nursing home population.

On April 8, 2021, CMS published a proposed rule that, among other things, proposes the adoption of a "COVID–19 Vaccination Coverage among Healthcare Personnel" quality measure. This would require Skilled Nursing Facilities (SNF) to report on COVID–19 vaccination of staff. Under the proposal, SNFs would begin reporting vaccination data through CDC's NHSN beginning October 1, 2021, and the quality measure would be adopted beginning in fiscal year 2023. We will continue to monitor CMS's actions responding to these two recommendations.

Question. The South African and Brazilian variants continue to circulate in the United States. What are issues Congress should consider in regards to the danger that these and other COVID–19 variants may pose to nursing homes, particularly residents who have been most vulnerable to the disease?

Answer. As we noted in our March 2021 CARES Act report (see GAO–21–387), the emergence of new COVID–19 variants underscores the need to remain vigilant in efforts to contain the spread of the virus. For example, one expert we interviewed noted that different variants could increase the number of COVID–19 cases and deaths and reduce health care systems' ability to care for patients. Because nursing home residents are at high risk for COVID–19 infection and death, due to the virus's high mortality rate among elderly adults and those with underlying conditions, continued vigilance is especially important for nursing homes.

As we reported in the same March 2021 report, several experts told us that it is important for the federal government to help the public and stakeholders understand how to use its

COVID–19 data, and one expert specifically highlighted the importance of doing so for data on COVID–19 variants. While CDC already makes data available on case numbers for COVID–19 variants, this expert told us that it is also important for the federal government to explain how to interpret these numbers and describe how stakeholders, including State and local public health officials, could use these data to inform their efforts to respond to the pandemic. This could include how data could be used to inform response efforts in nursing homes.

Additionally, collecting more complete data on COVID–19 vaccinations in nursing homes, as we recommended in our March 2021 CARES Act report (see previous response), could help with understanding whether vaccinated residents may be vulnerable to infection by COVID–19 variants. Similarly, demographic data, such as race and ethnicity data, for COVID–19 in nursing homes could help with understanding whether COVID–19 variants may have a disproportionate effect on a particular group. In our September CARES Act report (see GAO–20–701), we made three recommendations related to the collection of demographic data for COVID–19, including data on race and ethnicity; these recommendations remain open.

Question. Is additional surveillance necessary to detect the spread of viral variants? What types of surveillance, if any, should be implemented in regards to the nursing home industry specifically?

Answer. Surveillance is important for understanding the transmission of the virus, including variants. More complete data on COVID–19 in nursing homes, including data on COVID–19 vaccinations and demographic data, may help with understanding the impact of COVID–19 variants on nursing home residents. CMS and CDC could begin to gather more complete data on COVID–19 in nursing homes by implementing our recommendations.

Question. In the event that additional vaccinations and/or booster shots are needed to protect against variants, what lessons can be drawn from the experience of the CVS Walgreen Long-Term Care Partnership?

Answer. While we have not done a full evaluation of the Pharmacy Partnership for Long-Term Care Program, we noted in our March 2021 CARES Act report (see GAO–21–387) that a key challenge was the decentralization of the partnership program. Originally designed to be a federal program, each State was ultimately responsible for activating the partnership and allocating doses to the partnership. According to State and nursing home association officials, this resulted in more than 50 different plans for implementation, which caused confusion among jurisdictions' health departments, nursing homes, and pharmacy partners and hampered communication and vaccine education efforts. The officials said a more centralized distribution model may have created a more efficient approach to vaccinating the nursing home population.

Question. The GAO has issued numerous recommendations related to nursing homes over the years. Please provide a list of all outstanding recommendations that relate to the Centers for Medicare and Medicaid Services and remain open.

Answer. The following recommendations related to nursing homes and CMS remain open. We maintain that implementing these recommendations could improve HHS's oversight of nursing homes both generally and during a pandemic.

1. The Secretary of HHS should ensure that the Administrator of CMS, in consultation with CDC, requires nursing homes to offer COVID–19 vaccinations to residents and staff and design and implement associated quality measures.
Source: GAO–21–387, published March 31, 2021.
2. The Administrator of CMS should quickly develop a plan that further details how the agency intends to respond to and implement, as appropriate, the 27 recommendations in the final report of the Coronavirus Commission on Safety and Quality in Nursing Homes, which CMS released on September 16, 2020. Such a plan should include milestones that allow the agency to track and report on the status of each recommendation; identify actions taken and planned, including areas where the CMS determined not to take action; and identify areas where the agency could coordinate with other federal and non-federal entities.
Source: GAO–21–191, published November 30, 2020.
3. The Secretary of HHS, in consultation with CMS and CDC, should develop a strategy to capture more complete data on confirmed COVID–19 cases and deaths in nursing homes retroactively back to January 1, 2020, and to clarify the extent to which nursing homes have reported data before May 8, 2020. To the extent feasible, this strategy to capture more complete data should incorporate information nursing homes previously reported to CDC or to State or local public health offices.
Source: GAO–20–701, published September 21, 2020.
4. The administrator of CMS should require that abuse and perpetrator type be submitted by State survey agencies in CMS's databases for deficiency, complaint, and facility reported incident data, and that CMS systematically assess trends in these data.
Source: GAO–19–433, published June 13, 2019.
5. The administrator of CMS should require State survey agencies to immediately refer complaints and surveys to law enforcement (and, when applicable, to Medicaid Fraud Control Units) if they have a reasonable suspicion that a crime against a resident has occurred when the complaint is received.
Source: GAO–19–433, published June 13, 2019.
6. The administrator of CMS should develop and disseminate guidance—including a standardized form—to all State survey agencies on the information nursing homes and covered individuals should include on facility-reported incidents.
Source: GAO–19–433, published June 13, 2019.
7. The administrator of CMS should conduct oversight of State survey agencies to ensure referrals of complaints, surveys, and substantiated incidents with reasonable suspicion of a crime are referred to law enforcement (and, when applicable, to Medicaid Fraud Control Units) in a timely fashion.
Source: GAO–19–433, published June 13, 2019.
8. The administrator of CMS should develop guidance for State survey agencies clarifying that allegations verified by evidence should be substantiated and reported to law enforcement and State registries in cases where citing a federal deficiency may not be appropriate.

Source: GAO–19–433, published June 13, 2019.

9. The administrator of CMS should provide guidance on what information should be contained in the referral of abuse allegations to law enforcement.
Source: GAO–19–433, published June 13, 2019.
10. CMS should evaluate State survey agency processes in all States to ensure all State survey agencies are meeting federal requirements that State survey agencies are responsible for investigating complaints and facility-reported incidents alleging abuse in nursing homes, and that the results of those investigations are being shared with CMS.
Source: GAO–19–313R, published April 15, 2019.
11. CMS should identify options for capturing information from Oregon's Adult Protective Services investigations of complaints and facility-reported incidents of abuse and incorporate this information into oversight of Oregon nursing homes.
Source: GAO–19–313R, published April 15, 2019.
12. To help improve the Five-Star System's ability to enable consumers to understand nursing home quality and make distinctions between high- and low-performing homes, the Administrator of CMS should add information to the Five-Star System that allows consumers to compare nursing homes nationally.
Source: GAO–17–61, published November 18, 2016.
13. To improve the accessibility and reliability of SNF expenditure data, the Acting Administrator of CMS should take steps to improve the accessibility of SNF expenditure data, making it easier for public stakeholders to locate and use the data.
Source: GAO–16–700, published September 7, 2016.
14. To improve the accessibility and reliability of SNF expenditure data, the Acting Administrator of CMS should take steps to ensure the accuracy and completeness of SNF expenditure data.
Source: GAO–16–700, published September 7, 2016.
15. To improve consumers' access to relevant and understandable information on the cost and quality of health care services, the Secretary of HHS should direct the Administrator of CMS to include in the CMS Compare websites, to the extent feasible, estimated out-of-pocket costs for Medicare beneficiaries for common treatments that can be planned in advance.
Source: GAO–15–11, published October 20, 2014.
16. To improve consumers' access to relevant and understandable information on the cost and quality of health care services, the Secretary of HHS should direct the Administrator of CMS to organize cost and quality information in the CMS Compare websites to facilitate consumer identification of the highest-performing providers, such as by listing providers in order based on their performance.
Source: GAO–15–11, published October 20, 2014.
17. To improve consumers' access to relevant and understandable information on the cost and quality of health-care services, the Secretary of HHS should direct the Administrator of CMS to include in the CMS Compare websites the capability for consumers to customize the information presented, to better focus on information relevant to them.
Source: GAO–15–11, published October 20, 2014.

18. To improve consumers' access to relevant and understandable information on the cost and quality of health-care services, the Secretary of HHS should direct the Administrator of CMS to develop specific procedures and performance metrics to ensure that CMS's efforts to promote the development and use of its own and others' transparency tools adequately address the needs of consumers.
Source: GAO–15–11, published October 20, 2014.
19. To ensure that information entered into CMS's complaints database is reliable and consistent, the Administrator of CMS should identify issues with data quality and clarify guidance to States about how particular fields in the database should be interpreted, such as what it means to substantiate a complaint.
Source: GAO–11–280, published April 7, 2011.
20. To strengthen CMS's assessment of State survey agencies' performance in the management of nursing home complaints, the Administrator of CMS should conduct additional monitoring of State performance using information from CMS's complaints database, such as additional timeliness measures.
Source: GAO–11–280, published April 7, 2011.
21. To strengthen and increase accountability of State survey agencies' management of the nursing home complaints process, the Administrator of CMS should clarify guidance to the State survey agencies about the minimum information that should be conveyed to complainants at the close of an investigation.
Source: GAO–11–280, published April 7, 2011.
22. To strengthen and increase accountability of State survey agencies' management of the nursing home complaints process, the Administrator of CMS should provide guidance encouraging State survey agencies to prioritize complaints at the level that is warranted, not above that level.
Source: GAO–11–280, published April 7, 2011.

Questions Submitted by Hon. Elizabeth Warren

Question. Please provide a full list of all GAO recommendations related to CMS's Provider Enrollment, Chain, and Ownership System (PECOS) that the agency has yet to complete and identify which recommendations have not been implemented by CMS or other relevant regulators.

Answer. GAO does not currently have any open recommendations targeted to CMS's Provider Enrollment, Chain, and Ownership System (PECOS). However, we have made recommendations targeted to PECOS in the past, several of which were closed as implemented (see, for example, GAO–15–448). At least one recommendation targeted to PECOS—from our 2010 report on private investment in nursing homes, GAO–10–710—was closed as not implemented:

1. To improve the usability and accuracy of the ownership and control information collected and stored in PECOS, the Administrator of CMS should examine State systems to identify best practices for the collection and public dissemination of nursing

home ownership and chain information, including ways in which States make the hierarchy among owners more apparent.

- In 2012, CMS told GAO that it had recently implemented an automated provider screening system and that it was continuing to have internal discussions and explore data sources that can provide nursing home information for that system. However, CMS said it had no further updates and that it considered the matter closed.

Question. What recommendations, if any, does GAO have for the executive branch to improve its visibility into the ownership of private-equity-owned nursing homes?

Answer. GAO does not have any open recommendations related to private-equity-owned nursing homes. However, GAO currently has ongoing work related to the quality of nursing homes with chain ownership, including private equity owners.

Question. GAO has analyzed nursing homes through the lens of the COVID–19 pandemic and provided Congress with a series of recommendations. Are any of GAO's COVID–19-related recommendations specifically targeted at or relevant for for-profit facilities, including private-equity-owned facilities? Did the COVID–19 pandemic reveal any differences in the ability of for- and non-profit facilities to provide high-quality care to residents or to protect them from pandemics?

Answer. None of the four COVID–19-related nursing homes recommendations from our CARES Act reporting are specifically targeted to for-profit facilities; however, each of the four recommendations is relevant to all nursing homes, which would include for-profit facilities (see Lankford question, later in this response, for a list of these recommendations).

GAO currently has ongoing work looking at which nursing home characteristics, if any, affect the likelihood that a home experienced a COVID–19 outbreak. We are also aware of ongoing work from the HHS Office of Inspector General (OIG) that will describe the characteristics of the nursing homes that were hardest hit by the pandemic (OEI–02–20–00490).

Additionally, although not specific to the COVID–19 pandemic, we have previously reported on the intersection of nursing home characteristics and nursing home quality:

- In May 2020, we reported that, over a 5-year period, while nursing homes owned by for-profit organizations comprised about 68 percent of all surveyed nursing homes, they accounted for 72 percent of nursing homes that had infection prevention and control deficiencies cited in multiple years but only about 61 percent of nursing homes with no infection prevention and control deficiencies cited (see GAO–20–576R).
- In 2015, we reported that the poorest performing nursing homes were more likely to be for-profit or large homes (greater than 100 beds) compared to homes that performed well; this was consistent with a 2009 GAO analysis on the most poorly performing nursing homes (see GAO–16–33, GAO–09– 689).
- In 2011, we reported that private investment and other for-profit nursing homes had more total deficiencies than nonprofit homes, both before and after acquisition by private investment firms (see GAO–11–571).

Questions Submitted by Hon. John Barrasso

Question. Through the years, nursing homes in my State have reported they have lost the ability to train their own CNAs. According to an article published in Health Affairs, this is because nursing homes with a civil monetary penalty greater than $10,000 lose the ability to conduct CNA training for 2 years. In rural communities, where the nursing home is often the sole source of training for CNAs, this creates a tremendous burden. Please comment on the impact losing the ability to train CNAs has on nursing homes.

Answer. GAO does not currently have any ongoing work or open recommendations focused on CNA training, including in rural communities, but, if you would like, we would be happy to follow up with your staff to further discuss this issue.

We note that the Coronavirus Commission on Safety and Quality in Nursing Homes—which we refer to as the Nursing Home Commission and which was appointed by CMS—reported that the COVID–19 pandemic has disrupted CNA training, "leading to serious CNA workforce deficits." The Nursing Home Commission recommended that CMS catalyze interest in the CNA profession through diverse recruitment vehicles; issue guidance for on-the-job CNA training, testing, and certification; and create a national CNA registry.[148]

In our November 2020 CARES Act report (see GAO–21–191), we recommended that the Administrator of CMS quickly develop a plan that further details how the agency intends to respond to and implement, as appropriate, the 27 recommendations in the final report of the Nursing Home Commission. As of February 2021, this recommendation had not been implemented. However, we maintain the importance of this recommendation, as developing a plan for whether CMS will proceed with the Nursing Home Commission 's recommendations—and, if so, how it will do so— would improve the agency's ability to systematically consider the recommendations going forward, to include the recommendation related to CNAs.

Question. Can you provide suggestions on how to address this situation, especially in rural communities?

Answer. See previous response.

Question. Please discuss the impact of staffing turnover on the quality of care provided in nursing homes.

Answer. GAO has ongoing related work examining the relationship between staffing levels and the rate of critical incidents at skilled nursing facilities prior to the pandemic. If you would like, we would be happy to follow up with your staff to further discuss this issue.

Question. Specifically, do you believe turnover rates from nursing homes should be made more readily available for public review?

---

[148] MITRE, *Coronavirus Commission on Safety and Quality in Nursing Homes: Commission Final Report,* PRS Release Number 20–2382, September 2020.

Answer. GAO does not have any recommendations on this issue. However, we are aware that the HHS OIG recently made a related recommendation. In March 2021, HHS OIG reported that federal law requires CMS to provide data on staffing turnover and tenure on Care Compare, but that CMS has not yet done so. CMS told HHS OIG that the agency was delayed by the COVID–19 pandemic. HHS OIG recommended that CMS provide data to consumers on nurse staff turnover and tenure, as required by federal law.[149]

Questions Submitted by Hon. Todd Young

Question. What are some lessons learned from the public health emergency in terms of the integration of technology in nursing homes-both in helping residents visit virtually with loved ones and in accessing health care services?

Answer. GAO currently has ongoing work that may address the use of technology in nursing homes for telehealth and other purposes.

For example, as part of our ongoing work examining nursing home challenges associated with the COVID–19 pandemic, we have interviewed officials from three State long-term care ombudsman programs, some of whom have utilized or plan to utilize technology to connect with residents during the pandemic.

Additionally, we have ongoing work examining the use of telehealth in Medicare and Medicaid. This includes HHS's use of statutory and regulatory flexibilities to temporarily waive or modify Medicare telehealth provisions in response to COVID– 19, as well as how States have used telehealth in Medicaid to respond to the pandemic. While this work is focused on Medicare and Medicaid broadly, it is also relevant to nursing homes specifically, because these waivers permit telehealth visits in nursing homes.

Finally, in our January CARES Act report (see GAO–21–265, Veterans Health Care enclosure), we discussed the Department of Veterans Affairs' (VA) use of telehealth. Again, while not specific to nursing homes, this work is relevant because VA provides or pays for nursing home care in various settings. Among other things, we reported that VA's Veterans Health Administration (VHA) has several ongoing efforts aimed at removing technology barriers to telehealth use among veterans; for example, VHA has directed facilities to establish programs to help veterans become familiar with telehealth technology.

Question. How do you anticipate this type of technology continuing to be used beyond the pandemic?

Answer. Our ongoing work on telehealth in Medicare and Medicaid, mentioned earlier, may address this question. For example, as part of our ongoing work examining HHS's Medicare telehealth waivers, we plan to examine the perspectives of beneficiaries, providers, and payers on Medicare telehealth services and on the idea of making some Medicare telehealth waivers permanent.

---

[149] Department of Health and Human Services, Office of Inspector General, *CMS Use of Data on Nursing Home Staffing: Progress and Opportunities To Do More*, OEI–04–18–00451 (Washington, DC: March 2021).

Question. Based on your oversight of CMS's infection prevention protocols and emergency preparedness standards, what further steps should the Federal Government take to encourage proper antibiotic stewardship in nursing homes?

Answer. Last year, we issued a report on additional federal actions needed to reduce the impact of antibiotic resistant bacteria broadly, not limited to nursing homes (see GAO–20–341). In that report, we credited federal agencies for actions already taken to encourage proper antibiotic stewardship in nursing homes. For example, we noted that CMS published requirements for nursing homes and skilled nursing facilities to establish antibiotic stewardship programs by December 4, 2017, which experts credited as being a powerful lever for promoting the appropriate use of antibiotics. We also noted that, since 2014, CDC has published a series of guidance documents called the Core Elements of Antibiotic Stewardship, which are tailored to nursing homes and other settings. However, challenges remain, such as in collecting antibiotic use data from nursing homes, which less commonly use electronic health record systems that would facilitate data access. The Federal Government could further encourage proper antibiotic stewardship generally, including in nursing homes, by implementing that report's eight recommendations, all of which remain open.

Additionally, the Federal Government could address the one remaining open recommendation from our 2017 report on Food and Drug Administration (FDA) efforts to encourage the development of new antibiotics (see GAO–17–189). Specifically, we recommended that FDA develop and make available written guidance on the qualified infectious disease products (QIDP) designation that includes information about the process a drug sponsor must undertake to request the fast track designation, and about how the agency is applying the market exclusivity incentive. As of August 2020, FDA reported that it is working to finalize draft guidance issued in January 2018 that describes the QIDP designation.

Questions Submitted by Hon. John Cornyn

Question. GAO has noted the challenge of staff shortages that nursing homes have faced during the pandemic. Reports have noted the use of staffing agencies, shared staff with other providers, and the use of emergency waivers to hire nurse aides who have yet to complete their certification. What steps can be taken to provider greater flexibility to nursing homes to maintain necessary staff levels without negatively impacting resident care?

Answer. We note that the Nursing Home Commission, which was appointed by CMS, made five recommendations (with more than 20 associated action steps) related to stopgap measures to support the nursing home workforce.[150] This included actions such as assessing federal relief funds for hazard pay options and updating interstate compact language addressing public health emergencies to support a surge-staffing pool in viral hotspots.

In our November 2020 CARES Act report (see GAO–21–191), we recommended that the Administrator of CMS quickly develop a plan that further details how the agency intends to respond to and implement, as appropriate, the 27 recommendations in the final report of the Nursing Home Commission. As of February 2021, this recommendation had not been

[150] MITRE, *Commission Final Report,* 41–47.

implemented. However, we maintain the importance of this recommendation, as developing a plan for whether CMS will proceed with the Nursing Home Commission's recommendations—and, if so, how it will do so— would improve the agency's ability to systematically consider the recommendations going forward, to include the recommendations related to stopgap measures to support the nursing home workforce.

Additionally, GAO currently has ongoing work examining the use of contract staff in nursing homes.

Along similar lines, HHS OIG reported in August 2020 that many nursing homes were not meeting required staffing levels even prior to the COVID–19 pandemic. In an analysis of 2018 data, HHS OIG found that 14 percent of nursing homes reported 16 or more days where staffing was below required levels in 2018; another 40 percent reported between 1 and 15 days where staffing was below required levels.[151] HHS OIG noted that in April 2018, CMS announced it would automatically down-grade nursing homes' Staffing Star Ratings on Nursing Home Compare if they reported at least 7 total days with no reported registered nurse time during a quarter; according to OIG, 27 percent fewer nursing homes reported days with no registered nurse time following this announcement. However, OIG noted that there were still nursing homes falling short of meeting staffing requirements in ways not addressed by this penalty. HHS OIG recommended that CMS enhance its efforts to ensure nursing homes meet daily staffing requirements, such as by expanding the agency's use of Payroll Based Journal data to identify understaffed nursing homes and target them for further oversight.

Question. GAO has also noted a reluctance in some nursing home staff to receive the COVID–19 vaccine. Are there specific recommendations to improve address this reluctance?

Answer. In our March CARES Act report (see GAO–21–387), we shared that State and nursing home association officials had indicated that COVID–19 vaccine takeup rates among staff were lower than among residents. They attributed this to several factors, including underlying issues of government mistrust and myths spread on social media. However, because CDC does not have complete data on vaccines administered in nursing homes outside of the Pharmacy Partnership for Long-Term Care Program, and because CDC publicly reports vaccination information collected through that program only for all long-term care facilities (rather than nursing homes specifically), it is unclear how successful efforts have been to vaccinate nursing home staff.

While GAO does not have specific recommendations to address nursing home staff reluctance to receive the COVID–19 vaccine, our March report's recommendations relating to nursing home COVID–19 vaccination data and associated quality measures could, if implemented, better ensure that the necessary information is available to improve ongoing and future vaccination efforts for nursing home staff. Additionally, they could help ensure that data on staff vaccination rates are available to help manage the risk of COVID–19 outbreaks in nursing homes and serve as an important source of information for consumers about quality of care. We note that, on April 8, 2021, CMS published a proposed rule related to these recommendations (see previous response to Wyden Q3).

---

[151] Department of Health and Human Services, Office of Inspector General, *Some Nursing Homes' Reported Staffing Levels in 2018 Raise Concerns; Consumer Transparency Could Be Increased,* OEI–04–18–00450 (Washington, DC: August 2020).

Questions Submitted by Hon. James Lankford

Question. What, in your opinion, does the nursing home industry need most to solve some of the problems that are consistently discussed surrounding nursing home facility underreporting, fraudulent reporting, and instances of abuse? Would you suggest different staff requirements and/or enhanced CMS oversight?

Answer. GAO has several recommendations related to reporting (and under-reporting) of abuse and COVID–19 data in nursing homes. By implementing these recommendations, Federal agencies could improve their oversight of nursing homes both generally and during a pandemic.

We last reported on instances of abuse in nursing homes in November 2019 (see testimony GAO–20–259T and related report GAO–19–433). We made six recommendations in GAO–19–433 (see Wyden Q5 earlier in our response, #4 through 9). CMS agreed with these recommendations, but they all remain open. The risk of residents being abused, and of that abuse going unreported, is higher than it needs to be because CMS has not yet implemented these recommendations.

As we first reported in our September 2020 CARES Act report (see GAO–20–701), COVID–19 cases and deaths in nursing homes are likely underreported in CMS and CDC data because, among other reasons, CMS does not require nursing homes to report data prior to May 8, 2020. As a result, the data do not provide HHS with a complete picture of the extent of the pandemic and its effect on nursing homes. To address this issue, we recommended that the Secretary of HHS—in consultation with CMS and CDC—develop a strategy to capture more complete data on confirmed COVID–19 cases and deaths in nursing homes retroactively to January 1, 2020. As of February 2021, this recommendation had not been implemented. We maintain that implementing this recommendation could help fill important gaps in the Federal Government's understanding of, and transparency around, data on COVID–19 in nursing homes.

Similarly, in our March CARES Act report (see GAO–21–387), we noted that HHS does not publicly report data showing vaccination rates specifically for nursing homes and does not have complete vaccination data for nursing homes not participating in the Pharmacy Partnership for Long-Term Care Program. As a result, it is unclear to what extent efforts to vaccinate nursing home residents have been successful, and it may be difficult to use these data to improve ongoing and future vaccination efforts for the nursing home population. We made two recommendations to address this issue:

1. The Secretary of HHS should ensure that the Director of the CDC collects data specific to the COVID–19 vaccination rates in nursing homes and makes these data publicly available to better ensure transparency and that the necessary information is available to improve ongoing and future vaccination efforts for nursing home residents and staff.
2. The Secretary of HHS should ensure that the Administrator of CMS, in consultation with the CDC, requires nursing homes to offer COVID–19 vaccinations to residents and staff and design and implement associated quality measures.

We note that, on April 8, 2021, CMS published a proposed rule related to these recommendations (see previous response to Wyden Q3).

Question. It has been noted that a nursing home's star rating has little to no correlation to its COVID infection rates. Nursing homes across the country have been overwhelmingly shut down for the larger part of the past year. However, about a third of COVID deaths in the U.S. have been from within largely closed facilities. It is also widely noted that isolation of nursing home residents had little to do with infection control, and that the best indicator of COVID in a nursing home was simply community spread. Mr. Dicken, what are your preliminary recommendations to protect long-term care residents from nearly the same impacts of COVID community-spread of those outside a nursing facility?

Answer. We maintain the importance of our four CARES Act report recommendations related to nursing homes for improving the Federal response to COVID–19 in nursing homes and protecting nursing home residents from the impacts of COVID–19. These recommendations, which remain open, are:

1. The Secretary of HHS should ensure that the Director of the CDC collects data specific to the COVID–19 vaccination rates in nursing homes and makes these data publicly available to better ensure transparency and that the necessary information is available to improve ongoing and future vaccination efforts for nursing home residents and staff.
Source: GAO–21–387, published Mar. 31, 2021.
2. The Secretary of HHS should ensure that the Administrator of CMS, in consultation with the CDC, requires nursing homes to offer COVID–19 vaccinations to residents and staff and design and implement associated quality measures.
Source: GAO–21–387, published Mar. 31, 2021.
3. The Administrator of CMS should quickly develop a plan that further details how the agency intends to respond to and implement, as appropriate, the 27 recommendations in the final report of the Nursing Home Commission, which CMS released on September 16, 2020. Such a plan should include milestones that allow the agency to track and report on the status of each recommendation; identify actions taken and planned, including areas where the CMS determined not to take action; and identify areas where the agency could coordinate with other Federal and nonfederal entities.
Source: GAO–21–191, published Nov. 30, 2020.
4. The Secretary of HHS, in consultation with CMS and CDC, should develop a strategy to capture more complete data on confirmed COVID–19 cases and deaths in nursing homes retroactively back to January 1, 2020, and to clarify the extent to which nursing homes have reported data before May 8, 2020. To the extent feasible, this strategy to capture more complete data should incorporate information nursing homes previously reported to CDC or to State or local public health offices.
Source: GAO–20–701, published Sept. 21, 2020.

Additionally, GAO currently has ongoing work looking at which nursing home characteristics, if any, affect the likelihood that a home experienced a COVID–19 outbreak. If you would like, we would be happy to follow up with your staff to further discuss this issue. We are also aware of ongoing work from HHS OIG that will describe the characteristics of the nursing homes that were hardest hit by the pandemic (OEI–02–20–00490). This work should help provide clarity regarding factors associated with nursing home COVID–19 outbreaks, as studies published to date have had mixed results.

Questions Submitted by Hon. Robert P. Casey, Jr.

Question. To receive Medicare and Medicaid funding, nursing homes must meet minimum Federal quality and safety standards and must also submit annual cost reports. According to the Government Accountability Office (GAO), these "cost reports are the only publicly available source of financial data for many [nursing facilities]." In 2016, GAO found that while the Centers for Medicare and Medicaid Services collects information on nursing home revenue, it is not doing enough to ensure that the information is both accurate and accessible to the public.

In light of the pandemic, and the importance of ensuring that Federal dollars are spent on things like resident care, infection control, and ensuring an adequate workforce, how important is this cost information and what can we do to ensure that it is accurately and adequately reported?

Answer. As the question notes, GAO's 2016 report (GAO–16–700) made two recommendations related to the issue of Skilled Nursing Facility (SNF) expenditure data. Both of these recommendations remain open and have not been implemented by CMS (see below). GAO maintains the importance of making these data more accurate and accessible to the public. While we have not specifically reviewed these issues in the context of the COVID–19 pandemic, in our COVID–19 work we have made similar recommendations that, if implemented, would improve the transparency of nursing home information to the public, including nursing home data on COVID–19 vaccinations of residents and staff.

Recommendation 1: To improve the accessibility and reliability of SNF expenditure data, the Acting Administrator of CMS should take steps to improve the accessibility of SNF expenditure data, making it easier for public stakeholders to locate and use the data.

Status: The agency concurred with this recommendation in 2016 and Stated that it would review the feasibility of increasing the accessibility of this data. However, in August 2017, HHS told GAO that it now believes that the cost of implementing this recommendation would outweigh its benefits. HHS confirmed in July 2019 that its position on this recommendation has not changed. GAO continues to maintain that data on SNFs' relative expenditures should be readily accessible to the public to ensure transparency in SNF expenditures. As of November 2020, HHS officials have not informed us of any actions taken to implement this recommendation.

Recommendation 2: To improve the accessibility and reliability of SNF expenditure data, the Acting Administrator of CMS should take steps to ensure the accuracy and completeness of SNF expenditure data.

Status: CMS did not concur with this recommendation. HHS reported in 2016 that the amount of time and resources to verify the accuracy and completeness of SNF expenditure data could be substantial, without assurance of benefit to the agency and the public. However, during the course of our work, GAO found that CMS uses this expenditure data to update overall SNF payment rates, in addition to using it for more general purposes. Without taking steps to ensure the accuracy and completeness of expenditure data, CMS risks developing SNF payments rates that are based on unreliable data. As of November 2020, HHS officials have not informed us of any actions taken to implement this recommendation.

Prepared Statement of David Gifford, M.D., MPH, Chief Medical Officer, American Health Care Association/National Center for Assisted Living

Chairman Wyden, Ranking Member Crapo, and distinguished members of the Senate Finance Committee, thank you for making nursing homes and long-term care (LTC) providers a priority as you examine how COVID–19 has impacted the Nation. The American Health Care Association and the National Center for Assisted Living (AHCA/NCAL) appreciates the opportunity to share our perspective regarding caring for seniors in nursing homes amid the current COVID–19 crisis.

AHCA/NCAL represents more than 14,000 non-profit and proprietary nursing homes, assisted living communities, and homes for individuals with intellectual and developmental disabilities. The 2.5 million Americans served in LTC facilities every day are some of the most threatened by the SARS–coV–2 coronavirus (COVID–19).

LTC facilities (including nursing homes and other congregate facilities for older adults) have been considered the epicenter of the pandemic. As a geriatrician and the chief medical officer for AHCA/NCAL, I can attest that COVID–19 is the greatest tragedy to impact our residents and their families. Over 635,000 nursing home residents have been infected and more than 130,000 have died.[152] This virus has also affected health care workers, with over half-a-million nursing home staff becoming infected and over 1,600 having succumbed to the virus to-date.[153]

In addition, the pandemic has taken an emotional and physical toll on residents, patients and staff. For nearly a year, family members were unable to visit. Residents could not leave their rooms. They could not see the smiles of the nurses and aides caring for them, hidden behind masks. Our dedicated staff members did everything they could to keep residents safe, engaged, and happy. But at the same time, they constantly worried about becoming ill and/or infectingtheir loved ones at home or their residents. Undoubtedly, this virus will leave psychological scars for many that will last a lifetime.

It is critical that we figure out what happened, why it happened, and what we can do to keep it from ever happening again.

The Nature of the Virus

Nursing home residents are at the highest risk for complications due to COVID–19. More than half are over the age 85 and suffer from multiple chronic diseases, including dementia. According to the Centers for Disease Control and Prevention (CDC), compared to younger individuals, the risk of COVID–19 infections among the age group of our residents is two times higher, but the risk of hospitalization is 80 times higher, and the risk of death is 7,900 times higher.[154]

---

[152] CDC Nursing Home COVID–19 Data Dashboard. Accessed on March 13, 2021 at *https://www.cdc.gov/nhsn/covid19/ltc-report-overview.html*.

[153] CDC Nursing Home COVID–19 Data Dashboard. Accessible at *https://www.cdc.gov/nhsn/covid19/ltc-report-overview.html*.

[154] CDC Risk for COVID–19 Infection, Hospitalization, and Death By Age Group. Updated February 18, 2021. Accessed on March 13, 2021 at *https://www.cdc.gov/coronavirus/2019-ncov/covid-data/investigations-discovery/hospitalization-death-by-age.html*.

Nursing home residents experienced a 20-percent mortality rate with COVID– 19—the highest of any other infection or disease we have ever faced. A similarly high rate of infection and death was seen around the world among older adults living in LTC facilities. Researchers tracking COVID–19 data in the United States[155] and world-wide[156] consistently found that LTC residents made up a small percentage of total cases yet were a disproportionate share of each country's deaths in 2020.

It is important to understand the nursing home setting. Residents depend on our nurses, aides, housekeepers, dietary staff and therapists to help them with daily activities like eating, getting dressed and bathing, and this care assistance often requires very close contact for prolonged periods. Social distancing was not an option in long-term care.

As we now know, COVID–19 does not act like most respiratory viruses. It commonly spreads through asymptomatic and pre-symptomatic carriers,[157] making it extremely difficult for providers to prevent its entry and spread in LTC facilities. The incubation period for the virus is longer than most viruses (up to 14 days). The length of a person's infectious period (i.e., the ability to spread to others) is also longer than typical respiratory viruses (up to 10 days). Worst of all, it was found to have an airborne component of spread.[158] All these characteristics were not known early on during the pandemic. As a result, many early recommendations from public health officials were incorrect and therefore, ineffective at preventing spread.

Changing and Conflicting Government Guidance

The Centers for Medicare and Medicaid Services (CMS) and the CDC tried to keep pace with the evolving information about COVID–19, issuing numerous requirements and guidance to nursing homes at an unprecedented speed. Since the implementation of the public health emergency,

CMS and CDC combined have released 55 major new requirements or guidance to nursing homes in the areas of infection control, testing and the use of personal protective equipment (PPE), or on average, at least one per week. (This does not count the frequent minor updates or modifications to guidance, nor all the Medicare and Medicaid payment changes. Additionally, it does not include all the CMS guidance related to 1135 waivers, the Five-Star rating system, and survey frequency. There was also myriad guidance from other agencies, such as the Department of Labor and the Occupational Health and Safety Administration.)

In addition, many States issued orders and recommendations, which often conflicted with other States or Federal guidance. This ever evolving and conflicting guidance, scattered across

---

155 Kaiser Family Foundation. COVID–19: Long-term Care Facilities. Accessed on March 13, 2021 at CDC, Risk for COVID–19 Infection, Hospitalization, and Death By Age Group. Updated February 18, 2021. Accessible at *https://www.cdc.gov/coronavirus/2019-ncov/covid-data/investigations-discovery/hospitalization-death-by-age.html*.

156 Mathews A.W., Douglas J., Kamp J., and Yoon D. COVID–19 Stalked Nursing Homes Around the World. *Wall Street Journal.* Published online on December 31, 2020. Accessed at *https://www.wsj.com/articles/covid-19-stalked-nursing-homes-around-the-world-11609436215.*

157 Johansson M.A., Quandelacy T.M., Kada S., et al. SARS–CoV–2 Transmission From People Without COVID–19 Symptoms. *JAMA Network Open.* 2021;4(1):e2035057; doi:10.1001/jamanetworkopen.2020.35057.

158 CDC Science Brief: SARS–CoV–2 and Potential Airborne Transmission, updated Oct. 5, 2020, accessible at *https://www.cdc.gov/coronavirus/2019-ncov/more/scientific-brief-sars-cov-2.html.*

multiple websites and hundreds of pages, made it nearly impossible for providers to follow consistent best practices to mitigate the spread of the virus.

Even though public health officials constantly churned out new guidance, it was often too late and outdated by the time it was issued. The timing of some of the major recommendations made by CMS and CDC are depicted in the attached timeline (see last page) relative to the number of cases and deaths in nursing homes. Early on, the public health recommendations focused on a symptoms-based approach. CMS required that staff be screened for symptoms and asked staff to stay home if they had any one symptom suggestive of COVID–19. However, screening only for symptoms meant missing asymptomatic staff who could unwittingly spread the virus in the facility. Masks were not recommended for use by all staff throughout the facility until almost 4 months into the pandemic in late June. This allowed the virus to spread amongst staff members outside of designated COVID patient care areas. Early on and without adequate testing available, residents were cohorted based on symptoms, which sometimes resulted in asymptomatic or pre-symptomatic residents spreading the virus in what were believed to be COVID-free units or rooms.

Lack of Testing

Nursing home providers found it challenging to access affordable, reliable, and timely tests until many months into the pandemic. Due to the country's limited testing capabilities in beginning, LTC residents were not made a priority for testing. Even when they were made a priority by the CDC at the end of April, it was only for residents and staff with symptoms, and tests were rarely available. When they were available, it often took 5 days or more to receive the results. Testing kits and supplies were not sent to nursing homes until August. Routine surveillance testing was not required until September, six months after the start of the pandemic.

The lack of adequate and timely testing impaired the ability of providers to keep the virus at bay, as asymptomatic and pre-symptomatic spread could continue undetected. Even when testing kits became available in the fall of 2020, the initial lack of guidance and then changing guidance on how to interpret test results between the polymerase chain reaction (PCR) and antigen tests further compounded the effectiveness of testing to prevent spread.

Personal Protective Equipment Shortages

Despite caring for the most vulnerable population when it comes to COVID–19, LTC facilities were not made a priority for necessary equipment. Even after numerous calls for help,[159] it took months for LTC residents and staff to be made the highest priority for PPE. Worldwide supply chain issues left providers scrambling to find and purchase quality PPE, such as N95 masks, gowns, and gloves. Many suppliers delayed or limited the size of providers' orders, and many providers got taken by scammers pretending to have legitimate PPE. In addition, prices soared.

In many circumstances, staff had to use their ingenuity to make their own masks, gowns and face shields. I recall getting calls one night asking which type of material would be best for

[159] COVID–19 Timeline, accessible at *https://saveourseniors.org/timeline/;* accessed on March 13, 2021.

masks, and on a weekend asking if rain ponchos work better as gowns than trash bags. Academic research found that this lack of PPE was correlated with more cases and deaths in nursing homes reporting PPE shortages.[160]

In May, the Federal Emergency Management Agency (FEMA) organized two shipments of PPE supplies that would each cover the needs of a nursing home for one week.[161] The first shipment arrived in mid-May to early June, and the second shipment in July. These two shipments were an amazing logistical feat but did not start until 10–12 weeks into the pandemic. Also, they did not contain any N95 masks given the continued worldwide shortages. For many, the PPE was welcomed and life-saving, but there were several shipments that included PPE that either could not be used,[162,163] was past its expiration date, or did not meet CDC or CMS standards.[164] In one case a provider relayed to me, CMS inspectors would not use the PPE when offered to them during their on-site infection control inspection.

The Impact of Community Spread

Due to the nature of how COVID–19 spreads, the lack of PPE and testing, and ever shifting guidance, it is not surprising that the principal factor leading to COVID–19 outbreaks in nursing homes has been repeatedly shown to be related to the amount of spread in the surrounding community. Even the best nursing homes with the most rigorous infection control practices could not stop this highly contagious, invisible enemy.[165] Academic experts at Harvard University,[166] Brown University[167] and the University of Chicago[168,169] all found that the primary predictor of a nursing home experiencing an outbreak is the prevalence of COVID–19 in the surrounding community. Other factors that predicted outbreaks related to increased

---

160 McGarry B.E., Grabowski D.C., Barnett M.L. Severe Staffing and Personal Protective Equipment Shortages Faced By Nursing Homes During the COVID–19 Pandemic. *Health Affairs* (Millwood). 2020 Oct;39(10):1812–1821; doi: 10.1377/hlthaff.2020.01269. Epub 2020 Aug 20. PMID: 32816600.

161 FEMA press release. "Coronavirus pandemic response: PPE packages for Nursing Homes," released May 2, 2020. Accessed on March 14, 2021 at *https://www.fema.gov/fact-sheet/coronavirus-pandemic-response-ppe-packages-nursing-homes.*

162 Joran Rau. "Federal Help Falters as Nursing Homes Run Short of Protective Equipment." Kaiser Health News, posted June 11, 2020; accessible at *https://khn.org/news/federal-help-falters-as-nursing-homes-run-short-of-protective-equipment/.*

163 Priscilla Alvarez and Daniella Diaz. "Nursing homes receive defective equipment as part of Trump administration supply initiative." *CNN Politics*, updated Thursday June 11, 2020; accessible at *https://www.cnn.com/2020/06/10/politics/nursing-homes-ppe-defective-equipment-fema/index.html.*

164 Katie Smith Sloan, CEO of LeadingAge, Letter to Vice President on June 11, 2020; accessible at *https://www.leadingage.org/sites/default/files/LeadingAge%20Pence%20Letter%20611 20_final.pdf.*

165 Opinion by David C. Grabowski, R. Tamara Konetzka, and Vincent Mor. Opinion: We can't protect nursing homes from COVID–19 without protecting everyone. *Washington Post.* Published June 25, 2020; available at *https://www.washingtonpost.com/opinions/2020/06/25/we-cantprotect-nursing-homes-covid-19-without-protecting-everyone/.*

166 Abrams H.R., Loomer L., Gandhi A., Grabowski D.C. Characteristics of U.S. Nursing Homes With COVID–19 Cases. *J Am Geriatr Soc.* 2020 Aug;68(8):1653–1656; doi: 10.1111/jgs.16661. Epub 2020 Jul 7.

167 White E.M., Kosar C.M., Feifer R.A., Blackman C., et al. Variation in SARS–CoV–2 Prevalence in U.S. Skilled Nursing Facilities. *J Am Geriatr Soc.* 2020 Oct;68(10):2167–2173; doi: 10.1111/jgs.16752. Epub 2020 Aug 21. PMID: 32674223 PMCID: PMC7404330 DOI: 10.1111/jgs.16752.

168 Konetzka R.T., Gorges R.J. Nothing Much Has Changed: COVID–19 Nursing Home Cases and Deaths Follow Fall Surges. *J Am Geriatr Soc.* 2021 Jan;69(1):46–47; doi: 10.1111/jgs.16951. Epub 2020 Nov 20.

169 Gorges R.J., Konetzka R.T. Factors Associated With Racial Differences in Deaths Among Nursing Home Residents With COVID–19 Infection in the U.S. *JAMA Network Open.* 2021 Feb 1;4(2):e2037431; doi: 10.1001/jamanetworkopen.2020.37431. PMID: 33566110.

human-to-human interaction, which clearly increases the chance the virus can spread. These factors meant larger facilities, especially those in urban areas where there is higher proportion of minority residents, were more likely to experience outbreaks.

The same academic researchers could not find an association with COVID–19 outbreaks and other characteristics, such as the facility's Five-Star Rating on Nursing Home Compare; whether the facility had a prior violation related to infection control; or whether it was for-profit, part of a chain, or had a high Medicaid census. This relationship of COVID–19 cases in nursing homes mirroring the prevalence in the community continued through the fall based on analyses by the Kaiser Family Foundation[170] and CDC.[171]

With hindsight it is easy to criticize public officials and health care providers for failures during the pandemic. This is unfair, given the lack of knowledge about this virus. However, what was evident was that the LTC community was left behind, forgotten, or even blamed. This further demoralized our health care heroes in LTC who were giving their all and risking their lives as well as their family members' lives but received inadequate support.

It is critical that we figure out what we can do to prevent such tragedy from ever happening again. But in order to move forward, we must also reflect on the long-standing challenges within the LTC profession that COVID–19 exposed and exacerbated. Providers acknowledge that we can and need to do better to meet the needs of our Nation's seniors—continuous quality improvement is part of who we are.

Let me take a moment to highlight several historical challenges facing long term care that the pandemic further exposed. These include staffing, health care disparities, infection control, and reimbursement.

Workforce Crisis

Long-term care was already dealing with a workforce shortage prior to COVID, and the pandemic has only magnified the crisis due to staff members getting sick, having to isolate, or a lack of childcare options. At the same time, the pandemic required numerous new tasks (e.g., screening all personnel upon entry, reporting cases daily, serving meals in rooms, donning PPE for every resident) and more one-on-one care to help prevent spread, all requiring more staff. We commonly heard the phrase "all-hands-on deck" to help meet the residents' needs and new recommendations and guidance.

During the pandemic, AHCA/NCAL urged governors to help address the workforce shortage by outlining strategies in a roadmap for States in May 2020.[172] We also developed free online courses to help train temporary caregivers (nurse aides and feeding assistants) to help fill the gap the pandemic created. Additionally, AHCA/NCAL urged Congress and the administration to direct financial aid to long term care facilities, so that providers could use those resources to respond to the crisis, including by hiring more staff and offering hero pay.

---

[170] Priya Chidambaram and Rachel Garfield. Patterns in COVID–19 Cases and Deaths in Long-Term Care Facilities in 2020. Kaiser Family Foundation. Coronavirus. Published: January 14, 2021; *https://www.kff.org/coronavirus-covid-19/issue-brief/patterns-in-covid-19-cases-and-deaths-in-long-term-care-facilities-in-2020/.*

[171] Bagchi S., Mak J., Li Q., et al. Rates of COVID–19 Among Residents and Staff Members in Nursing Homes—United States, May 25–November 22, 2020. *MMWR Morb Mortal Wkly Rep* 2021;70:52–55; doi: *http://dx.doi.org/10.15585/mmwr.mm7002e2.*

[172] AHCA/NCAL Long Term Care Workforce Roadmap for Governors and States; *https://www.ahcancal.org/Survey-Regulatory-Legal/Emergency-Preparedness/Documents/COVID19/AHCANCAL-Workforce-Roadmap.pdf.*

In a survey of nursing home providers conducted in November 2020, 70 percent of nursing homes had hired additional staff and nine out of 10 asked staff to work overtime and provided hero pay.[173]

We need ongoing staff support as this pandemic continues, but we also need a more long-term solution. AHCA/NCAL has been highlighting this workforce crisis for years, including testifying to Congress twice in 2019. It is time that we address this. We need a comprehensive strategy to recruit more health care heroes to serve in long-term care.

Infection Control

As described earlier, prior infection citations have not been shown to be associated with COVID–19 outbreaks or cases. However, nursing homes have been cited for infection control practices historically.[174] These trends led CMS to issue an extensive set of new regulations in November 2016 phased in over 3 years, including the requirement for a designated infection preventionist in every nursing home starting in November 2019.[175] These new requirements and regulations were just taking effect when the pandemic hit.

Unfortunately, many infection preventionists became ill or had to isolate following exposure or presenting with symptoms. This highlighted the importance of having the infection preventionist position met not by a single person but adjusted based on the size and needs of the facility. A large nursing home with 300 residents has different infection control demands than a small, rural nursing home with 20 residents. AHCA supported the infection preventionist regulations and developed a certification program to train over 3,000 infection preventionists before they went into effect. However, the nursing shortage continues to make it challenging to identify infection preventionists, as many are hired away by hospitals. To meet the need for infection preventionists, we need help with recruiting and retaining registered nurses (RNs) to serve in this role.

Disparities in Care

The pandemic has disproportionately impacted minority populations more than others. This has been no different in nursing homes.[176,177] The disparities in care outcomes were known prior to

---

[173] AHCA Survey State of the Nursing Home Industry; *https://www.ahcancal.org/News-and-Communications/Fact-Sheets/FactSheets/State-of-Nursing-Home-Industry_Dec2020.pdf.*

[174] GAO. Infection Control Deficiencies Were Widespread and Persistent in Nursing Homes Prior to COVID–19 Pandemic. GAO–20–576R. Published: May 20, 2020. Publicly Released: May 20, 2020; *https://www.gao.gov/products/gao-20-576r.*

[175] Medicare and Medicaid Programs: Reform of Requirements for Long-Term Care Facilities. A Rule by the Centers for Medicare and Medicaid Services on 10/04/2016 published in Federal Register; available at *https://www.federalregister.gov/documents/2016/10/04/2016-23503/medicare-and-medicaid-programs-reform-of-requirements-for-long-term-care-facilities.*

[176] Gorges R.J., Konetzka R.T. Factors Associated With Racial Differences in Deaths Among Nursing Home Residents With COVID–19 Infection in the U.S. *JAMA Network Open.* 2021 Feb 1;4(2):e2037431; doi: 10.1001/jamanetworkopen.2020.37431. PMID: 33566110.

[177] Li Y., Cen X., Cai X., Temkin-Greener H. Racial and Ethnic Disparities in COVID–19 Infections and Deaths Across U.S. Nursing Homes. *J Am Geriatr Soc.* 2020 Nov;68(11):2454-2461; doi: 10.1111/jgs.16847. Epub 2020 Sep 28.

COVID.[178] Academic experts who have analyzed the differences in outcomes among African American and Latino residents in long-term care find the disparities to be related to both the overall quality of the facility and the Medicaid reimbursement challenges.[179,180] This has led several academic and policy experts to call for more resources and changes to Medicaid to address these disparities.[181,182] As a country, we need to step up and make sure that minority populations have equitable health-care coverage and supports, including in long-term care. This in part, means properly funding health-care programs like Medicaid, so that long-term care providers who care for people of color have the staffing and other resources needed to meet their residents' needs.

Financial Crisis

Prior to the COVID–19 pandemic, Medicaid underfunding plagued nursing homes for years. More than 60 percent of all nursing home residents rely on Medicaid to cover their daily care. However, Medicaid reimbursements only cover 70 to 80 percent of the actual cost of care in a nursing home. The intense needs of our residents require dedicated staff to provide hands-on care and consequently, labor makes up an enormous proportion of everyday expenses (roughly 70 percent). The chronic Medicaid underfunding makes it challenging for providers to offer competitive wages and benefits and make other investments in their workforce.

Over the last year, long-term care facilities have faced skyrocketing costs. Providers have dedicated extensive resources to fighting COVID–19. The costs associated with routine testing, PPE, and staffing have pushed many facilities to the brink. The Provider Relief Fund created by Congress has been a lifeline, allowing nursing homes to stay open and providers to purchase resources to protect their residents and staff. However, nursing homes only received approximately $13 billion from the Provider Relief Fund, or roughly 7 percent of the fund's total. This is less than half of what nursing homes spent on PPE and additional staffing alone in 2020 ($30 billion), and these additional costs are expected to continue in 2021 as the pandemic lingers.

In addition, revenue has significantly declined due to fewer patients coming from the hospital as well as fewer potential residents seeking long term care. Nationally, nursing home occupancy significantly dropped from 80.2 percent in January 2020 to 68.2 percent in March 2021.[183] This has resulted in $11.3 billion in losses to nursing homes in 2020 and is projected

[178] Mack D.S., Jesdale B.M., Ulbricht C.M., Forrester S.N., Michener P.S., Lapane K.L. Racial Segregation Across U.S. Nursing Homes: A Systematic Review of Measurement and Outcomes. *Gerontologist.* 2020 Apr 2;60(3):e218–e231; doi: 10.1093/geront/gnz056. PMID: 31141135.

[179] Campbell L.J., Cai X., Gao S., Li Y. Racial/Ethnic Disparities in Nursing Home Quality of Life Deficiencies, 2001 to 2011. *Gerontol Geriatr Med.* 2016 Jun 6;2:2333721416653561; doi: 10.1177/2333721416653561. eCollection 2016 Jan–Dec. PMID: 27819015.

[180] Barton Smith D., Feng Z., Fennell M.L., et al. Separate and unequal: Racial segregation and disparities in quality across U.S. nursing homes. *Health Aff* (Millwood). Sep–Oct 2007;26(5):1448–58; doi: 10.1377/hlthaff.26.5.1448. PMID: 17848457 DOI: 10.1377/hlthaff.26.5.1448.

[181] *Ibid* #27.

[182] Grabowski D.C. Strengthening Nursing Home Policy for the Postpandemic World: How Can We Improve Residents' Health Outcomes and Experiences? Commonwealth Fund; issue briefs August 20, 2020; *https://www.commonwealthfund.org/publications/issue-briefs/2020/aug/strengthening-nursing-home-policy-postpandemic-world.*

[183] AHCA analysis of CDC NHSN data; accessible at *https://www.ahcancal.org/Data-and-Research/Pages/default.aspx;* downloaded on March 14, 2021.

to increase in 2021 to $22.6 billion. AHCA/NCAL did an extensive analysis estimating nursing home financials and found that in combining anticipated COVID costs and projected losses, the industry expects to lose $94 billion over a 2-year period (2020–2021).[184]

Today, thousands of LTC facilities are on the verge of collapse, with more 1,600 nursing homes in danger of closing their doors this year. This has real consequences for residents and their families. Again, most residents are older adults living with multiple underlying health conditions, and they require a high-level of specialized care. Closures leave residents displaced from their long-standing communities and loved ones. Closures also reduce options for quality care, especially in rural areas.

In order to protect access to long-term care for vulnerable seniors and improve staffing issues, Medicaid reimbursement needs to be reformed as numerous academic experts have advised.[185,186,187] Medicaid reimbursement rates must catch up with the cost of care. Nursing homes need adequate funding and resources in order to provide quality care. We urge policy-makers and stakeholders to work toward long-term solutions that tackle this systemic issue.

How We Move Forward: The Care for Our Seniors Act

The pandemic has led the nursing home sector to reflect what can be done to prevent such tragedy from ever happening again and how to address longstanding challenges COVID–19 exposed. After reviewing the evidence, expert recommendations, and the Commission for Safety and Quality in Nursing Homes report,[188] AHCA and LeadingAge announced the Care for Our Seniors Act.[189] This is a comprehensive plan aimed at offering solutions that will improve the quality of care in our Nation's nursing homes as we begin to look towards a post COVID–19 environment. This plan recommends policies and steps to improve clinical care, strengthen and support our workforce, improve oversight, and modernize our physical structures. Specifically, we are supporting:

Clinical—Enhance Quality Care

- 24-hour R.N.: We support a new Federal requirement that each nursing home have an R.N. on staff 24 hours a day and provide recommendations on how to effectively implement this requirement.

---

[184] AHCA Issue Brief: Protect Access to Long Term Care for Vulnerable Residents; *https://d3dkdvqff0zqx.cloudfront.net/groups/ahca/attachments/protect%20access%20to%20long%20 term%20care_ib.pdf.*

[185] Grabowski D.C., Mor V. Nursing Home Care in Crisis in the Wake of COVID–19. *JAMA.* 2020 Jul 7;324(1):23–24; doi: 10.1001/jama.2020.8524. PMID: 32442303 DOI: 10.1001/jama.2020.8524.

[186] Grabowski D.C. Strengthening Nursing Home Policy for the Postpandemic World: How Can We Improve Residents' Health Outcomes and Experiences? Commonwealth Fund; issue briefs August 20, 2020; *https://www.commonwealthfund.org/publications/issue-briefs/2020/aug/strengthening-nursing-home-policy-postpandemic-world.*

[187] R. Tamara Konetzka, Caring for Seniors Amid the COVID–19 Crisis. Testimony Before the United States Senate Special Committee on Aging. May 21, 2020; accessible at *https://www.aging.senate.gov/imo/media/doc/SCA_Konetzka_05_21_20.pdf.*

[188] Independent Nursing Home COVID–19 Commission Findings Validate Unprecedented Federal Response. Issued on September 16, 2020; available at *https://www.cms.gov/newsroom/press-releases/independent-nursing-home-covid-19-commission-findings-validate-unprecedented-federal-response.*

[189] AHCA and Leading Age's Care For Our Seniors Act; available at *www.ahcancal.org/solutions.*

- Enhanced infection preventionist: We will help establish an updated guideline for staffing infection preventionists in each nursing home based on proven, successful strategies. This includes proper funding and workforce availability to effectively implement meaningful, sustained changes.
- Minimum 30-day supply of PPE: We support efforts to require a minimum supply of PPE in nursing homes, which will be supported by ongoing Federal/State stockpiles with PPE that is acceptable for health-care use.

Workforce—Strengthen and Support Front-line Caregivers:

- Recruit and retain more long-term care workers: We support implementing a multi-phase tiered approach leveraging Federal, State, and academic entities. This includes loan forgiveness for new graduates who work in LTC, tax credits for licensed LTC professionals, programs for affordable housing and childcare assistance, and increased subsidies to professionals' schools whose graduates work in nursing homes for at least 5 years.

Oversight—Improve Systems to Be More Resident-Driven

- Survey improvements for better resident care: We support development of an effective oversight system and processes that promote improved care and protect residents, consistent with CMS standards.
- Chronic poor-performing nursing facilities: The survey system needs a process to help turn chronic poor-performing facilities around or close the facility. We are proposing a five-step process to address such facilities.
- Publicly report customer satisfaction: Nursing homes are the only health-care setting in which CMS collects and publicly reports quality data that does not include customer satisfaction. We recommend adding this measure to the government's Five-Star rating system to help monitor the quality of a nursing home for family members and guide consumer choice.

Structural—Modernize for Resident Dignity and Safety

- Shift to private rooms: The average nursing home is around 40 to 50 years old. The traditional care models are no longer considered appropriate to provide person-centered care. One central aspect of this shift is a greater emphasis on autonomy, dignity and privacy. Private rooms also support infection control best practices. We support the development of a national study producing data on conversion costs and a recommended approach to make this shift.

Long-lasting transformation that will protect our residents requires a considerable investment in the LTC profession. As a health-care provider that relies almost entirely on government reimbursement (Medicare and Medicaid), nursing homes cannot make substantial reforms on their own. They need the support of Federal and State policy-makers and resources.

Conclusion

Long-term care providers welcome a national discussion regarding how we can improve in light of the COVID–19 pandemic. We urge the Senators of this committee and the entire Congress to recognize the nature of this virus and that we need a collaborative approach to address longstanding challenges in our Nation's nursing homes.

Focusing solely on regulations fails to recognize the cause of this crisis, nor does it help solve it. The reality is that many of these outbreaks have occurred because nursing homes were located in communities with high rates of spread and because long-term care residents and staff were not prioritized by public health officials, leaving providers scrambling for testing, PPE, and staffing resources. Just like hospitals, we called for help from the very beginning. But unlike hospitals, our calls often went unanswered or came too late. In our case, it has been difficult to get anyone to listen. Prioritizing long-term care facilities in emergency situations is key, as we have seen in other emergencies, such as natural disasters.

Despite a year of tragedy, a virus that will linger well into the future, and historic challenges within long-term care, I remain optimistic. We have three remarkably safe and effective vaccines. Nursing home residents and staff were made a priority to receive the vaccine by the CDC and the vast majority of Governors. As a result, nursing home cases and deaths have declined dramatically since mid-December and faster than the general population. This has allowed CDC and CMS to update guidance to allow more in-person visitations. We are elated to see families and residents reunited. Making our nursing homes a top priority for the vaccine demonstrates the power of putting long-term care and our Nation's seniors first.

I want to end by saying that our hearts go out to the residents and their family members who have suffered through the past year, separated from each other—in some cases forever. Our thoughts also go to the long-term caregivers who have given their all this past year, often without the recognition they deserve.

I have spoken with providers, families and other stakeholders who all agree that the health-care system needs to be better aligned to achieve the outcomes we all want. If any good can come out of the pandemic, we are hopeful that it can serve as the catalyst needed to institute meaningful change.

On behalf of the residents, their families and the staff in nursing homes across the country, thank you for your dedication and leadership to tackle the long-term care needs of our seniors and individuals with disabilities. Your ongoing help and support mean more now than ever before. Ensuring that essential and necessary resources are provided to long-term care providers is critical to protecting our Nation's most vulnerable. We look forward to having constructive discussions on solutions with you to combat COVID–19 and usher in a stronger long-term care system.

Timeline: COVID–19 and Nursing Homes

Despite repeated calls for help, nursing homes did not receive resources or priority for months. Even then, the high amount of spread in surrounding communities made it impossible for nursing homes to prevent the virus from entering their facilities. This timeline identities major regulatory, policy and resource supports skilled nursing facilities (SNFs) received during the pandemic, as compared to the timing of cases and deaths.

The Federal Government began collecting and reporting nursing home cases and deaths in May 2020. Since the implementation of the public health emergency, CMS and CDC combined have released 55 (or on average at least one per week) major new requirements or guidance in areas of infection control, testing and PPE use. This does not count minor guidance updates or modifications nor payment changes.

Questions Submitted for the Record to David Gifford, M.D., MPH

Questions Submitted by Hon. Ron Wyden

Question. The Centers for Medicare and Medicaid Services (CMS) issued an interim final rule last year that required nursing homes to report COVID–19 data to the Centers for Disease Control and Prevention on a weekly basis beginning May 17, 2020. These data included COVID–19 infections, COVID–19 deaths, and the availability of key equipment and workers at individual nursing homes. The data have proved to be helpful for the public, policy-makers, and industry stakeholders to track the pandemic, and related issues, in these care settings. However, to date, CMS has *not* required nursing homes to provide such data prior to May 8, 2020, despite calls from Senate Democrats to do so. In September 2020, the Government Accountability Office (GAO) noted that "by not requiring nursing homes to submit data from the first 4 months of 2020, HHS is limiting the usefulness of the data in helping to understand the effects of COVID–19 in nursing homes." GAO went on to recommend that "HHS, in consultation with CMS and CDC, develop a strategy to capture more complete data on COVID–19 cases and deaths in nursing homes retroactively back to January 1, 2020."

Do you support GAO's recommendation? Why or why not? Please briefly explain.

Answer. COVID–19 cases among resident and staff were reported by nursing homes to State or local public health agencies since the beginning of the pandemic. As pointed out by the GAO, these data systems did not readily communicate with CDC or integrate to create a national database. As a result, CMS issued an interim final rule mandating all Medicare or Medicaid certified nursing homes to submit case counts on a weekly basis to the CDC's National Healthcare Safety Network (NHSN) system starting in May 2020. This resulted in duplicate reporting requirements for nursing homes all because State and Federal systems could not communicate effectively.

We support States making the data they have on COVID–19 case counts prior to May 2020 available to the CDC or other Federal agencies for research purposes to learn about the pandemic and how to better combat the spread of COVID–19. We are not supportive of asking providers to go back through their medical records to identify cases and provide data they have already provided solely because State and Federal systems are not integrated. This would take an extensive amount of time and resources away from resident care, shifting the burden of data collection onto providers at a time staff are already stretched thin due ongoing workforce challenges and the pressures of the pandemic.

A lesson that should be addressed from this pandemic has been that State and Federal public health data systems are underfunded, underdeveloped and undermaintained. The public health infrastructure needs more Federal funding to modernize their data systems and make sure they are integrated. We are currently experiencing the same problem with State immunization registries. They do not integrate with Federal data systems and long-term care

(LTC) pharmacies and providers are having to enter duplicate immunization data in State immunization registries and CDC Federal registries. This is not a good use of health-care staff's time. They should be devoted to making sure residents and staff receive the vaccine and monitoring their reaction, not entering the same data into multiple systems because the States and Federal Governments are not collaborating cohesively.

Question. A recent paper published by the National Bureau of Economic Research noted that people who receive treatment in nursing homes owned by private equity firms have worse health outcomes than those living in facilities under other ownership structures.[190] This paper adds evidence to reports of worse outcomes associated with private equity's investment in the nursing home industry. Nursing homes have also become popular investments for real estate investment trusts (REITs), which often lease back properties to private equity firms or other related parties. The involvement of private equity in the nursing home industry has been of interest to the Finance Committee for more than a decade, and the role of private equity and for-profit ownership in the nursing home industry was raised in testimony and questions at the hearing. Several reports from Federal agencies have suggested the need for more thorough information on facility ownership.[191,192]

Please provide a list of all private equity firms and real estate investment trusts (REIT) that are currently members of AHCA, or have been within the last 5 years. In your response, please include instances in which a subsidiary (or an otherwise related party) of a private equity firm or REIT—e.g., a nursing home chain owned by a private equity company, or that leases a large portion of its facilities from a REIT—is an AHCA member, noting the parent company, controlling entity, or related party.

Answer. AHCA does not collect information from our members nor have access to CMS's Medicare Provider Enrollment, Chain, and Ownership System (PECOS) data on private equity, REIT or controlling party involvement with nursing homes or "chain-owned" nursing homes.

Question. Section 6101 of the Affordable Care Act (ACA) sought to increase ownership transparency within the industry, but to date, the provision has not been fully implemented or enforced by the Centers for Medicare and Medicaid Services. Does AHCA support the full implementation of section 6101?

Answer. AHCA's background and position on section 6101 of the ACA is outlined in our policy memo available at *https://www.ohca.org/uploads/old/ppac_disclosure_of_ownership.pdf.* However, clarity on definitions and using existing reporting requirements need to be taken into consideration so that duplicative reporting is not required. CMS did implement transparency reporting requirements in 2011, which nursing homes comply with (see: *https://www.cms.gov/Medicare-Medicaid-Coordination/Fraud-Prevention/Medicaid-Integrity-Education/Downloads/ebulletins-providerenrollment-disclosureownership.pdf*). We are supporttive of making this information more easily accessible than CMS and many States currently offer.

---

[190] *https://www.nber.org/papers/w28474.*

[191] *https://oig.hhs.gov/oei/reports/oei-04-11-00591.pdf.*

[192] *https://www.gao.gov/assets/gao-10-710.pdf.*

Question. Beyond the provisions of section 6101, does AHCA support additional transparency into nursing home ownership, financial arrangements, use of government funds, and worker pay?

Answer. AHCA is supportive of transparency on ownership. We believe much of the transparency data that many members of the public, policy-makers and the media are asking for are currently collected. We should use the existing data before mandating additional and potentially unnecessary data collection efforts.

Also, we believe the most important issue for residents and their families is transparency on the quality of the care being provided, regardless of ownership. Proper resources should be devoted to assuring that nursing home residents' care is met, which should be reflected in transparency of quality outcomes. Creating additional reporting and bureaucracy that diverts resources away from resident care is not helpful.

Question. COVID–19's toll on nursing homes has not been limited to viral infections. Residents have suffered mentally and physically, and had less access to family members and patient advocates. On March 10, 2021, the Centers for Medicare and Medicaid Services issued new guidance that allows for residents to more easily receive visitors. On the same day, the Centers for Disease Control and Prevention issued Updated Healthcare Infection Prevention and Control Recommendations in Response to COVID–19, which stated "quarantine is no longer recommended for residents who are being admitted to a post-acute care facility if they are fully vaccinated and have not had prolonged close contact with someone with SARS–coV–2 infection in the prior 14 days." The committee has received written testimony for this hearing from medical experts raising concerns that the new guidance may be overly permissive, and could put nursing home residents in danger, particularly if COVID–19 variants breakthrough vaccine protections. On the other hand, some advocates have called for more permissive visitation guidelines.

As a trained physician, do you have any concerns about the guidance that was issued?

Answer. As with all medical care decisions, there are risks and benefits to each decision, medication, test or procedure ordered for a patient. One needs to balance the risks and benefits, which may not be interpreted the same between two different individuals with the same situation. In the case of allowing or not allowing visitations, we have faced this same dilemma. Allowing visitors could increase the chances of viral spread, but not allowing visitors increases the risk of isolation and decline in residents. The new guidance we believe takes the risks and benefits into consideration. As with each new guidance, there remains unanswered questions about how to apply the guidance to specific situations. Nursing homes have demonstrated good faith efforts to implement each new guidance but will need clarity from time to time from CDC. Getting that clarity or not taking into consideration good faith efforts to adoption new guidance has been a frustration we have heard over and over again from providers.

Question. Do nursing homes and long-term care facilities need additional guidance to properly dial visitation?

Answer. As we learn more about how the virus spreads, how effective preventive measures are as well as the effectiveness of being vaccinated, we need CMS and CDC to update their guidance about how residents can participate in communal dinning, activities, travel outside the facility as well as family visitation. In addition, screening and testing procedures currently in place are predicated on what we knew last summer and fall prior to vaccination and variants.

We need CMS and CDC to update guidance on a regular basis but also to provide enough lead time for providers to change their practices. For example, the reopening guidance went into effect immediately. As a result, we had family members showing up at the facility that same day demanding entry when the facility perhaps did not have personal protective equipment (PPE) for visitors or procedures in place to allow safe visitation described in the CMS guidance document.

Question. Preliminary research conducted by Columbia University researchers suggests that the Pfizer and Moderna vaccines were up to 12 times less effective at neutralizing the B.1.351 COVID–19 variant ("South African variant") than earlier strains of the coronavirus.[193] The researchers also found that convalescent plasma was 9 times less effective against the South African variants, leading them to write "[t]aken together, the overall findings are worrisome, particularly in light of recent reports that both Novavax and Johnson & Johnson vaccines showed a substantial drop in efficacy in South Africa."[194] The researchers went on to write, "mutationally, this virus is traveling in a direction that could ultimately lead to escape from our current therapeutic and prophylactic interventions directed to the viral spike. If the rampant spread of the virus continues and more critical mutations accumulate, then we may be condemned to chasing after the evolving SARS–CoV–2 continually, as we have long done for influenza virus."[195] The Centers for Disease Control and Prevention (CDC) has previously found suspected cases of reinfection among nursing home residents who previously tested positive for COVID–19.[196] Similarly, a paper published earlier this year in *The Lancet* suggested that a resurgence in COVID–19 cases in the Brazilian city of Manaus may have been due to a new variant (known as P1 or "Brazilian variant") that "may evade immunity generated in response to previous infections."[197]

Question. The South African and Brazilian variants continue to circulate in the United States.[198] What is your level of concern about the danger that these and other COVID–19 variants may pose to nursing homes, particularly residents who have been most vulnerable to the disease?

Answer. The variants pose a significant concern to both vaccine effectiveness and the current infection control practices. The lack of widespread genetic testing also makes understanding how these viruses are spreading in long term care and if they are more virulent difficult to determine. Funding to State public health laboratories is needed to expand genetic testing and to also evaluate residents who test positive after vaccination. Currently, our

---

193 *https://www.nature.com/articles/s41586-021-03398-2_reference.pdf?utm_medium=affiliate&utm_source=commission_junction&utm_campaign=3_nsn6445_deeplink_PID100024933&utm_ content=deeplink.*

194 *https://www.nature.com/articles/s41586-021-03398-2_reference.pdf?utm_medium=affiliate&utm_source=commission_junction&utm_campaign=3_nsn6445_deeplink_PID100024933&utm_ content=deeplink.*

195 *https://www.nature.com/articles/s41586-021-03398-2_reference.pdf?utm_medium=affiliate&utm_source=commission_junction&utm_campaign=3_nsn6445_deeplink_PID100024933&utm_ content=deeplink.*

196 *https://www.cdc.gov/mmwr/volumes/70/wr/mm7008a3.htm.*

197 *https://www.thelancet.com/article/S0140-6736(21)00183-5/fulltext.*

198 *https://www.cdc.gov/coronavirus/2019-ncov/transmission/variant-cases.html.*

members routinely hear that the vaccines are not 100-percent effective, so we expect to see some residents who are fully vaccinated test positive. There is little evaluation being conducted to determine if these post-vaccination infections are the result of variants or not. Similarly, we do not know if PPE recommendations and source control masks are as effective with this new variant and if the airborne component of spread is more prevalent. Funding to NIH and CDC to support more rapid research is needed.

Question. Is additional surveillance necessary to detect the spread of viral variants? What types of surveillance, if any, should be implemented in regards to the nursing home industry specifically?

Answer. Yes, as mentioned above, more funding is needed to public health and research institutions to expand genetic testing and contact tracing of residents and staff who test positive, particularly those who have been fully vaccinated. CDC and CMS also need to update their testing surveillance guidance that takes into consideration vaccination status but also persistent low levels of viral shedding at non-infectious levels causing PCR positive tests. These "false positive" PCR tests trigger changes in visitation, testing and cohorting procedures in nursing homes that may not be necessary. Understanding persistent long-term viral particle shedding is needed to understand how to use PCR and Antigen testing in LTC.

Question. What steps has the industry taken to prepare itself for the possible need for rapidly distributing booster shots to protect against variants? In your view, what would be the best model to accomplish such a rollout, and what would be a reasonable amount of time?

Answer. We are working with a coalition of LTC pharmacy providers, LTC provider associations and national associations representing State public health and immunization programs to develop a more efficient way to enroll LTC pharmacies and LTC providers in State immunization programs and registries. This would streamline the process for nursing homes and other long-term care facilities to offer booster shots to residents and staff on-site, which is a critical component of any vaccination effort in long-term care. AHCA/NCAL also plans to build upon its existing #GetVaccinated campaign *(https://getvaccinated.us/)* to educate and encourage LTC staff to get a booster shot when made available to them.

One challenge is the inability of State immunization registries to interface effectively with CDC and other Federal databases. Funding is desperately needed to improve the public health infrastructure at CDC and State public health agencies with respect to immunization registries and infection disease reporting. The inability of these systems to share data coupled with its dated, inefficient infrastructure does not allow easy modifications to facilitate tracking during an epidemic or pandemic. This has been a significant hinderance and source of frustration for many during the COVID–19 pandemic. This can be explained by years of poor public health funding for adequate infrastructure. Congressional support to modernize CDC's and State public health databases would make a significant difference.

Additionally, funding to help CMS build data systems to track key leadership positions in skilled nursing facilities (SNFs) is needed to get information out quickly. CMS currently lacks a data system to collect information from States on the SNF administrator, director of nursing, infection preventionist or medical director, four positions required by regulations. States maintain these lists but rarely in a readily accessible digital format and not in ways that can be easily shared with CMS or other Federal agencies. As a result, rapid communication of new information and guidance is not possible. If a booster shot is required, communication with these four positions will be critical.

Question. What lessons can be drawn from the experience of the CVS-Walgreen Long-Term Care Partnership?

Answer. This partnership in many ways was an amazing success story. In less than 3 months, a national program was created to distribute, administer, and report on vaccine administration to more than 15,000 nursing homes and 30,000 other long-term care facilities, such as assisted living.

One criticism is the delegation to States, which in some ways helped, but mainly added confusion and overly complicated the program. States decided when the program would start, which vaccine to use, and if nursing homes should start first or simultaneously with assisted living and other LTC facilities. This crated scheduling challenges.

Moreover, the lack of a database on the four professional positions described above required collecting primary contact information for all SNFs, which resulted in challenges reaching the individual if there were any errors or typos. This resulted in difficulties for CVS and WAG in contacting facilities to schedule clinics. Having an up-to-date database on the four leadership positions (administrator, director of nursing, infection preventionist and medical director) is desperately needed at CMS. This of course will require funding to CMS to develop and maintain such a database.

Question Submitted by Hon. Elizabeth Warren

Question. Private equity facilities own approximately 11 percent of nursing homes nationwide.[199] For years, reports have highlighted that private equity owned facilities provide worse care than other nursing homes. According to one 2014 study, private equity-owned facilities generally "deliver poorer quality of care" than other chain-affiliated for-profit facilities; are likely to try to reduce cost by "substituting expensive but skilled RNs with cheaper and less skilled nurses"; and "report significantly higher number of deficiencies" that climb with more years of private equity ownership.11[200] A study released last month similarly showed found that private equity ownership of nursing homes "increases the short-term mortality of Medicare patients by 10 percent, implying 20,150 lives lost due to [private equity] ownership over [a] 12-year sample period."[201] Private equity ownership was also associated with "declines in other measures of patient well-being, such as lower mobility" and taxpayer spending-per-episode increases of 11 percent.[202] Meanwhile, an Americans for Financial Reform analysis of

---

[199] Skilled Nursing News, "COVID–19 Brings Private Equity Investment in Nursing Homes Into the Spotlight," Alex Spanko, March 19, 2020, *https://skillednursingnews.com/2020/03/covid-19-brings-private-equity-investment-in-nursing-homes-into-the-spotlight/.*

[200] *Journal of Health Care Finance,* "Private equity ownership of nursing homes: Implications for quality, June–July 2014," Rohit Pradhan et al., October 2015, *http://healthfinancejournal.com/index.php/johcf/article/view/12.*

[201] National Bureau of Economic Research, "Does Private Equity Investment in Healthcare Benefit Patients? Evidence From Nursing Homes," Atul Gupta, Sabria T. Howell, Constantine Yannelis, and Abhinav Gupta, February 2021, *https://www.nber.org/system/files/working_papers/w28474/w28474.pdf.*

[202] *Id.*

long-term care facilities in New Jersey found higher rates of COVID–19 infection and death at PE-run sites.[203] However, it is challenging to identify specific ownership structures of nursing homes based on existing CMS data.[204]

Answer. AHCA represents more than 14,000 member facilities, including both for-profit and not-for-profit nursing homes and assisted living facilities. How many of these facilities are nursing homes? What percentage of these facilities are owned or controlled by private equity entities? For all nursing homes, what is the average percentage of nursing home revenue that is spent on direct patient care? For the private equity-owned or controlled facilities, what is the average percentage of nursing home revenue that is spent on direct patient care?

AHCA membership includes approximately 10,000 of the Nation's 15,000 nursing homes, 4,000 of the estimated 30,000 assisted living communities, and 200 intermediate care facilities for individuals with intellectual and development disabilities (ICF/ID). Among nursing homes, we represent approximately two-thirds of for-profit facilities, half of not-for-profit facilities, and half of government facilities. We do not have information nor access to CMS PECOS data on number owned or controlled by private equity. We also do not collect or calculate the proportion of revenue spent on direct patient care.

Questions Submitted by Hon. Patrick J. Toomey

Question. Prior to the COVID–19 pandemic, I worked alongside my Pennsylvania colleague Senator Casey to address the quality of care for nursing homes residents. We were successful in pressing the Centers for Medicare and Medicaid Services (CMS) to publicize both participants and candidates affiliated with the Special Focus Facility (SFF) program, which provides more frequent oversight of facilities that consistently fail to meet Federal safety and care requirements.

Specific to this issue, Senator Casey and I reintroduced the Nursing Home Reform Modernization Act (S. 782) on March 16, 2021, which would expand the SFF program to ensure that all facilities nominated as candidates for the program receive additional oversight. Our legislation would also increase educational resources for underperforming facilities and create an independent advisory panel to inform CMS on how best to rank nursing home performance.

As you know, part of our bill would allow nursing homes to reinvest their civil monetary penalties (CMP) to make improvements and remedy the root causes contributing to consistent deficiencies. Financial penalties can be an effective tool to incentivize compliance with Federal requirements. However, if the ultimate goal is to help a facility improve and keep residents in their homes—at what point do the penalties make it more challenging for a consistently poor performing nursing home to improve?

---

[203] Americans for Financial Reform, "Report: The Deadly Combination of Private Equity and Nursing Homes During a Pandemic," August 6, 2020, *https://ourfinancialsecurity.org/2020/08/report-3-private-equity-nursing-homes-coronavirus/*.

[204] *Health Affairs*, "These Administrative Actions Would Improve Nursing Home Ownership and Financial Transparency in the Post COVID–19 Period," Charlene Harrington et al., February 11, 2021, *https://www.healthaffairs.org/do/10.1377/hblog20210208.597573/full/*.

Answer. By the time a SNF finds itself on the Special Focus Facility list, it has often had repeated citations but also CMPs over the preceding two to 3 years. At this point, further citations and CMPs are very unlikely to remedy the underlying problem. Also, at this point, the facility needs to invest in additional resources which may be staff, equipment, or environmental changes. Further citations and CMPs would no longer be helpful at this point and would only make matters worse. Having access to capital, like the money collected through CMPs would remedy the situation by helping these facilities acquire the resources needed to address underlying issues. The Care For Our Seniors Act, a package of major reforms for the nursing home industry we developed with LeadingAge, includes a proposal on how to address chronic poor performing nursing homes *(https://www.ahcancal.org/Advocacy/Documents/Poor-Performing-Facilities.pdf)*.

Question. Can you describe a situation in which a poor-performing nursing home and its residents would benefit from the facility being able to reinvest its CMPs into quality improvement initiatives?

Answer. Facilities often find themselves on the SFF list due to lack of staffing, equipment or outdated physical environment. Rural facilities especially often need access to clinical expertise that is not available, and the cost to upgrade to broad band Internet and offer telemedicine are not possible without access to additional funds. This is where access to the CMP funds would be helpful. Additionally, chronically poor-performing facilities may need help addressing low staffing levels, and CMPs funds could assist in recruiting caregivers and offering them signing bonuses. Fundamentally, taking more resources away from an already under resourced facility for whatever the reasons does not make sense. Providing access to CMP funds or allowing further CMPs to be used to reinvest in needed changes to remedy the root cause leading to the chronic poor performance would help avoid closure of these facilities.

Questions Submitted by Hon. John Barrasso

Question. Wyoming nursing facilities are mostly located in rural and frontier communities. These nursing homes are often attached to a rural hospital. These facilities provide training for Certified Nursing Assistants (CNAs), which are the back-bone of the nursing home workforce. Through the years, nursing homes in my State have reported they have lost the ability to train their own CNAs. According to an article published in *Health Affairs,* this is because nursing homes with a civil monetary penalty greater than $10,000 lose the ability to conduct CNA training for 2 years. In rural communities, where the nursing home is often the sole source of training for CNAs, this creates a tremendous burden.

Please comment on the impact losing the ability to train CNAs has on nursing homes.

Answer. Finding and recruiting staffing at all levels but particularly among CNAs has become a greater and greater challenge. Developing a training program has been an effective strategy to recruit and retain CNAs. These programs require an investment in resources and staff. However, current statutory language requires these training programs to be suspended for 2 years for any citation resulting in substandard quality or CMPs greater than $10,000. Even when the facility has quickly remedied the situation leading to the CMP so that they are in full compliance, the CNA program is suspended for 2 years. This has not only resulted in the closure of many programs but also inhibits many providers from investing in the creation of these programs for fear of suspension. Once suspended, the ability to recruit and train additional staff becomes even more challenging. Often more staff are needed, yet the solution to the problem is hindered by this statutory language.

Question. Can you provide suggestions on how to address this situation, especially in rural communities?

Answer. It is understandable that a facility found to be seriously out of compliance with Medicare or Medicaid standards should not be training CNAs, but once the facility has remedied the situation and attained substantial compliance, the suspension of the CNA program should be lifted. This requires a change to the statute, which AHCA has advocated for over the past several years. We would be happy to work with your office and the Senate Finance Committee to address this problem.

Question. A top concern of Wyoming nursing facilities is making sure there are enough staff to care for residents. Many Wyoming nursing homes provide professional development and other educational opportunities to attract and maintain their staff.

Can you discuss solutions related to workforce development you believe will improve the ability of nursing facilities to attract and maintain direct care staff?

Answer. There are two principal challenges with recruiting and retaining staff in nursing homes. First, there are not enough nurses and other health professionals being trained in the Nation to meet the needs of older adults seeking care from all types of providers, including hospitals, physician offices, home health agencies, etc. Second, hospitals and other provider settings are able to offer more competitive wages and benefits as they are less dependent on Medicaid funds. In SNFs, two-thirds of the residents are covered by Medicaid, which MedPAC has shown under reimburses for the actual cost of care in nursing homes. As a result, nursing homes cannot compete with hospitals for nurses and other staff.

What is desperately needed is for Congress to provide additional funding to nursing schools and other schools training our health-care workforce but to make the funding tied to having graduates work in long-term care. This is similar to funding to medical schools linked to training primary care providers. Without this requirement, we have seen new graduates seek employment in hospitals and other provider settings. Another approach is to provide financial incentives to health-care professionals to work in long-term care. Two mechanisms would include loan forgiveness and tax incentives. Many graduates including nurses, pharmacists, therapists and social workers graduate with enormous student debt. Having loan forgiveness for each year working in long-term care would help increase the workforce in nursing homes. Similarly, tax credits to health-care professionals who work in long-term care would also help.

There are other strategies we are happy to discuss with you and your staff but these two approaches we believe are most effective. You may also view more of our ideas to address workforce challenges in long-term care through our specific proposal in our Care for Our Seniors Act, a package of major reforms for the nursing home industry we developed with LeadingAge *(https://www.ahcancal.org/Advocacy/Documents/Workforce-Strategies.pdf)*.

Question. An article in the March edition of *Health Affairs* points out that although staff turnover is an important indicator of nursing home quality, this has never been included on the Nursing Home Compare website, maintained by Medicare.

Please discuss the impact of staffing turnover on the quality of care provided in nursing homes.

Answer. Staff turnover has been shown to be associated with quality outcomes in numerous academic studies. In fact, turnover has a stronger association with quality outcomes than staffing levels. When staff leave, it's hard to assure consistent compliance with policies and procedures as you are always training new staff. Also, new staff are less familiar with the residents and therefore, may miss subtle changes in their condition that signify a problem. We have made staff turnover and retention a center piece of the AHCA Quality Initiative but were hampered by the lack of a Federal measure on turnover and retention.

Question. Specifically, do you believe turnover rates from nursing homes should be made more readily available for public review?

Answer. Yes, AHCA has supported CMS moving to calculate and publicly report staff turnover and retention. AHCA made turnover and retention a core measure and goal of our Quality Initiative. We believe, as the literature has shown, that turnover and retention are more important measures than staffing levels.

Questions Submitted by Hon. Todd Young

Question. Workforce issues, including high staff turnover, have been a long-standing issue for nursing homes. Research suggests that high nursing staff turnover can have a negative impact on the quality of care for residents; it has been connected with increases in patient rehospitalizations and the use of physical restraints, and it can also affect the spread of infections within nursing homes.

The COVID–19 pandemic has only exacerbated this problem. Nursing homes lost nearly 10 percent of their workforce in 2020. And a significant percentage of nursing homes nationwide—including nearly 16 percent in my State of Indiana—are still reporting shortages of nursing staff.

Dr. Gifford, one of AHCA/NCAL's recommendations to governors early on in the pandemic was to temporarily waive existing State regulations and allow medical professionals to work across State lines. Are these State licensing barriers something that could be streamlined or otherwise addressed on a more permanent basis to respond to workforce issues in nursing homes?

Answer. State licensing laws for physicians, nurses, administrators, pharmacists, and other health-care professionals are similar in concept but differ in specific details. This makes it difficult for professionals moving from State to State. CMS used the public health emergency to issue 1135 waivers allowing health-care professionals who bill for and work in Medicare-certified facilities in any State as long as they were licensed in good standing in one State. However, this does not supersede State licensing requirements. During emergencies such as a pandemic, natural disaster, etc. this limits the ability of health-care professionals to cross State lines to help when workforce shortages exist relative to the emergency.

Two potential solutions exist. First, each State as part of their emergency preparedness plans should have model executive orders for governors to waive State licensing restrictions to allow health care professionals from other States to assist during the emergency. While this need arises during nearly every emergency, such model orders are not part of each State's emergency preparedness plans. Second, States can participate in "compact" agreements that allow the easy transition between States for individuals with licensure in good standing. This may require State legislation to participate. Many States have such agreements for nurses and physicians but not all.

Without such, States are reinventing the wheel to develop executive orders and rushing to their State legislatures to get approval during each emergency. This is not something that States should be waiting until an emergency happens before addressing.

Question. How can the Federal Government better support partnerships between nursing homes and academic entities whose graduates may be interested in joining the long-term care workforce?

Answer. The Federal Government can emphasize the need for more State cooperation in allowing health-care professionals with licensure of good standing to move between States, particularly during emergencies. Congress should link Federal emergency planning funding and other Federal funding to making sure States have these programs in place before emergencies happen.

Question. As outlined in many of your testimonies, the visiting restrictions and isolation necessitated by the COVID–19 pandemic took a heavy toll on the emotional and mental health of many nursing home residents separated from their family members and other loved ones. Fortunately, with increased vaccination and declining COVID–19 deaths, many of these restrictions have been lifted.

While we hope that restrictions of this scale will not be necessary again, it is worth examining ways to alleviate the negative emotional and mental health effects that isolation may have on nursing home residents. The use of technology, for one, has allowed residents to interact virtually with family and other loved ones from whom they are otherwise separated. Expanded use of telehealth has also helped residents access routine health-care services while limiting spread of the coronavirus.

What are some lessons learned from the public health emergency in terms of the integration of technology in nursing homes—both in helping residents visit virtually with loved ones and in accessing health-care services?

Answer. Video-conferencing in nursing homes is a technology that we need to build upon and expand. Prior to the pandemic, communication with family and friends was challenging. In-person visitation often only happened when family or friends lived close by and could travel. Anecdotally, we hear that nearly half of residents never have in-person visits due to family or friends living far away or their inability to travel to the facility. The pandemic exposed this limitation when all visitors were restricted.

The restriction of all visitors required the use of digital and video technology which often does not exist in many long-term care facilities due either to inadequate Internet infrastructure as well as technological devices to support video conferencing. As a result, many staff turned to their personal smart phones or tablets to help family communicate with residents. CMS did allow facilities to apply for a limited amount of funds from the CMP accounts to purchase equipment to facilitate video conferencing. While this was helpful, it was woefully inadequate and took substantial time to complete the application and review process.

The use of telemedicine was critical during the pandemic. The risk of spread of the virus increased with each human-to-human interaction. Use of telemedicine allowed health-care professionals to provide care to residents without being physically present. This was facilitated by CMS waiving Medicare payment regulations through 1135 waivers; however, these waivers will cease when the public health emergency expires. There are benefits to telemedicine for patients even after the pandemic. Bills such as S. 368, the Telehealth Modernization Act, led by Senator Scott, would make those waivers permanent, and we support this legislation.

Question. Do you anticipate this type of technology continuing to be used beyond the pandemic?

Answer. Yes, I do. As mentioned, in-person visitation was often a challenge prior to the COVID. The need for better and more frequent communication between family members and friends is needed. The familiarity and expansion in its use will likely continue after the pandemic but will require building the appropriate infrastructure.

Many rural facilities have inadequate access to broadband Internet to facilitate video conferencing. Communication at popular times of the year, such as holidays, often overwhelms a facility's bandwidth. Additionally, telemedicine can help provide life-improving care to residents, especially in rural communities, where the availability of health-care professionals is scarce. Telemedicine could help fill the gap where workforce shortages exist. Also, the technology is continually evolving and improving, and nursing homes do not always have the resources to keep up with the latest technology even though it could be beneficial to residents.

Congress should fund the expansion of Internet infrastructure (bandwidth and Wi-Fi technology) to allow strengthen communication between residents and their families and friends as well as further develop telemedicine. The constant upgrading necessary to keep abreast of the latest technology will also be critical to better patient care, avoid problems over time, and prepare for the next emergency.

Questions Submitted by Hon. Maggie Hassan

Question. We have heard repeatedly from long-term care facility workers that the lack of access to paid sick leave is keeping some individuals from choosing to take the COVID–19 vaccine. Widespread vaccinations within long-term care facilities is our most effective tool in protecting workers and residents, so we must eliminate any barriers that are impacting vaccine uptake at this critical time.

Approximately what percentage of your member facilities currently provide paid sick leave to workers?

Answer. We do not have that information available among our membership.

Question. Among those workers who receive paid sick leave, how many hours does each worker receive annually?

Answer. We do not have that information available among our membership.

Question. What additional paid sick leave policies have your member organizations established for workers since the beginning of the COVID–19 pandemic?

Answer. Anecdotally, we have heard many providers provided various additional wages and benefits to staff including "hero" or bonus pay, childcare, assistance programs for things like groceries, and paid time off, whether to receive the vaccine or if they had to isolate due to symptoms of or exposure to COVID.

Question. What additional paid sick leave policies have your member organizations established for workers the relationship between access to paid leave and COVID–19 vaccination rates became apparent?

Answer. As mentioned above, we have heard anecdotally that providers provided paid time off to staff to receive the COVID–19 vaccine if they were unable to attend one of the three on-site clinics offered at the facility by CVS or Walgreens. Similarly, we heard they offered paid time off should they develop any symptoms following the vaccine that limited their ability to work.

Question. In addition to being an important near-term protection during the COVID–19 pandemic, do you believe that widespread access to annual paid sick leave for workers in long-term care facilities would reduce the prevalence of influenza and other illnesses that pose risks to residents in these facilities?

Answer. AHCA does not have information on paid sick leave for our members. Health insurance and paid sick leave are important for all workers in the country including health-care workers but are not always consistently offered to employees. Efforts to provide paid sick leave should also be coupled with increase childcare services for long-term care health-care workers. These would help with control of infectious outbreaks, epidemics and pandemics. We would support efforts by Congress to make these services available and affordable to health-care workers and other staff who provide vital services in nursing homes.

It is important to keep in mind that all health-care settings, especially long-term care, must delicately balance ensuring that there are enough caregivers to properly aide residents and patients, while also making sure sick employees do not create unnecessary, additional risks to residents. This means we need additional support to help prevent workforce shortages and that long term care receives the necessary resources to further invest in their staff.

We have been calling for help with the long-term care workforce shortage and chronic underfunding of nursing homes for years. If policy-makers wish to expand paid sick leave or other benefits to health-care workers, we also need your support in funding such benefits and in recruiting more caregivers to long-term care. Our Care for Our Seniors Act *(www.ahcancal.org/solutions)* offers meaningful proposals to address workforce and funding challenges that could help encourage more providers to offer or expand pick sick leave benefits.

Questions Submitted by Hon. John Cornyn

Question. We've heard from nursing homes and long-term care facilities that experienced difficulty staying up to date with public health guidance as they were released. You've noted the challenge of guidance being outdated by the time they were released.

Did AHCA members experience issues with guidance coming from State and local public health officials conflicting with CDC and CMS guidance? What recommendations do you have to improve the process of new guidance being pushed out to congregate care providers?

Answer. While CMS and CDC worked at unprecedent pace to issue new guidance, it was still often slow and outdated by the time it was issued, often due to this being a novel coronavirus. In some circumstances, the clearance process delayed issuing of guidance further. Notice that Federal guidance was forthcoming was not consistently shared or was misstated due to clearance delays that took longer than anticipated. As a result, States stepped in to develop their own guidance which invariably would conflict with Federal guidance when issued and/or conflict with other States' guidance. This added to confusion among providers.

The linking of guidance to strict enforcement actions also exacerbated the challenges. Facilities using a "good faith" effort to follow guidance would find themselves being cited for non-compliance. This led providers to ask for detailed guidance for every scenario, which further bogged down the Federal agencies. Further complicating the confusion was the fact that the multitude of guidance was located on multiple different webpages and issued by numerous agencies. Also, early on changes to guidance documents and webpages were made without any notation, making it hard to locate changes and ensure providers were accessing the most updated version. CDC eventually added a date indicating when the webpage was last updated and provides a short summary of the changes made at the top of the page. This has been extremely helpful.

Guidance is needed from the Federal agencies. It needs to be issued quickly and located in a centralized location—ideally on single page encompassing guidance from all relevant agencies. Notations need to be made on any changes being made to existing guidance that is updated. CMS continues to issue its guidance in QSO memos, and one cannot find a single page pulling together all the guidance in one place.

Strict enforcement needs to be limited to those who are blatantly non-compliant. Those who are aware of the guidance and making a good faith effort to comply but may be doing not as intended should not be cited, fined, or sued.

Question. AHCA called for reforms to Medicaid reimbursement to adequately fund care in nursing homes. Can you elaborate on what steps you believe are necessary to improve care for residents?

Answer. For years, nursing homes have been underfunded by Medicaid, significantly impacting their ability to invest in their workforce, clinical practices, and infrastructure. COVID–19 exacerbated these financial challenges, as the industry has dedicated tens of billions of dollars to fight the virus with PPE, testing and additional staff support. This pandemic has pushed nursing homes to the financial brink, and more than 1,000 facilities are in danger of closing this year, threatening access to long-term care for vulnerable seniors and individuals with disabilities. With 60 percent of residents relying on Medicaid for their daily care, the program must fund nursing homes for the actual cost it takes to provide high-quality care.

To address chronic Medicaid underfunding, AHCA and LeadingAge propose the following short and long-term investment strategies for nursing homes through our Care for Our Seniors Act *(www.ahcancal.org/solutions)*:

- *Enhanced FMAP (EFMAP)* to States to for the mandatory nursing facility benefit with requirements that additional Federal funds be used for nursing facility (NF) rates. Additions to NF rates will cover the costs of new quality and clinical provisions to improve patient care and staff safety;
- *Federal Framework for "Allowable Cost" or "Reasonable Cost"* would establish Federal guidelines for State allowable cost definitions. Currently, State definitions of "allowable cost" vary widely and, without a Federal framework, will continue to limit Medicaid reimbursable care and other nursing facility costs. Specifically, AHCA would require States to cover 100 percent of costs up to the 90th percentile; and
- *Medicaid Rate Adequacy Requirement* that rates are brought up to the cost of care and, subsequently updated regularly to keep pace with increases in costs of care. Currently, Medicaid contains no requirement that Medicaid rates be updated to keep pace with increases in the cost or care, ensuring quality or administrative burden. Under AHCA's proposed policy, States would undertake a two-step process: (1) conduct a cost of care study comparing market costs and reimbursement with Medicaid reimbursement levels and increase reimbursement to the new "allowable cost" benchmark; and (2) conduct a Medicaid rate update and rebase annually replicating step one, above.

Additionally, AHCA proposes that States be required to form a Nursing Facility Value-Based Purchasing (VBP) Committee. State Nursing Facility VBP Committees would be charged with developing a State-specific Nursing Facility VBP Design Concept which must be submitted to CMS 2 years after the end of the Public Health Emergency.

Questions Submitted by Hon. James Lankford

Question. There has been heightened discussion about the nursing home survey process regarding what it accomplishes and perhaps what it misses.

What is your opinion on the current process, and what do you think can be done to ensure better resident care?

Answer. The current nursing home survey process is not serving residents' best interests. The goal of the nursing home survey process is to assure basic levels of quality and safety for all patients, residents and clients receiving care from Medicare and Medicaid certified providers. However, the same modes of citation and penalty have been used for decades and have not evolved to reflect the science of quality improvement nor a current understanding of how to effectively use oversight to create change and achieve desired outcomes. The punitive nature of the process continues to drive good staff members and leaders out of long-term care and into other health-care jobs where the oversight process focuses on supporting a culture of safety and continuous quality improvement. Multiple stakeholders—including nursing home staff, consumer advocates, Congress, and CMS—are dissatisfied with the survey and enforcement process and results.

For instance, the same top issues are cited year after year, which shows that the current oversight process is not successfully driving improvements in these areas as it is meant to do. At the same time, with more than 200 distinct citations or "F-tags" that may be issued, half are cited less than 1 percent of the time. This shows the survey process is trying to measure too many things and is not focused on the most important areas impacting resident care.

In addition, the current survey process does not effectively identify providers' systemic strengths and weaknesses, nor are these strengths and weaknesses communicated clearly and effectively to consumers. The survey and enforcement process centers around inspection and control which is not driving improved results for quality of care and quality of life for residents. The impact and success of the survey/regulatory system is frequently measured by rates of penalties imposed and performing more frequent surveys, rather than by the quality improvements that have been achieved and sustained through the oversight process. This approach makes it difficult for providers to correct problems and sustain compliance while preventing consumers from making more informed choices that also help drive quality improvement.

Within this system, CMS spends much of its survey budget on addressing poor performing nursing homes, yet the current process and use of resources is not effective in improving care among struggling providers. At the same time, too much time is spent on surveying providers that are consistently high performers. The extensive investment of time, money and energy by State survey agencies, the Federal Government, nursing home staff as well as other stakeholders in the survey process is not delivering an equal or better return on investment to benefit the residents the system is intended to serve.

The goal of the survey process should be to get as many providers to be in substantial compliance all the time. AHCA recommends a more modern, efficient, and effective survey process that focuses on what matters most to residents to support high quality of care and quality of life. This includes reforming the survey process based on understanding when citation and enforcement is helpful in driving compliance andimprovement and when it is important to recognize and support providers' good faith efforts; implementing changes to better help turn around chronic poor performing nursing homes; and adding customer satisfaction to the Five-Star rating system to help monitor the quality of a facility for family members and guidance consumer choice.

AHCA and LeadingAge's Care for Our Seniors Act outlines these proposed reforms to the oversight system *(www.ahcancal.org/solutions)*.

Question. Do you think that adding customer satisfaction information to the "nursing home compare" website may be helpful in providing accountability?

Answer. Yes, customer satisfaction should be added to Nursing Home Compare. Customer satisfaction is well-excepted and a critical type of quality measure. Nursing homes are the only Medicare provider that does not have customer satisfaction collected and publicly reported by

CMS. During the pandemic, we have heard of the importance of communication with family and residents about what is happening. We believe one way to examine how facilities responded would have been to collect satisfaction data but unfortunately, despite our repeated calls for this information to be collected and reported, this has not happened.

AHCA and LeadingAge included adding customer satisfaction to Nursing Home Compare among our many reform proposals in the Care for Our Seniors Act *(https://www.ahcancal.org/Advocacy/Documents/Customer-Satisfaction.pdf)*.

Prepared Statement of R. Tamara Konetzka, Ph.D., Louis Block Professor, Department of Public Health Sciences, Biological Sciences Division, University of Chicago

Chairman Wyden, Ranking Member Crapo, and distinguished members of the committee, thank you for the opportunity to testify today on the topic of COVID– 19 in nursing homes.

My name is Tamara Konetzka. I am a professor of health economics and health services research at the University of Chicago. I have been conducting research on long-term and post-acute care for more than 25 years. I have led numerous studies that examine the quality of nursing home care and how public policy might improve it, how Medicare and Medicaid policy influence care access and quality, and how increasing provision of services in home- and community-based settings impacts health. I serve on the technical expert panel that advises the Centers for Medicare and Medicaid Services on the Nursing Home Compare 5-star rating system that publicly reports nursing home quality.

Almost 40 percent of all COVID–19 deaths in the United States have been linked to long-term care facilities.[205] The scope of this problem became apparent early in the pandemic, generating widespread media attention and public alarm. Almost a year ago, a *New York Times* article referred to nursing homes as "death pits,"[206] due to seemingly uncontrollable COVID–19 spread within these facilities. This devastation continued during subsequent surges.[207]

The circumstances that led to this tragedy, often referred to as a "perfect storm,"[208] start with the attributes of the novel coronavirus itself. The coronavirus that causes COVID–19 is airborne, can be spread asymptomatically, and is particularly dangerous for older adults with underlying health conditions. It is therefore no surprise that nursing home residents, with their demographic and clinical profile, suffered disproportionately high rates of cases, hospitalizations, and deaths.

The nursing home setting exacerbates this risk. Many facilities house, in close quarters, dozens or sometimes hundreds of residents who require hours of handson care on a daily basis. Many residents share rooms with others. Physical distancing is extremely difficult given the realities of congregate care settings. Finally, asymptomatic spread means that residents and staff can cause an outbreak without knowing it. This was especially lethal early in the pandemic

---

[205] About 40 percent of U.S. Coronavirus Deaths Are Linked to Nursing Homes. *The New York Times.* 2020.

[206] Stockman F., Richtel M., Ivory D., Smith M. "They're Death Pits": Virus Claims at Least 7,000 Lives in U.S. Nursing Homes. *New York Times.* April 17, 2020.

[207] Konetzka R.T., Gorges R.J. Nothing Much Has Changed: COVID–19 Nursing Home Cases and Deaths Follow Fall Surges. *J Am Geriatr Soc.* 2020.

[208] Ouslander J.G., Grabowski D.C. COVID–19 in Nursing Homes: Calming the Perfect Storm. *J Am Geriatr Soc.* 2020.

when there was less known about asymptomatic transmission and less widespread testing of asymptomatic individuals.

At long last, there is cause for optimism. Overall COVID–19 cases and deaths have declined nationwide in recent months.

The sharpest declines are occurring in nursing homes. The weekly number of new COVID–19 cases and deaths in nursing homes are at their lowest since national data collection began last May. Reported deaths among nursing home residents have declined by more than 80 percent since the new year. It is still difficult at this early date, and without the necessary data, to rigorously assess the causes of the decline.

We do know that the vast majority of nursing home residents have been vaccinated. This has almost certainly played a large role. Trends in nursing home cases and deaths, after closely matching trends in community cases and deaths throughout the pandemic, started to diverge mid-January, when a much higher percent of nursing home residents had been vaccinated than community residents.

Increased vaccination and declining COVID–19 deaths have brought other physical and emotional benefits for nursing home residents. These made possible new CDC/CMS recommendations that nursing homes fully open to visitors, a hugely important development for residents and their families.

Despite this welcome progress, there remains need for caution, and particularly the need to resist complacency. First, not all residents and staff are vaccinated. Whereas most nursing home residents were eager to be vaccinated, take-up has been much lower among staff, by some reports 37 percent.[209] Second, many facilities face high staff and resident turnover. This dynamic will produce declining vaccination rates in many facilities over time without ongoing efforts. Third, COVID–19 infection is still possible after vaccination, a risk that may increase with new coronavirus variants. If the U.S. experiences a new surge in cases this spring as public health measures are relaxed, it will provide a real test of the effectiveness of vaccination efforts in nursing homes in avoiding the new surge.

Even if vaccination proves to be wildly successful, there is still much to be learned from this pandemic to help prepare for the next one.

Evidence on Predictors of Nursing Home Cases and Deaths

Policy-makers and researchers alike have examined attributes of nursing homes associated with better and worse outcomes from the pandemic, looking for clues as to organizational best practices, opportunities for intervention, and where to assess blame. The results are clear and consistent, and not what many expected. A large body of evidence, some produced by our team at the University of Chicago[210] and some by others, shows that the two strongest and most consistent predictors of worse COVID–19 outcomes are *nursing home size,* with larger facilities being more at risk, and *COVID–19 prevalence in the surrounding community.* Given an

---

209 Gharpure R., Guo A., Bishnoi C.K., et al. Early COVID–19 First-Dose Vaccination Coverage Among Residents and Staff Members of Skilled Nursing Facilities Participating in the Pharmacy Partnership for Long-Term Care Program—United States, December 2020–January 2021. *MMWR Morb Mortal Wkly Rep.* 2021;70(5):178–182.

210 Rebecca J. Gorges was my collaborator on this research. I also thank Xiaoxuan (Stephen) Yang for research assistance.

outbreak, nursing homes in the highest quintile of community prevalence averaged five more deaths per facility than similar nursing homes in the lowest quintile.

Related studies examined the role of staff in inadvertently bringing the virus into nursing homes. One analysis used cell phone data to track staff movements in and out of facilities[211] and another examined the ZIP codes where nursing home staff live;[212] they found that staff traffic between facilities and in and out of areas with high virus prevalence was associated with more cases and deaths in the nursing homes where they worked. Nursing assistants in nursing homes usually work for minimum wage, few or no benefits, and no sick leave. To make ends meet, they often work multiple jobs in multiple facilities.[213,214] Without sick leave, staff may have felt compelled to work even when symptomatic or after a COVID–19 exposure. These conditions likely exacerbated the risk of outbreaks.

Equally important are nursing home attributes that are *not* linked with COVID–19 outcomes. Multiple rigorous studies have found no meaningful association between COVID–19 outcomes and standard nursing home quality metrics—usually measured by the Nursing Home Compare star ratings.[215,216,217,218] (Studies that did find an association often failed to control for community virus prevalence or had very small samples.) Beyond the star ratings, several studies examined specific and salient aspects of quality such as prior infection control citations. Perhaps surprisingly, these were also not associated with poor COVID–19 outcomes.[215,219]

Such results do not imply that we should ignore traditional nursing home quality and infection control measures. Rather, they suggest that high quality and good infection control are not enough. The reality is that staff enter and leave daily. When COVID–19 is prevalent in surrounding communities, even nursing homes that are of high quality and that implement recommended infection control procedures remain at risk.

The numbers bear this out. At this point, more than 99 percent of nursing homes in the Nation have had at least one COVID–19 case among residents or staff. More than 80 percent have had at least one COVID–19 death. This is not a "bad apples" problem, and no subset of nursing homes has found a magic bullet to keep the virus out. Despite the emergence of best practices and regulatory inspections for infection control, nursing home cases and deaths closely matched trends in community cases and deaths not only in spring but throughout the summer and fall surges.

---

211 Chen M.K., Chevalier J.A., Long E.F. Nursing home staff networks and COVID–19. *Proc Natl Acad Sci U S A.* 2021;118(1).

212 Shen K. Relationship between nursing home COVID–19 outbreaks and staff neighborhood characteristics. *medRxiv preprint.* 2020.

213 Baughman R.A., Stanley B., Smith K.E. Second Job Holding Among Direct Care Workers and Nurses: Implications for COVID–19 Transmission in Long-Term Care. *Med Care Res Rev.* 2020:1077558720974129.

214 Van Houtven C.H., DePasquale N., Coe N.B. Essential Long-Term Care Workers Commonly Hold Second Jobs and Double- or Triple-Duty Caregiving Roles. *J Am Geriatr Soc.* 2020;68(8):1657–1660.

215 Abrams H.R., Loomer L., Gandhi A., Grabowski D.C. Characteristics of U.S. Nursing Homes With COVID–19 Cases. *J Am Geriatr Soc.* 2020.

216 Chatterjee P., Kelly S., Qi M., Werner R.M. Characteristics and Quality of U.S. Nursing Homes Reporting Cases of Coronavirus Disease 2019 (COVID–19). *JAMA Network Open.* 2020;3(7):e2016930.

217 Dean A., Venkataramani A., Kimmel S. Mortality Rates From COVID–19 Are Lower In Unionized Nursing Homes. *Health Aff (Millwood).* 2020;39(11):1993–2001.

218 Gorges R.J., Konetzka R.T. Staffing Levels and COVID–19 Cases and Outbreaks in U.S. Nursing Homes. *J Am Geriatr Soc.* 2020.

219 White E.M., Kosar C.M., Feifer R.A., et al. Variation in SARS–CoV–2 Prevalence in U.S. Skilled Nursing Facilities. *J Am Geriatr Soc.* 2020.

This reality underscores a key oversight and lesson of the past year. Many of us have been asking: What should nursing homes be doing differently? How can they do better? Alongside these questions, we must ask with equal urgency: What should our entire communities be doing? Put differently: The single most important thing we could have done as a Nation to reduce the tragedy in nursing homes over the past year was to use public health measures to control the spread of the virus in the general population. That will be true this coming year, as well.

Racial Disparities in Nursing Home Cases and Deaths

It is now well-known that the pandemic has disproportionately harmed communities of color. Disparities in COVID–19 cases and deaths are also clear in the nursing home sector. We recently examined these differences in nursing homes nation-wide, in a study published in *JAMA Network Open.*[220] Because we lacked individual-level data, we focused on the racial distribution of residents in each facility, categorizing nursing homes by the percent of residents who are white. The differences are striking: Nursing homes serving more (>40 percent) non-white residents experienced more than three times as many COVID–19 cases and deaths as those serving primarily white residents.

In unpacking the reasons for such disparities, we found that race was correlated with two strong predictors of COVID–19 outcomes, nursing home size and COVID– 19 prevalence in the surrounding community. Non-white residents are more likely to live in larger facilities in neighborhoods where COVID–19 is prevalent. They face correspondingly greater risk of becoming infected or dying from COVID–19. Of note, although non-white residents tend to be in lower-quality nursing homes, these quality differences do not appear to explain disparities in COVID–19 outcomes, consistent with the broader research I described above. And although our measures of facility case-mix were limited, facility differences in residents' prior underlying health do not appear to explain COVID disparities, either.

As we consider ways to reduce risk and improve outcomes for COVID–19 and for future public health threats, reducing these disparities by race should be a prominent goal.

The Importance of Staffing

The key predictors of nursing home cases and deaths—size and location—leave little room for immediate and direct intervention by nursing homes themselves. Our team took a nuanced look at the role of staffing using national data, in the hope of identifying factors that might be more under the control of nursing homes and more amenable to policy changes. Other researchers have found complementary results in smaller studies.[221,222]

---

[220] Gorges R.J., Konetzka R.T. Factors Associated With Racial Differences in Deaths Among Nursing Home Residents With COVID–19 Infection in the U.S. *JAMA Netwrk Open.* 2021;4(2):e2037431.

[221] Figueroa J.F., Wadhera R.K., Papanicolas I., et al. Association of Nursing Home Ratings on Health Inspections, Quality of Care, and Nurse Staffing With COVID–19 Cases. *JAMA.* 2020;324(11):1103–1105.

[222] Li Y., Temkin-Greener H., Shan G., Cai X. COVID–19 Infections and Deaths Among Connecticut Nursing Home Residents: Facility Correlates. *J Am Geriatr Soc.* 2020;68(9):1899–1906.

In the often-contentious world of nursing home policy, it is difficult to find things that everyone agrees on—researchers, policy-makers, advocates, and nursing homes themselves. Here's one thing everyone agrees on: On average, nursing homes lack sufficient numbers of staff to provide the quality care we would all want to receive. Having enough staff is arguably the single most important element in delivering high-quality care. Providing hands-on assistance to residents is at the heart of what nursing homes do. A large body of research confirms the importance of staffing to nursing home outcomes.

It became clear during the pandemic that having enough staff was critical to implementation of best practices in preventing or containing COVID–19 outbreaks. These staffing-intensive practices include: testing of all residents, the physical separation of COVID-positive and COVID-negative residents, and the assignment of dedicated staff to each group to avoid traffic between the two. At the same time, the ability of nursing homes to attract and retain sufficient staffing has been exacerbated by the pandemic: Staff were getting sick with COVID. Others were afraid of becoming infected, or of bringing the virus home to families, especially in the absence of adequate PPE. Some staff members had to stay home with children who were suddenly learning online. And it was difficult to find new staff to hire, for these same reasons and due to competition with hospitals for additional health care personnel. In the week ending February 21st, almost 17 percent of nursing homes reported a shortage of staffing.

We specifically examined whether nursing homes that had higher staffing ratios just prior to the pandemic had better COVID–19 outcomes. Having more staff did not reduce the probability of an initial outbreak. However, *higher baseline staffing ratios were helpful in stemming an outbreak once it started: Nursing homes with the highest staff hours per resident-day experienced fewer cases and deaths than those at the bottom of the distribution.* I should note that the effects of staffing are dwarfed by the effects of community spread,14 but increasing staffing represents a clear intervention that could improve care and can save lives, during the pandemic and beyond.

Recommendations

My research and the experiences in which I have been immersed for the past year suggest several policy recommendations moving forward:

1. First, CMS policies implemented during the past year that aim to "incentivize" nursing homes to handle the pandemic well (rewarding facilities that have few deaths and/or fining those that have many) are misguided. Some of these policies are valuable long-term strategies to encourage quality improvement. These are not appropriate in the midst of a crisis, particularly given the loose connection between nursing home actions and COVID–19 deaths. At the time of an outbreak, what is needed is not incentives or blame but rather assistance, especially to those facilities that are struggling with outbreaks and may be experiencing shortages of PPE, lack of access to rapid testing, or insufficient staffing. I therefore strongly support the allocation of American Rescue Plan funds to States for "strike teams" to rapidly fill these gaps during an outbreak.
2. Second, we must provide greater assistance to large facilities in communities of color. Such facilities do not typically earn performance bonuses. If we are not careful, incentive policies intended to promote best practices will instead exacerbate racial and

ethnic disparities by depriving under-resourced facilities—and thus their patients and staff—of critically needed resources. All policies need to be evaluated in the light of equity concerns.

3. Third, data collection and wide availability are essential to assemble an accurate evidence base, to rapidly mobilize the clinical and policy research community, and to formulate effective policy. We would not have the evidence I discussed today without the data Congress mandated that the CDC and CMS collect and disseminate beginning last spring. Large gaps remain. Researchers cannot access facility-specific data on vaccination dates and rates or COVID–19 cases and deaths by race within nursing homes. This precludes rigorous analyses of the effects of vaccines, for example, or a patient-level analysis by race. Consumers who are considering nursing home care also have a right to know what percent of residents and staff have been vaccinated. These data need to be made available quickly.
4. Fourth, the COVID–19 pandemic underscores both the necessity and the limitations of traditional infection control measures and metrics. The American Rescue Plan puts substantial emphasis and funding into improving nursing home infection control practices. It is clear that these practices have been neglected and must be improved. At the same time, this is a solution to a relatively narrow set of problems, a solution that would not have avoided the tragedy of the past year. This brings me to my final and arguably most important recommendation.
5. Fifth, direct-care staffing in nursing homes needs to be increased. Even perfect infection control procedures will not improve safety of nursing home residents without the staff to implement them. In addition to low pay and few benefits, the job of direct-care nursing home staff is difficult, often dangerous, and emotionally and physically taxing. Add the risk of a potentially fatal infectious disease, and it's amazing they show up and that they stay. Addressing these challenges requires resources.

Despite broad agreement that nursing home understaffing is a problem, there is less agreement about the root causes, and from where the resources should come. Many argue, and I largely agree, that America's long-term care system is under-funded. Nursing homes that rely on Medicaid cannot afford to increase staffing without additional reimbursement. At the same time, the dominance of for-profit ownership, the growing role of private equity, cross-subsidization from Medicare, and complex ownership arrangements such as related-party transactions make it difficult to see where taxpayer money is being spent, and what profit margins truly are. Greater transparency about these ownership structures is urgently needed. We only know that under current structures, the problem of understaffing has existed for decades; something is not working.

In the short run, understaffed nursing homes cannot solve their shortages when faced with a COVID–19 outbreak. They need direct help in the form of strike teams. In the long run, resolving and moving beyond the debate about root causes of under-staffing to improve these jobs and actually increase staffing is essential. This is, admittedly, a much harder problem to solve, but it is an essential one. We can't forget about this problem when the current pandemic is contained. We will never achieve adequate nursing home quality unless we find a way to attract and support the workforce providing the hands-on care. Addressing this challenge is the best way to honor the memory of more than 1,900 nursing home workers and more than

130,000 nursing home residents who have died from COVID thus far. We can't turn back the clock to prevent the tragedy of the past year. We can at least take steps to learn from it.

Thank you for this opportunity to share my thoughts and expertise on the critical issue of the tragedy of the COVID–19 pandemic in nursing homes.

Questions Submitted for the Record to R. Tamara Konetzka, Ph.D.

Questions Submitted by Hon. Ron Wyden

Question. The Centers for Medicare and Medicaid Services (CMS) issued an interim final rule last year that required nursing homes to report COVID–19 data to the Centers for Disease Control and Prevention on a weekly basis beginning May 17, 2020. These data included COVID–19 infections, COVID–19 deaths, and the availability of key equipment and workers at individual nursing homes. The data have proved to be helpful for the public, policy-makers, and industry stakeholders to track the pandemic, and related issues, in these care settings. However, to date, CMS has *not* required nursing homes to provide such data prior to May 8, 2020, despite calls from Senate Democrats to do so. In September 2020, the Government Accountability Office (GAO) noted that "by not requiring nursing homes to submit data from the first 4 months of 2020, HHS is limiting the usefulness of the data in helping to understand the effects of COVID–19 in nursing homes." GAO went on to recommend that "HHS, in consultation with CMS and CDC, develop a strategy to capture more complete data on COVID–19 cases and deaths in nursing homes retroactively back to January 1, 2020."

Do you support GAO's recommendation? Why or why not? Please briefly explain.

Answer. I support GAO's recommendation. Having accurate data is essential not only to fighting a pandemic but to analyzing which practices and policies worked and which did not. I note that the issue is not only that nursing homes were not required to report COVID–19 cases and deaths prior to May 8, 2020, but that they were not required even to specify whether they were including those earlier cases and deaths; thus, we cannot distinguish true zeroes from missing data. Analyses to date have had to make assumptions about how to handle those early months. Rigorous analyses based on more accurate data will help to fight the remaining challenges of this pandemic and to prepare better for the next one.

Question. Residents and loved ones deserve to know whether a nursing home is safe when deciding where to receive their care. Such knowledge is more needed now than ever with the additional risk of COVID–19. The Five-Star rating system was created to do just that—provide clear and meaningful information on the quality of nursing homes. The recent story in *The New York Times* ("Maggots, Rape and Yet Five Stars: How U.S. Ratings of Nursing Homes Mislead the Public," March 13, 2021) was the latest evidence that this system needs to be fundamentally rethought. In many cases, research has shown that a facility that receives the system's top ratings does not necessarily provide better care or protection for nursing home residents when compared to lower-rated homes. Nursing homes may be able to game certain quality measures to keep or achieve high ratings while providing substandard care.

What changes do you recommend to the Five-Star system so it will better reflect patients' outcomes of care and inform residents and loved ones about the quality and safety of nursing homes?

Answer. I would like to start by pushing back a little against this characterization of the Five-Star system and adding some clarity about the evidence. While the system is certainly flawed and in need of constant refinement, I also believe it has substantial face validity. On average, 5-star nursing homes are significantly better than 1-star or 2-star homes in meaningful ways. Bad things sometimes happen in very good facilities, and some of the measures are susceptible to gaming, but this does not mean the entire rating system is fundamentally bad. After almost 2 decades of studying public reporting of nursing home quality, I can say that I would use (and have used) the Five-Star system myself to help choose a nursing home for family members. It should always be just a starting point for in-person visits and discussion.

That said, I agree that improvement is needed. I recently published a review of the evidence on Nursing Home Compare and the Five-Star system (Konetzka et al., 2020). We concluded that two key areas of quality are completely missing from Nursing Home Compare (now Care Compare) and should be added: (1) measures of resident experience and quality of life; and (2) end-of-life care. Although improved safety is critical, the lack of attention to quality of life is arguably a much more important problem both in practice and in terms of what we measure and report. For long-stay residents, the nursing home is where people live, and yet our current system of measurement focuses solely on physical health. To the existing measures of physical health and safety I would also now add the need for reporting of COVID–19 vaccination rates among residents and staff; prospective residents need to know those rates in order to assess their risk.

In terms of the accuracy of what is already reported, there are some issues to be solved. The most important component of the Five-Star rating is the inspection score, derived from State Medicare/Medicaid surveys for regulatory compliance. Although there are known problems with the survey system, it is considered the most objective because it is not based on facility-reported data. Suspicions of gaming usually focus on the staffing and the quality measures components. Our research shows nuanced evidence about this problem; blatant gaming exists, but the measures also lead to some true quality improvement (Davila et al., 2020; Konetzka et al., 2020; Perraillon et al., 2017). The Centers for Medicare and Medicaid Services (CMS) has made several key improvements in recent years to try to minimize gaming. In particular, the flawed data system for collecting staffing data was replaced with a more reliable and detailed payroll-based journal system, and several quality measures were added that are based on Medicare claims data rather than facility-reported assessment data. These have reduced, though not eliminated, the opportunities for gaming.

I think of quality measurement and reporting as an ongoing process of refinement; we will never reach a point where we think we have an ideal system. In terms of priorities in order to best inform consumers about the quality and safety of nursing homes, the addition of resident experience measures would address the most glaring problem with usefulness of the Five-Star system.

Question. Many stories of poor quality, abuse, and neglect in nursing homes start and end with chronic understaffing. This is an issue that has existed for decades and has yet to be adequately addressed. In recent years, more than half of facilities had lower staffing levels than those recommended by experts, and 75 percent of nursing homes almost never met staffing levels required by CMS.[223] The COVID–19 pandemic has exacerbated these existing issues, with nursing homes experiencing severe staffing shortages. Additionally, research shows that Black Medicare beneficiaries are more likely to be admitted to the lowest-quality nursing homes, which have lower ratios of nurses to residents.

In your written and oral testimony, you spoke about the impact of staffing on quality of care and the racial disparities in quality of care.

Would additional staffing requirements for Medicare, Medicaid, and certified nursing homes help to reduce racial disparities in the quality of care in these facilities?

Answer. We know from research that nursing home residents of color are more likely to be in low-quality nursing homes with the lowest staffing ratios (Konetzka and Werner, 2009; Mor et al., 2004). So, to the extent that additional staffing requirements are most binding for those facilities and succeed in raising the floor for minimal staffing, these requirements will directly help to reduce racial and ethnic disparities in the quality of nursing home care.

Question. What specific actions should Congress and/or CMS take to ensure that nursing facilities have a level of overall staffing that is concurrent with high quality care?

Answer. There are multiple possible ways to increase staffing in nursing homes. The most direct way is to mandate minimum staffing ratios that are substantially higher than current ratios. This will likely necessitate an increase in Medicaid reimbursement in order to cover the additional costs of hiring more staff and paying them more, based on two premises: (1) current Medicaid reimbursement is too low to make meaningful changes to staffing ratios; and (2) meaningful increases in hiring will be difficult without an expanded workforce, and that expansion would require more attractive compensation (including higher wages, sick pay, and some benefits including health insurance).

Several caveats apply to the need for higher reimbursement to increase staffing. First, the lack of transparency in the use of taxpayer dollars by nursing homes currently makes it difficult to assess the extent to which Medicaid rates currently have slack or need to be raised, although there seems to be general agreement and indirect evidence that they are too low. Thus, it would be helpful for any reimbursement increases to be tied to increased transparency about financial flows. Second, the increased reimbursement should be tied explicitly to spending on staffing.

A final note is that minimum staffing ratios are just that—minimal—and will likely be binding only for the lowest-quality facilities that currently have the most Medicaid residents and the fewest staff. Prioritizing these facilities makes sense. Substantially improving staffing across the entire industry would take more fundamental and multi-faceted rethinking of the way in which we deliver and pay for nursing home care.

Question. In your written testimony, you discussed your support for the nursing home strike teams policy included in the American Rescue Plan Act as a way to fill gaps that facilities may be experiencing during the pandemic. You also indicated that you oppose the approach taken under the Trump administration, whereby the Department of Health and Human Services

---

[223] *https://www.ncbi.nlm.nih.gov/pmc/articles/PMC7328494.*

distributed $2 billion in incentive payments to nursing homes from the Provider Relief Fund based on their relative rates of COVID–19 cases and deaths.

What information should HHS and States take into consideration when allocating these funds to ensure the facilities that need the most support preventing and responding to COVID–19 outbreaks receive it, and that racial disparities in nursing homes are taken into account?

Answer. Assistance during a crisis needs to be allocated based on risk and need, not on some notion of merit. Strike teams and other emergency assistance need to get to nursing homes on the verge of an outbreak immediately. First, this requires HHS and states to ensure that facilities have adequate testing supplies and are testing at least as often as recommended by CDC guidance. A critical step is that once one or more cases are identified, all residents and staff need to be tested, and those who test positive need to be physically separated from those who test negative. Low-resourced facilities may struggle to implement these necessary steps with the required speed and may benefit from strike teams for assistance. The roles of HHS and the state need to include ongoing, regular communication with facilities about testing supplies, turnaround time for results, and the identification of positive cases, as well as the ability to send in strike teams immediately. The key is speed and regular communication.

I don't believe it is necessary to specifically target nursing homes with more residents of color. Rather, policy-makers should prioritize areas and nursing homes at highest risk to make sure they get the assistance they need. Nursing home residents of color have been particularly hard hit during this pandemic because they are more likely to be in large nursing homes in areas where COVID–19 rates are high. If policy-makers focus assistance on areas and homes with the highest COVID–19 risk, the assistance will go disproportionately to residents of color, working to reduce the disparity.

Finally, I repeat from my testimony that addressing a crisis should not be viewed in the same way as long-run efforts to improve the quality of nursing home care. Addressing a crisis may entail providing assistance to nursing homes that policymakers view as "undeserving" due to underlying quality problems or for-profit status. The assistance can be in-kind or come with strings to make sure it is used for the intended purpose, but a crisis is not the time to implement an incentive and reward system, or the residents may pay the price.

Question. A recent paper published by the National Bureau of Economic Research found that people who receive treatment in nursing homes owned by private equity firms have worse health outcomes than those living in facilities under other ownership structurers. This paper adds evidence to reports of worse outcomes associated with private equity's investment in the nursing home industry. Nursing homes have also become popular investments for real estate investment trusts (REITs), which often lease back properties to private equity firms or other related parties. The involvement of private equity in the nursing home industry has been of interest to the Finance Committee for more than a decade, and was a topic of interest for members during this hearing. In your testimony, you noted the urgent need for greater transparency regarding nursing home ownership structurers in light of "the dominance of for-profit ownership, the growing role of private equity, cross-subsidization from Medicare, and complex ownership arrangements such as related-party transactions," making it "difficult to see where taxpayer money is being spent, and what profit margins truly are." Please answer the following.

If you have any other examples of issues associated with these ownership arrangements, please provide them.

Answer. The paragraph above captures the essence of this problem. I do not have additional examples, but would like to describe my broader perspective on the role of private equity in the nursing home industry. The main advantage to society of a private-equity takeover in any sector is, in theory, the creation of efficiencies. The firm that is bought might have untapped potential for cost-cutting or a more profitable organizational structure, which private equity owners then capitalize on. Investors get a return and the resulting firm is leaner. In the nursing home sector, it is not clear that this is a desirable goal, even if health outcomes did not suffer. Efficiencies may be created, but they accrue neither to the taxpayer funding the care, nor to the patient getting the care. So, what great advantage does this increased efficiency bring? In a sector where the main challenge has been quality, for a population that often cannot advocate for itself, I don't see any advantage of private equity buyouts—with many potential downsides.

Question. You noted the need for greater transparency in your testimony. Please provide specific recommendations about the types of transparency measures you suggest the Congress consider.

Answer. First, requirements to clearly report all owners involved in related party transactions need to be enforced. Second, I would recommend improving financial transparency by (1) reinstating the requirement that nursing homes receiving Federal funding file annual Medicare cost reports; (2) requiring similar financial reporting across all related parties, such that profits and losses for the entire entity can be assessed; and (3) requiring similar financial reporting for chains as a whole. This type of reporting is a first step in calculating two critical data points for related policies—the percent of Medicare and Medicaid dollars spent on patient care, and the adequacy or inadequacy of Medicaid reimbursement rates.

Transparency is not the end goal, but a necessary step to inform appropriate policy. At the same time, requiring transparency may reduce some of the incentive to engage in complex ownership arrangements.

Question. Are you aware of any evidence or data that show residents or staff of facilities owned by private equity firms have fared worse or experienced worse outcomes during the COVID–19 pandemic?

Answer. There have been two studies that I know of that directly examined this question (Braun et al., 2020; Gandhi et al., 2020). Somewhat surprisingly to many, neither of the studies found that nursing homes owned by private equity firms had worse COVID–19 outcomes; in fact, results of the more rigorous study suggested that private-equity-owned nursing homes had better outcomes (Gandhi et al., 2020).

These findings are consistent with the rest of the evidence on COVID–19 outcomes which found that the underlying quality of the nursing home had little influence. One possible interpretation for the lack of an association is that the attributes of a nursing home required for providing high-quality care in normal times are not exactly the same attributes required for responding to a crisis. Anecdotally, especially early in the pandemic, containing an outbreak had more to do with procurement connections (to obtain testing and PPE) than with quality. It is possible that private-equity owners did not see large numbers of COVID–19 deaths being in the interest of profitability and that they possibly even assisted with procurement. Indeed, the article by Gandhi and colleagues found that private-equity-owned nursing homes were less likely to have experienced shortages in PPE. Of note, outcomes were more negative for nursing homes that had been owned by private equity in the past, suggesting that once private-equity owners sell a nursing home, any resource-related advantages disappear.

Question. Section 6101 of the ACA sought to increase transparency of nursing home ownership structures. To date, CMS has not fully implemented or enforced this section of the ACA, although the agency does have existing reporting mechanisms for nursing home ownership that provide a certain amount of information to the public. As the committee considers the impacts of the changing ownership landscape in the nursing home industry, would implementing section 6101 provide sufficient transparency? Are there additional measures the committee should consider?

Answer. Implementing and fully enforcing section 6101 would be helpful in identifying the parties involved in these complex ownership arrangements, which seems necessary but not sufficient. It is not clear to me that section 6101 would enable a financial analysis of where the money flows once these parties are identified. This broader financial analysis is critical to assessing the two issues I noted above: the percent of Medicare and Medicaid dollars spent on patient care, and the adequacy or inadequacy of Medicaid reimbursement rates. Estimates of these are essential for any policies aimed at improving the quality of nursing home care.

Questions Submitted by Hon. Elizabeth Warren

Question. Private equity facilities own approximately 11 percent of nursing homes nationwide.[224] For years, reports have highlighted that private equity owned facilities provide worse care than other nursing homes. According to one 2014 study, private equity-owned facilities generally "deliver poorer quality of care" than other chain-affiliated for-profit facilities; are likely to try to reduce cost by "substituting expensive but skilled RNs with cheaper and less skilled nurses"; and "report significantly higher number of deficiencies" that climb with more years of private equity ownership.[225] A study released last month similarly showed found that private equity ownership of nursing homes "increases the short-term mortality of Medicare patients by 10 percent, implying 20,150 lives lost due to [private equity] ownership over [a] 12-year sample period."[226] Private equity ownership was also associated with "declines in other measures of patient well-being, such as lower mobility" and taxpayer spending-per-episode increases of 11 percent.[227] Meanwhile, an Americans for Financial Reform analysis of long-term care facilities in New Jersey found higher rates of COVID–19 infection and death at

[224] *Skilled Nursing News*, "COVID–19 Brings Private Equity Investment in Nursing Homes Into the Spotlight," Alex Spanko, March 19, 2020, *https://skillednursingnews.com/2020/03/covid-19-brings-private-equity-investment-in-nursing-homes-into-the-spotlight/*.

[225] *Journal of Health Care Finance,* "Private equity ownership of nursing homes: Implications for quality, June–July 2014" Rohit Pradhan et al., October 2015, *http://healthfinancejournal.com/index.php/johcf/article/view/12.*

[226] National Bureau of Economic Research, "Does Private Equity Investment in Healthcare Benefit Patients? Evidence From Nursing Homes," Atul Gupta, Sabria T. Howell, Constantine Yannelis, and Abhinav Gupta, February 2021, *https://www.nber.org/system/files/working_papers/w28474/w28474.pdf.*

[227] *Id.*

PE-run sites.[228] However, it is challenging to identify specific ownership structures of nursing homes based on existing CMS data.[229]

In studying the quality of care provided at American nursing homes, what challenges, if any, exist in identifying facility owners? How do those challenges affect researchers' ability to assess quality of care differences between for-profit and non-profit nursing homes, including homes owned by private equity firms?

Answer. Enormous challenges remain in identifying nursing facility owners. Some progress has been made following provisions in the Affordable Care Act requiring nursing homes to reveal ownership structures, but these data are incomplete and unaudited. Depending on the research question, this is sometimes an impediment to conducting research on nursing home quality; it is not an impediment to comparisons of for-profit to nonprofit nursing homes but is an impediment when comparing chain-owned facilities by chain or with independent facilities. More importantly, it is a major impediment to assessing the flow of taxpayer money, the percent being spent on patient care, and the adequacy of payment rates.

Question. What additional information, if any, could the Centers for Medicare and Medicaid Services collect on nursing home ownership that could aid regulators or researchers studying quality of care issues, or families seeking high quality nursing homes?

Answer. It would be helpful to regulators and researchers to have more complete and audited data on ownership structures and cost reports that allow an assessment of the flow of taxpayer dollars, the percent that is being spent on patient care, and profit margins that take into account all related parties. It seems to me that not having these assessments presents a serious obstacle to meaningful policy change aimed at increasing the quality of nursing home care. If we don't know what the money is being used for, how can we tell if it is adequate or how much additional reimbursement is needed to produce the desired level of quality?

It is less clear how families seeking high-quality nursing homes would use the ownership information, assuming they do not have strong prior beliefs about which ownership structures are associated with higher quality. We know that consumers sometimes view nonprofit status as a signal for quality, and that information is already available. As the research on these more complex ownership structures becomes clearer, the information could become more useful.

Question. What improvements, if any, could the Centers for Medicare and Medicaid Services make in the presentation and public availability of nursing home ownership data—for example, in terms of formatting, update frequency, etc.—to help regulators or researchers studying quality of care issues, or families seeking high-quality nursing homes?

Answer. For decades, it has been arduous or impossible to identify which nursing homes belong to which chains; the chain indicator available in CMS data reflects joint ownership of

[228] Americans for Financial Reform, "Report: The Deadly Combination of Private Equity and Nursing Homes During a Pandemic," August 6, 2020, *https://ourfinancialsecurity.org/2020/08/report-3-private-equity-nursing-homes-coronavirus/*.

[229] *Health Affairs,* "These Administrative Actions Would Improve Nursing Home Ownership and Financial Transparency in the Post COVID–19 Period," Charlene Harrington et al., February 11, 2021, *https://www.healthaffairs.org/do/10.1377/hblog20210208.597573/full/*.

two or more facilities, not a very useful demarcation, and the chain name field is so inconsistent as to be useless. This makes rigorous research on chains difficult, and presents a barrier to the assessment of overall quality for particular chains. CMS could solve this issue by posting chain status and a consistently worded chain name on Care Compare, with updates as they occur.

Question. What, if anything, has the COVID–19 pandemic revealed about the role of private equity in the U.S. nursing home industry and the safety of residents in private-equity-owned facilities?

Answer. There have been two studies that I know of that directly examined this question (Braun et al., 2020; Gandhi et al., 2020). Somewhat surprisingly to many, neither of the studies found that nursing homes owned by private equity firms had worse COVID–19 outcomes; in fact, results of the more rigorous study suggested that private-equity-owned nursing homes had better outcomes (Gandhi et al., 2020).

These findings are consistent with the rest of the evidence on COVID–19 outcomes, which found that the underlying quality of the nursing home had little influence. One possible interpretation for the lack of an association is that the attributes of a nursing home required for providing high-quality care in normal times are not exactly the same attributes required for responding to a crisis. Anecdotally, especially early in the pandemic, containing an outbreak had more to do with procurement connections (to obtain testing and PPE) than with quality. It is possible that private-equity owners did not see large numbers of COVID–19 deaths being in the interest of profitability and that they possibly even assisted with procurement. Indeed, the article by Gandhi and colleagues found that private-equity-owned nursing homes were less likely to have experienced shortages in PPE. Of note, outcomes were more negative for nursing homes that had been owned by private equity in the past, suggesting that once private-equity owners sell a nursing home, any resource-related advantages disappear.

Question. What steps do you believe the U.S. Congress should take to minimize risks to patients living in private-equity-owned nursing facilities, including but not limited to risks related to staffing, infection control, and future pandemics?

Answer. I do not believe that private equity should have a role in owning nursing homes, so some steps on the part of the U.S. Congress are warranted. There are several ways to reduce the growth in private-equity ownership. One is to simply ban these leveraged buyouts; given the extent of public funding for nursing home care, this could be justified. Another is to make the nursing home sector much less attractive to private equity. This might be achieved through policies that simultaneously work to improve the quality of care and would serve to protect those already living in facilities owned by private equity: requiring minimum staffing ratios and requiring that a certain percentage of revenues be spent on patient care.

Questions Submitted by Hon. John Barrasso

Question. An article in the March edition of *Health Affairs* points out that although staff turnover is an important indicator of nursing home quality, this has never been included on the Nursing Home Compare website, maintained by Medicare.

Please discuss the impact of staffing turnover on the quality of care provided in nursing homes.

Answer. A fairly large body of evidence suggests that nursing homes with higher staff turnover have lower quality of care. The research is of mixed quality, with two main challenges. First, national data on turnover have not been available until very recently with the implementation of the payroll-based journal system, the data used in the *Health Affairs* article. Thus, most studies of turnover are small and localized. Second, while high turnover is associated with poor quality, the causal connections are unclear. Does high turnover lead to poor outcomes, or do nursing homes with low quality just have more trouble retaining staff? In any case, there is face validity to a causal relationship: If staff members do not stay long enough to get to know residents and their needs, problems and changes may go unnoticed and communication may be lost in the frequent transitions.

Question. Specifically, do you believe turnover rates from nursing homes should be made more readily available for public review?

Answer. I would not prioritize it, though it could do some good. Public reporting has two main goals: to provide information to consumers and to incent improvement by providers. For consumers, the question I would ask is: Would posting turnover rates tell them anything new? As established in the *Health Affairs* article, turnover rates are highly correlated with the overall star ratings in the direction one would expect. Thus, adding turnover rates to the system would be unlikely to change consumers' choices, though perhaps some consumers would be particularly interested in this measure. I would be much more enthusiastic about adding patient experience measures, which are central to how we think about quality in long-term care but are completely missing from Care Compare.

Even if not very useful to consumers, publicly reporting turnover rates could lead providers to pay more attention to turnover and to try to reduce it. For this reason, there may be some benefit to public reporting of turnover rates. I still believe the need for it is outweighed by the compelling need to add patient experience measures.

Questions Submitted by Hon. Todd Young

Question. As outlined in many of your testimonies, the visiting restrictions and isolation necessitated by the COVID–19 pandemic took a heavy toll on the emotional and mental health of many nursing home residents separated from their family members and other loved ones. Fortunately, with increased vaccination and declining COVID–19 deaths, many of these restrictions have been lifted.

While we hope that restrictions of this scale will not be necessary again, it is worth examining ways to alleviate the negative emotional and mental health effects that isolation may have on nursing home residents. The use of technology, for one, has allowed residents to interact virtually with family and other loved ones from whom they are otherwise separated. Expanded use of telehealth has also helped residents access routine health-care services while limiting spread of the coronavirus.

What are some lessons learned from the public health emergency in terms of the integration of technology in nursing homes—both in helping residents visit virtually with loved ones and in accessing health-care services?

Answer. The expanded use of technology has been one of the silver linings of this pandemic across health-care sectors, even though it cannot fully substitute for in-person interaction and contact. This has been true in nursing homes as well, with some caveats. One caveat is that many older adults, especially those with dementia, are uncomfortable with these technologies. Another caveat, related to the first, is that using them requires time and effort of nursing home staff to facilitate. Nursing homes have exhibited understaffing for decades and this was exacerbated during the pandemic, so facilitating video visits became another task on the list competing for staff time. Nonetheless, while I am not aware of large-scale studies examining the effects of video visits in nursing homes, it seems safe to say that they mitigated the effects of social isolation to some extent and allowed family members some ability to monitor the mental and physical well-being of the resident.

Question. How do you anticipate this type of technology continuing to be used beyond the pandemic?

Answer. I expect that the use of technology to facilitate video visits with family and health-care providers will become standard. Even without the need for social isolation, there are numerous situations in which an in-person visit is not possible or not advised, for example when a family member lives far away or is ill. Increased use of televisits may also reduce the need for some transfers of residents for routine health care. It could also enable more frequent monitoring and may be a cost-effective way to enable some to remain at home, and out of the nursing home, a little longer.

Question Submitted by Hon. John Cornyn

Question. Your testimony notes the lack of vaccine uptake by nursing home staff. This coupled with high turnover can lead to higher risks for residents.

What recommendations do you have to address the issue of vaccine reluctance and improving staff retention?

Answer. Vaccine hesitancy among nursing home staff is a significant problem. To the extent that some of the hesitancy is due to the vaccines being new and people wanting to gather evidence about how others have fared, rates should increase as time passes. There are also several things that policy-makers and nursing home managers can actively do: (1) continue to provide education and public health messaging about the safety and efficacy of the vaccines and the dangers of COVID–19; and (2) make the logistics of getting the vaccine easy, e.g., through repeated on-site vaccine clinics for staff and new residents. If staff who originally declined now have to find their own appointments for vaccines off-site, it will be a significant obstacle to increasing take-up. Other small nudges may also help, such as requiring unvaccinated staff to wear more protective equipment. While the vaccines are still under

Emergency Use Authorizations, any more significant nudges (such as bonuses) or mandates seem ethically questionable.

Improving staff retention is a bigger problem that will require fundamental policy reforms. It is difficult to imagine making anything but small, incremental progress unless we change the way we treat nursing home and home health caregivers. As long as they make minimum wage and often have no sick pay or benefits or promotion prospects while doing physically and mentally demanding work, there will be understaffing and there will be turnover; understaffing and turnover tend to move together. Increasing Medicaid reimbursement and tying it to increased staffing would be a start.

Questions Submitted by Hon. James Lankford

Question. During the hearing, you mentioned the benefits of States having essential caregiver programs.

What are other ways States and localities can encourage increased family engagement and oversight in order to ensure the proper safety of a facility for their loved one? In what ways can Federal entities like CMS ensure participants in family engagement programs, such as essential caregivers, are given the utmost access to information regarding their loved one?

Answer. Family engagement and oversight are critical to the well-being of nursing home residents, not just for safety but for quality of life. Although they are not always mutually exclusive, I believe that safety and clinical outcomes are too often prioritized over quality of life, in part because safety and clinical outcomes are what we measure and reward. During the pandemic, I believe that CMS should have encouraged (or even mandated) all States to adopt essential caregiver programs, while providing the testing and PPE resources to do so safely. Any increased COVID–19 risk (likely small) would have been outweighed by the benefits of these interactions.

I see two main impediments to full communication and resident engagement with family members, both of which exist in more normal times but were exacerbated by the pandemic. The first concerns fears of regulatory action or litigation if negative information is disclosed. A fear-based system is never conducive to openness; there should be some reward to being fully transparent and open, perhaps in the form of reduced risk of regulatory sanctions or litigation. The second main impediment is resources. Although families often help with care, full communication with families and the facilitation of family engagement requires time and effort on the part of nursing home managers and staff. We have a system of nursing home care in which, for many facilities, there seems to be a crisis every day. During the pandemic, this was the case for most facilities. When staffing is so short that basic care needs are being neglected, communication with families is unlikely to be prioritized. Solving this issue will require significant reforms, likely involving increased Medicaid reimbursement tied to higher staffing standards.

One additional way to improve openness and communication with families is to publicly report resident and family satisfaction with the level of communication. In a review of the evidence on Nursing Home Compare that I recently published (Konetzka et al., 2020), we identified resident and family experience and satisfaction as a critical gap in what we report, and communication would be an element of that addition. We know that providers tend to focus on what is measured and what is reported, so this could help, at least incrementally.

References

Braun, R. T., Yun, H., Casalino, L. P., Myslinski, Z., Kuwonza, F. M., Jung, H. Y., and Unruh, M. A. (October 1, 2020). Comparative Performance of Private Equity-Owned US Nursing Homes During the COVID–19 Pandemic. *JAMA Network Open,* 3(10), e2026702. *https://doi.org/10.1001/jamanetworkopen.2020.26 702.*

Davila, H., Shippee, T. P., Park, Y. S., Brauner, D., Werner, R. M., and Konetzka, R. T. (September 28, 2020). Inside the Black Box of Improving on Nursing Home Quality Measures. *Med Care Res Rev,* 1077558720960326. *https://doi.org/10.1177/1077558720960326.*

Gandhi, A., Song, Y., and Upadrashta, P. (August 28, 2020). Have Private Equity Owned Nursing Homes Fared Worse Under COVID–19? (August 28, 2020). Available at SSRN: *https://ssrn.com/=3682892* or *http://dx.doi.org/10.2139/ssrn.3682892.* SSRN preprint. *http://dx. doi.org/10.2139/ssrn.3682892.*

Konetzka, R. T., and Werner, R. M. (October 2009). Disparities in long-term care: Building equity into market-based reforms. *Med Care Res Rev,* 66(5), 491–521. *https://doi.org/1077558709331813* [pii] 10.1177/1 077558709331813.

Konetzka, R. T., Yan, K., and Werner, R. M. (2020). Two Decades of Nursing Home Compare: What Have We Learned? *Medical Care Research and Review* [published online ahead of print, June 13, 2020].

Mor, V., Zinn, J., Angelelli, J., Teno, J. M., and Miller, S. C. (2004). Driven to tiers: Socioeconomic and racial disparities in the quality of nursing home care. *Milbank Q,* 82(2), 227–256.

Perraillon, M. C., Brauner, D. J., and Konetzka, R. T. (August 1, 2017). Nursing Home Response to Nursing Home Compare: The Provider Perspective. *Med Care Res Rev,* 1077558717725165. *https://doi.org/10.11 77/1077558717725165.*

Prepared Statement of Quiteka Moten, MPH, CDP, State Long-Term Care Ombudsman, Commission on Aging and Disability, State of Tennessee

Biography

Quiteka "Teka" Moten works for the Tennessee Commission on Aging and Disability as the State Long-Term Care Ombudsman. Teka is from Memphis, TN and is a graduate of the University of Tennessee—Knoxville with a B.A. in interdisciplinary studies and a B.A. in sociology. Following undergrad, Teka worked as senior programs coordinator for the YWCA in Knoxville. Next, she managed programs and policy efforts for the Alzheimer's Association in South Central Tennessee. During this time, she worked to establish rural senior networks, train first responders, and manage early-stage engagement programs and respite grants.

Following her time with the Alzheimer's Association, Teka pursued her master of public health in behavioral sciences at Tennessee State University while working as a government contractor. Passionate about supporting caregivers, Teka has spent years assisting families affected by Alzheimer's and other dementias. Through providing hands-on training, care plan management, and respite referrals, Teka makes use of her Certified Dementia Practitioner and PAC Dementia Coach designations by training caregivers and health-care professionals. She has made appearances on several local television and radio programs throughout the State and southern region—most notably are her features in NPT's "Aging Matters" series.

Overview of the Ombudsman Program (OMB)

The Long-Term Care Ombudsman Program (LTCOP) is an essential component to the oversight of communities such as skilled nursing facilities, assisted care living facilities, and residential homes for the aged, or (SNFs, ACLFs, and RHAs). There are 1,362 staff Ombudsmen (FTE) including 50 States along with DC and Puerto Rico and 5,947 designated volunteer Ombudsmen in the Nation. For context's sake, there are 16,253 nursing facilities per NORS 2019, Total Counts.[230]

The structure of each State Long-Term Care Ombudsman Program varies based upon organizational criteria developed by NASUAD (National Association of States United for Aging and Disabilities).[231] Major activities of the Tennessee Long-Term Care Ombudsman Program include required visits, reporting, mandatory meetings with other State agencies, follow-up on facility-initiated discharges, and coordination of the volunteer Ombudsman programs (VORs).

The cases for the LTCOP are resolved through complaint investigations as laid out in the CMS State Operations Manual. LTCOP representatives investigate individual complaints and address concerns that impact residents in facilities. Long-Term Care Ombudsmen (LTCOs) can also address general concerns they personally observe during a visit (e.g., odors, concerns about the environment, staff not knocking on resident doors before entering rooms.) As LTCOPs are resident-directed, LTCOs cannot share information without resident consent. Investigations by LTCOP representatives are done to gather facts, but the main goal is to resolve the issue to the residents' satisfaction.

The LTCOP operates as a community-based, bedside advocacy program working to uphold residents' rights. The Nursing Home Reform Act established the following Residents' Bill of Rights:[232]

- The right to live in a caring environment free from abuse, mistreatment, and neglect.
- The right to live without the fear of enduring physical restraint.
- The right to privacy.
- The right to receive personal care that accommodates physical, medical, emotional, and social needs.
- The right to a social contact/interaction with fellow residents and family members.
- The right to be treated with dignity.
- The right to exercise self-determination.
- The right to exercise freedom of speech and communicate freely.
- The right to participate in the creation and review of one's individualized care plan.
- The right to be fully informed in advance of any changes to care plan or status of the nursing home.
- The right to voice grievances without discrimination or reprisal.

---

[230] See Aging, Independence, and Disability (AGID) Program Data Portal: *https://agid.acl.gov/DataGlance/NORS/.*

[231] State Long-Term Care Ombudsman Programs: Organizational Structure: *https://ltcombudsman.org/uploads/files/support/NASUAD-2016-Ombudsman-Rpt.pdf.*

[232] The 1987 Nursing Home Reform Act: *https://www.aarp.org/home-garden/livable-communities/info-2001/the_1987_nursing_home_reform_act.html.*

How COVID Impacted the OMB Program

COVID and the ensuing policies disrupted the Ombudsman Program's immediate access to residents (as provided for in the Code of Federal Regulations). The inability to have face-to-face meetings made it difficult to verify complaints, assure confidentiality and readily gain consent from residents and/or their medical surrogates. It also made it difficult to advocate for residents dealing with facility-initiated discharges (oftentimes leaving them in behavioral health or medical centers with the risk of losing Medicaid). Particularly affected by these issues were people living with dementia (PLWD); those who were aphasic or unable to speak; those who were deaf, hard of hearing or, have assistive technology needs; those without the manual dexterity to use a phone; and those without funds to purchase their own.

In addition, the workforce shortage in nursing homes was further exacerbated by COVID. Lack of staffing and an inability to be with their family had a major impact on residents. Some of the complaints received by the Tennessee Long-Term Care Ombudsman Program included:

- An overall decline in quality of care in many facilities;
- Unanswered call lights, not getting basic care/assistance, and dehydration;
- Issues with repositioning which left residents in bed resulting in an exponential increase in bed sores;
- Unchanged catheters and pressure sores resulting in sepsis and death;
- Issues of dignity and hygiene stemming from residents having to sit in their own urine and feces for hours;
- Delayed discharges to hospitals for treatment of serious conditions, facility-initiated hospice;
- Communication issues with facilities and privacy concerns by families;
- Resident isolation (resulting in emotional distress and leading to physical decline); and
- COVID infection cases, issues surrounding cohorting residents, and room changes.

Solutions

There are a few contemplations as the Tennessee State Long-Term Care Ombudsman:

1. There is a need to reform the strategy of recruiting and retaining staff support especially with a rapidly growing elderly population.
2. It's fair to make the argument that LTCOP's are an essential piece of the system that seeks to respond to and support the health, safety, and welfare of residents regardless of any status a State may have bestowed upon the program.
3. There is a need for more Geri-psych units. Residents are typically held for 2 weeks if sent out by nursing homes; that is usually not enough time for the medications residents received to cycle out of their systems and then hold the resident for observation.
4. There should be an established, uniform system for communicating with families in the event of a PHE or natural disaster.

Questions Submitted for the Record to Quiteka Moten, MPH, CDP

Questions Submitted by Hon. Ron Wyden

Question. The Centers for Medicare and Medicaid Services (CMS) issued an interim final rule last year that required nursing homes to report COVID–19 data to the Centers for Disease Control and Prevention on a weekly basis beginning May 17, 2020. These data included COVID–19 infections, COVID–19 deaths, and the availability of key equipment and workers at individual nursing homes. The data have proved to be helpful for the public, policy-makers, and industry stakeholders to track the pandemic, and related issues, in these care settings. However, to date, CMS has *not* required nursing homes to provide such data prior to May 8, 2020, despite calls from Senate Democrats to do so. In September 2020, the Government Accountability Office (GAO) noted that "by not requiring nursing homes to submit data from the first 4 months of 2020, HHS is limiting the usefulness of the data in helping to understand the effects of COVID–19 in nursing homes." GAO went on to recommend that "HHS, in consultation with CMS and CDC, develop a strategy to capture more complete data on COVID–19 cases and deaths in nursing homes retroactively back to January 1, 2020."

Do you support GAO's recommendation? Why or why not? Please briefly explain.

Answer. I agree with the recommendation by GAO to "develop a strategy to capture more complete data on COVID–19 cases and deaths in nursing homes retro-actively back to January 1, 2020." Unfortunately, this is needed because the cases and deaths in nursing homes often mirrored that of their counties/communities. By contrast, this was not the case in many hospitals and Emergency Department (or ED) settings. With that, exploration into the complete data would help better examine the transmission of COVID earlier on in skilled nursing facilities and other long-term care facilities. The standards for care in each State spell out required documentation that may assist in accomplishing data collection.

Question. During the hearing, several Senators and witnesses raised the importance of the Federal Government collecting and publishing information from individual nursing homes that show the rate of vaccinations for residents and staff. Since that time, a bipartisan group of senators have sent a letter to the U.S. Department of Health and Human Services calling on it to take steps to begin this data collection.

Do you support this type of information being made public? How would it help the work of Long-Term Care Ombudsmen and their role protecting the rights of residents in nursing homes and other congregate living facilities?

Answer. Information on residents' vaccination percentages should and have been made public through Federal Pharmacy Partnerships and respective QIOs. Allowing the publication of information on staff vaccination percentages, however, is a bit more difficult to weigh in on due to risk of exposing PHI (like HIPPA) and leaving staff vulnerable to pressures by other staff and their community as a result. Nonetheless, the Ombudsman Program and other pertinent State agencies should be privy to this information—even if aggregated—so that we have a better understanding of risks for residents and their families as well as our own. This would also help to inform conversations around re-entry practices and needs for targeting community education to encourage vaccination(s) where possible. In addition, for Ombudsman Programs and other stakeholders working on respective ad hoc State COVID committees, this information would assist in continuing to form expectations for visits as we hopefully move closer to herd immunity.

Question. In preparation for this hearing, Oregon's Ombudsman provided my office with reports documenting issues that long-term care residents in the State have faced over the last year. They read like a list of nightmares. The Oregon Ombudsman received reports of residents being left in soiled clothing for hours, patients that developed pressure sores that reached bone, and falls that went unreported by facilities. These types of problems aren't unique to Oregon. Yet, it's clear the pandemic has reduced basic protections of the Nation's most vulnerable.

How has the pandemic impacted your work looking out for the well-being of nursing home residents, and how did the pandemic affect the number and types of complaints your office received?

Answer. The pandemic impacted the mechanisms for consumer protection and advocacy of residents by hindering immediate access. Without the ability for families or the Ombudsman Program (and in some instances first responders) to readily gain facility access, instances of neglect, abuse, exploitation, and untreated medical conditions that did not rise to the level of immediate jeopardy, or IJs, often times went unreported. In addition, due to visitation restrictions, Ombudsmen were unable to make quarterly visits to skilled nursing facilities albeit a Federal requirement—and a source of many of the cases opened by virtue of in-person observation. With that, nationally, the Ombudsman Program saw a decrease in complaints throughout the first wave of COVID. However, our offices were inundated with calls and concerns for visitation and care questions that may not have risen to the level of opening a case/complaint resulting in an exponential increase in Information and Assistance calls to the Ombudsman Program.

Question. The Centers for Medicare and Medicaid Services issued new visitation guidance on March 10, 2021, that will make it easier for nursing home residents to receive visitors. Do you expect that the administration's policy will make it easier for you to do your job looking out for the safety of long-term care residents?

Answer. The new guidance visitation issued on March 10, 2021 was merely 3 days short of having been in place for an entire year, so the new guidance was obliging in many respects with a few reservations. The visitation guidance was helpful in reestablishing expectations for allowing residents their rights to visit (or guardrails if you will—especially in States that were no longer following State specific guidance). So, short answer—yes, it makes our job easier cause we finally have good news to share. In addition, what resulted from the guidance was hope for residents and families—but for facility staff and State government, its immediacy placed a strain on areas that were still experiencing high rates of positivity, COVID outbreaks, or staff testing positive. Lastly, there was seemingly vague language that went weeks without clarity until national webinars.

Question Submitted by Hon. John Barrasso

Question. A top concern of Wyoming nursing facilities is making sure there are enough staff to care for residents.

Many Wyoming nursing homes provide professional development and other educational opportunities to attract and maintain their staff.

Can you discuss solutions related to workforce development you believe will improve the ability of nursing facilities to attract and maintain direct care staff?

Answer. Perhaps the most polarizing issue for long-term care facilities during COVID was the workforce shortage. The concern speaks to a few issues—lack of childcare, education equity, corporate responsibility, and general fiduciary oversight, but most importantly—quality of care for residents. Providing care in a nursing home setting is tough! It requires physical strength and often mental restraint; we received a myriad of complaint calls from staff detailing just that.

Solutions for Workforce Development Include

- *Temporary CNAs progression:* Working through a process for temporary CNAs based on education and time in facility during the pandemic.
- *WIOA grants:* Consideration for collaboration with WIOA Eligible Training Programs to award additional funds to students working towards non-credit certifications who are willing to do both school and work in facilities.
- *Childcare provision:* Developing childcare centers in wings of facilities that are not at full census for staff who are single parents and/or may not qualify for assistance.
- *Student Loan Forgiveness:* Quite possibly the greatest way to attract almost anyone who has amassed quite a bit of debt.

Questions Submitted by Hon. Todd Young

Question. As outlined in many of your testimonies, the visiting restrictions and isolation necessitated by the COVID–19 pandemic took a heavy toll on the emotional and mental health of many nursing home residents separated from their family members and other loved ones. Fortunately, with increased vaccination and declining COVID–19 deaths, many of these restrictions have been lifted.

While we hope that restrictions of this scale will not be necessary again, it is worth examining ways to alleviate the negative emotional and mental health effects that isolation may have on nursing home residents. The use of technology, for one, has allowed residents to interact virtually with family and other loved ones from whom they are otherwise separated. Expanded use of telehealth has also helped residents access routine health-care services while limiting spread of the coronavirus.

What are some lessons learned from the public health emergency in terms of the integration of technology in nursing homes—both in helping residents visit virtually with loved ones and in accessing health-care services?

Answer. The major lesson of technology in nursing homes is that it is only as good as (1) the staff's familiarity with the software/hardware; and (2) their capacity to use it in a meaningful, person-centered way. While there are success stories as it pertains to telehealth and visitation, the reality is that many residents didn't reap the benefits of technology due to the shortage of staff to meet their care needs. For many in nursing homes, much of the care residents required was outside a facility and could not be provided via telehealth. And due to transmission-based protocols and fear of quarantine, many residents went without medical care to avoid a 2-week lockdown; in some instances, this included treatments like dialysis, dental appointments/denture fittings, eye appointments, and other medical circumstances that contribute to the quality of life for older and vulnerable people.

Technology, while great as a concept and expenditure, is up to the discretion of facilities. What we also learned about technology is that there was:

- An increase in use for end-of-life visits (especially for long-distance caregivers).
- An increase in use for cases in which APS, TBI, or VAPITs were involved.
- A contingency on its use depending on staffing capacity at nursing homes. In facilities where community transmission was mirrored, it meant that use of technology for communication took a back seat to pushing paperwork and water carts.
- There should be some consideration for standards on virtual care plans and facility-initiated medical transfers to keep families involved in the process and able to lay eyes on their loved ones amidst tough decisions being made if ever visitation restrictions are put back in place.

Question. How do you anticipate this type of technology continuing to be used beyond the pandemic?

Answer. Beyond the pandemic—as more baby boomers age into Medicare and the long-term care setting daily, I think there will be an uptick in technology use. For many of those working in the almost $80-billion elder care industry, it means the realization of a paradigm shift to accompany the next generation. This mean not only reconsidering the institution of skilled nursing facilities by design and activity offering, it means:

- Using technology for person-centered care of residents while protecting their Personal Health Information, or PHI. If I had a magic wand, there would be a means to personalize the experience of each resident based on their intake info and schedule including pre-loaded songs and movies that they genuinely enjoyed throughout childhood through to present day.
- Taking the opportunity to engage children and younger adults on an intergenerational level; they could assist with programming tablets and/or teaching residents how to work the equipment.

- Retrofitting facilities to accommodate the needs and wants of a generation who has a better grip on technology and a desire to have it daily; there are several Life and Safety considerations forthcoming for State departments of health.
- Welcoming a more vocal generation into facilities that is aware of technology and its many uses. This means conversations and State bill introductions about technological equipment like smart speakers, gadgets like smart displays for video chatting, and features like AI-infused smart camera and smart sound.

Question. You mentioned the need for a uniform system for communicating with families in the event of a public health emergency or natural disaster. Could you elaborate on this recommendation?

Answer. In May 2020, the first of many requirements to notify families of COVID was released by CMS. At that time, the guardrails issued to inform families were broad to say the least. A skilled nursing facility could select a myriad of ways to inform loved ones including phone calls, automated calling services, text services, and notices on facility/corporate home pages. Because novel coronavirus was just beginning to take its toll, there was not yet a system in place to deal with thoroughly explaining visitation restrictions/outbreaks, lack of immediate access, and an inability for families to present when needed to (1) interpret changed behavior, mood, or effect of loved ones; and (2) have face-to-face discussions on care plans—and ensure follow-through in person. This along with the workforce shortage led to many facility phones going unanswered due to amount of staff, repeat calls, calls from multiple family members of the same resident, request from media, etc.

As we inch closer to herd immunity, the reality is that we should use this time to devise a system by which families can readily communicate with loved ones in facilities during public health emergencies. Priority should be given to a system by which families are notified when there is a facility-initiated hospital or Geri-psych transfer along with facility-initiated hospice—none of these should come as a surprise to families or happen without their consent haphazardly unless it is a medical or behavioral emergency. This ideally would be executed through a text messaging alert system coordinated by Skilled Nursing Facilities, local health departments, QIOs, the Ombudsman Program, and State departments of health.

Prepared Statement of Adelina Ramos, Certified Nursing Assistant, SEIU District 1199 New England, Greenville, RI

Thank you to Chairman Wyden, Ranking Member Crapo, and members of the Senate Finance Committee for inviting me to speak today. My name is Adelina Ramos, and I'm a CNA at a nursing home in Greenville, RI. I am a proud immigrant to this country, having moved here from Cape Verde Islands off the western coast of Africa when I was child.

At my facility, I work with Alzheimer's patients. To be trusted by families in my community to care for their loved ones is a great privilege and honor. But over the past year, my days have been filled with fear and sadness.

I don't think anyone in my small Rhode Island community thought COVID–19 would arrive at our doorstep. But it did, and nursing homes were not prepared. When COVID first hit, we lost over 20-plus residents in just over a month. A CNA at my facility died too, and she was one of the first nursing home workers to die of COVID in Rhode Island.

As more and more people in my facility tested positive, we confronted management to let them know we didn't have the right PPE—and what we had wasn't enough to last—or training to keep our residents safe and prevent the virus from spreading in our facility.

We were extremely short-staffed too. At one point I was caring for 26 critically ill residents with only the help of one other CNA, a nurse and a housekeeper. My residents couldn't eat or drink without help. They couldn't move or get out of bed by themselves. They all required oxygen changes every 15 minutes. And because they had Alzheimer's, sometimes they would get very scared or angry.

It was horrifying. But management didn't seem to be too concerned when my co-workers and I told them what was going on. We pleaded for more staff on each shift, but they said they couldn't find anyone. And so our residents and staff kept getting sick. They kept dying.

On Mother's Day, I realized I couldn't smell my ginger tea. I thought it was because of my mask. I knew that was one of the symptoms of COVID, but I wasn't experiencing anything else. When the National Guard arrived to test people a few weeks later, I got the news I had been dreading for so long: I was COVID-positive. I was asymptomatic, and so I was unknowingly putting those around me at risk— at work and at home.

My in-laws live with us, and I serve as their caregiver. They are both in their late sixties and have preexisting conditions that put them at high risk of contracting a serious case of COVID–19. I was worried about infecting my husband, because then he wouldn't be able to see his parents.

As a mother, I never thought I'd have to tell my 15-year-old son to stay away from me. Don't touch me. Don't hug me. Don't get too close. I knew I would never be able to forgive myself if I passed this deadly virus on to my child. So I did what I had to do to keep him safe, even though it broke my heart into a million little pieces.

Today, I'm COVID-free and vaccinated, and I can finally hold my son close and care for my in-laws again. Things are looking up, but the physical and emotional trauma this pandemic caused can't be cured with a shot in the arm.

When I started working at a nursing home, I understood I'd have residents pass away. But when that happens, our job is to make sure they're comfortable, cared for and surrounded by loved ones in their final moments. But because of the pandemic, family members couldn't come into our facility to be with their dying parents, grandparents, siblings, or friends. Normally, when someone passes away, the funeral home comes to our facility to handle the body. But it wasn't safe for funeral homes to enter our facility because they didn't have enough PPE. So we became the morticians and had to put bodies into body bags.

Despite my years of training and the love I have for my residents, there was nothing I could do to help them. Our residents felt so alone. Because we were dressed head to toe in protective gear, they couldn't tell who we were. They deserved so much better than what we were able to provide with so few staff and resources. As they took their final, difficult breath, I hope they knew that we tried our best. I hope they knew that we loved them like family. I hope they knew that we didn't mean to fail them.

Between April and June of last year, nursing homes in Rhode Island received over $50 million dollars in State and Federal funding in response to the COVID–19 crisis. That was on top of a Federal stimulus payment of $2,500 per nursing home bed plus $50,000 per facility—

almost $26 million.[233] Still, Rhode Island has one of the worst records in the Nation for COVID–19-related nursing home deaths—six in 10 COVID–19 deaths were in long-term care settings.[234] Where did all that money go? How was this allowed to happen?

But the pandemic didn't cause the issues we've faced—it only made them worse. Rhode island currently ranks 41st in the country for the average number of hours nursing home residents receive. The starting wage for Rhode Island nursing home workers like me is just $12.34.[235] I am fortunate that I am a member of a union. My co-workers and I were able to work together through our union to negotiate higher wages and pandemic pay. I felt like I at least had an ability to advocate for myself and my residents and shine a light on all the wrongs in our care system, which COVID–19 exposed in the most tragic and deadly way. It didn't have to be like this.

If you ask any CNA what their top issues are on the job, it's low wages, unsafe staffing, and poor job quality. They are linked together. I feel a calling to do this work and care for others. But it is hard to do this job when you can't pay your bills, put dinner on the table or afford to take your child to the doctor. Some of us have to work two or three jobs, just to meet our basic needs. And all this is made harder by the fact that because of short staffing, we don't have the time to spend with residents when they need us.

One of my hardest days during COVID–19 was when one of my patients was slipping away and wanted me to sit at her bedside but I couldn't stay because there were twenty other residents who also needed me. This is the cycle we need to break.

Most nursing home workers are women and many of us are women of color and immigrants—just like me. Centuries of systemic racism and sexism have kept alive the false idea that care workers are unskilled, uneducated, and just there to clean up. We've been denied a living wage and crucial benefits like affordable health insurance and paid time off, and too many of us don't have a union to advocate for ourselves and our residents.

I am doing my part with my union and my coworkers. I was scared to get the vaccine—many of us are, we have felt so disposable for so long that there is a lack of trust—we didn't want to be test subjects. But I did my research, I knew how important it was and how it would keep me, my family, and my residents safe. And now I educate others about my experience with the vaccine. It is why the union matters and the worker voices matter—people in all communities need sources of information that feel like they have their best interest at heart.

Our country's COVID death toll is nearing 600,000. That's more than the populations of Baltimore, Atlanta, Miami and nearly three times the population of Rhode Island's capital city, Providence.

Though vaccination rates are going up, giving us all hope that soon, the infection rates will slow and the deaths will stop, the population of Americans in need of long term care is skyrocketing. This pandemic has shown us what happens when we're not prepared to meet the demands for care.

Every shift must be appropriately staffed so residents—our Nation's parents, grandparents and loved ones with disabilities—can live with dignity and get the care they deserve and depend on. We still need PPE. We need paid time off and affordable health care. We need livable wages

---

[233] Crossroads of Care: Repairing Rhode Island's Nursing Homes in the Wake of COVID–19, *https://drive.google.com/file/d/1uc3xZ9MxA1ubUDTI4fRa8Fkp3D7NzA9c/view.*

[234] *https://www.kff.org/coronavirus-covid-19/issue-brief/state-covid-19-data-and-policy-actions/.*

[235] *https://dlt.ri.gov/documents/pdf/lmi/oesnrcf.pdf.*

that allow us to provide for our families. And every nursing home worker must have a seat at the table to be able to negotiate a better life.

We refuse to be trapped in cycles of poverty and struggle to care for our own families. We refuse to continue on with the deadly status quo in this industry any longer. Change needs to happen *now,* and not just on the State level. It's why we must raise the minimum wage to at least $15 and make sure workers have the ability to join a union to advocate for our own futures. Congress has the power to take action and raise the standards in all nursing homes in the U.S. so that everyone— no matter where they are from, where they live or what they do for a living—can access high quality long term care provided by a skilled, strong workforce that is respected, protected, and paid.

Questions Submitted for the Record to Adelina Ramos

Questions Submitted by Hon. Ron Wyden

Question. The Centers for Medicare and Medicaid Services (CMS) issued an interim final rule last year that required nursing homes to report COVID–19 data to the Centers for Disease Control and Prevention on a weekly basis beginning May 17, 2020. These data included COVID–19 infections, COVID–19 deaths, and the availability of key equipment and workers at individual nursing homes. The data have proved to be helpful for the public, policy-makers, and industry stakeholders to track the pandemic, and related issues, in these care settings. However, to date, CMS has *not* required nursing homes to provide such data prior to May 8, 2020, despite calls from Senate Democrats to do so. In September 2020, the Government Accountability Office (GAO) noted that "by not requiring nursing homes to submit data from the first 4 months of 2020, HHS is limiting the usefulness of the data in helping to understand the effects of COVID–19 in nursing homes." GAO went on to recommend that "HHS, in consultation with CMS and CDC, develop a strategy to capture more complete data on COVID–19 cases and deaths in nursing homes retroactively back to January 1, 2020."

Do you support GAO's recommendation? Why or why not? Please briefly explain.

Answer. Yes, it is important for us to be able to look back at the beginning of the pandemic to see what went wrong so that we can make sure something like this does not happen again. Asking nursing homes to provide information about COVID– 19 infections, deaths, PPE, and staffing for the first 4 months of 2020 will help us to understand the timing of the pandemic's entrance into nursing homes and the nature of its progression over time. For example, if this data shows problems like low staffing levels or inadequate PPE, this means that measures need to be put in place ensure adequate staffing and adequate availability of PPE.

Question. Black women and immigrants make up a disproportionate share of Certified Nursing Assistants and other nursing home workers—all of whom have been hit hard by the COVID–19 pandemic. To date, more than 550,000 nursing home workers have been infected by COVID–19, and at least 1,600 have died. Under normal conditions, these direct care workers conduct strenuous work at low wages, and it is not uncommon for them to have to work double shifts, work at multiple facilities, or take two jobs simply to make ends meet.

In your testimony, you described how your facility's staffing issues were made worse when your coworkers were forced to stay home due to COVID–19. The American Rescue Plan Act that President Biden just passed provides funding for strike teams, which will provide support in the short term for facilities with staffing issues that have been worsened by COVID–19. However, this is a short-term solution and will not address the ongoing issue of low wages like an increased, national minimum wage would.

How would a $15 minimum wage help nursing home workers, and what would the benefit be for patients?

Answer. A national minimum wage of $15 would benefit all workers, including many who work in nursing homes. But from my experience we will need an even higher wage to truly address the staffing crisis among CNAs. Congress and the administration need to make sure that Medicare and Medicaid money going to these nursing homes actually goes to front-line staff.

First, higher wages can serve as an incentive to attract more workers to the profession, and higher wages can also work to encourage existing nursing home workers to stay in their positions. With more workers entering the workforce, and less workers leaving, staffing levels could presumably be improved. As I mentioned in my testimony, my facility was severely understaffed at times during the pandemic and those low staffing levels impacted resident care. Nursing home residents, and particularly those that are critically ill, require substantial amounts of hands-on care as they may be unable to perform essential tasks like eating or getting out of bed by themselves. Therefore, it is very important that CNAs are given enough time per resident to ensure that resident needs are properly met.

Higher wages might also make it less likely that nursing home workers have to work two or three jobs. The reason why many nursing home workers work multiple jobs in different nursing homes to earn the money necessary to provide for their families. If nursing home workers could earn a living wage by working only one job, a lot more of us would choose to only work one job. This would help residents because workers would be less likely to travel between facilities every day, decreasing the chance that a worker could carry an infection from one facility to another.

In addition to higher wages, nursing home workers also deserve pandemic pay or hazard pay during a global pandemic. During a pandemic, the job of a nursing home worker becomes more dangerous, and therefore deserving of additional pay. Sadly, one of my coworkers at my nursing home passed away from COVID–19 and I contracted COVID–19 as well—although my case was asymptomatic. Pandemic pay or hazard pay should be guaranteed for nursing home workers during a pandemic emergency period.

Question. During the hearing, several Senators and witnesses raised the importance of the Federal Government collecting and publishing information from individual nursing homes that show the rate of vaccinations for residents and staff. Since that time, a bipartisan group of senators have sent a letter to the U.S. Department of Health and Human Services calling on it to take steps to begin this data collection.

As a front-line nursing home worker, would knowing this type information affect whether you would feel comfortable working in a given facility?

Answer. Although I was a bit hesitant to get the vaccine at first, I am now fully vaccinated against COVID–19 and I encourage others to become vaccinated as well. However, I do understand why some of my colleagues are reluctant to be vaccinated. As a workforce of mostly women and many people of color, nursing home workers have been mistreated over the years, so it is not surprising that there are some workers who have yet to be vaccinated. As far as knowing the vaccination rate for a particular facility, I do think that information is important, but I do not think vaccination rates should be used to penalize nursing homes or nursing home workers. The vaccine should be made available to nursing home workers at no cost, but it should be their choice whether or not to take it.

Questions Submitted by Hon. Todd Young

Question. As outlined in many of your testimonies, the visiting restrictions and isolation necessitated by the COVID–19 pandemic took a heavy toll on the emotional and mental health of many nursing home residents separated from their family members and other loved ones. Fortunately, with increased vaccination and declining COVID–19 deaths, many of these restrictions have been lifted.

While we hope that restrictions of this scale will not be necessary again, it is worth examining ways to alleviate the negative emotional and mental health effects that isolation may have on nursing home residents. The use of technology, for one, has allowed residents to interact virtually with family and other loved ones from whom they are otherwise separated. Expanded use of telehealth has also helped residents access routine health-care services while limiting spread of the coronavirus.

What are some lessons learned from the public health emergency in terms of the integration of technology in nursing homes—both in helping residents visit virtually with loved ones and in accessing health-care services?

Answer. When it is absolutely necessary to limit visitation in nursing homes, video visitation technology can be useful, but its utility should not be overstated. Many of our residents have mental health conditions like Alzheimer's, and others have extremely limited mobility which can limit the benefits of video visitation. And as far as caring for residents, telemedicine can be useful, but we cannot forget the importance of hands-on care in a face-to-face setting.

Question. How do you anticipate this type of technology continuing to be used beyond the pandemic?

Answer. I anticipate video visitation and telemedicine to continue to be used beyond the pandemic, where appropriate, but I do not see these forms of technology taking the place of traditional resident care.

Prepared Statement of Hon. Tim Scott, a U.S. Senator from South Carolina

For the past year, nursing homes and other senior care providers have served on the front lines of our Nation's pandemic response efforts, working tirelessly to protect many of the most vulnerable Americans from the threats posed by COVID–19. From the earliest days of the pandemic, we have understood the heightened risks that this virus presents to older Americans, and senior care communities have borne a disproportionate burden. As of last month, more than one-third of COVID–19-related deaths in the U.S. were of long-term care facility residents and staff. For roughly a dozen States, these individuals have accounted for more than half of all pandemic-related fatalities. Fortunately, in many States, government officials, health experts, and providers have partnered to protect seniors, particularly in these facilities. In South Carolina, for instance, Governor McMaster and our health department acted quickly and decisively to prioritize nursing homes for comprehensive testing, as well as to collect and publish key data points on cases and fatalities in extended care facilities.

Unfortunately, credible evidence suggests that a number of State governments have taken actions that have undermined our ability to mount a response that can effectively target resources, supports, and interventions. By ordering or otherwise encouraging nursing homes to accept patients with active COVID–19 infections who were being discharged by hospitals, certain States put scores of lives at risk. To make matters worse, recent reports suggest that in New York, Governor Cuomo's advisors actively intervened to distort data on nursing home resident fatalities, downplaying the dire consequences of the Governor's actions and tainting crucial data points that informed the State's subsequent response efforts. In the case of New York, where deaths were initially under-counted by as much as 50 percent, inaccurate data reporting denied providers, public health experts, and families the clarity and transparency that they deserved.

We have a responsibility to investigate and ensure accountability for State-level actions that have jeopardized American lives and compromised the integrity of our pandemic response efforts. I was disappointed, earlier this year, when every Senate Democrat voted against my proposal to ensure accurate State reporting of nursing home resident and staff fatalities related to COVID–19. I was similarly disappointed, earlier this month, when Senate Democrats once again chose to oppose accountability, this time by voting against an amendment I drafted that would have tied a portion of nursing home strike team funding to accurate State data reporting. Every Senate Republican voted in support of both of these common-sense measures.

Moving forward, I hope that my Democratic colleagues will join us in advancing policies and initiatives that hold States accountable for actions that erode public trust and harm the most vulnerable Americans.

Prepared Statement of Hon. Ron Wyden, a U.S. Senator from Oregon

The U.S. is now a full year into the COVID–19 pandemic. Vaccinations are up. Americans are beginning to feel encouraged. Yet so many families—hundreds of thousands spread across the country—are unable to share in the sense of uplift about what's to come because they are mourning loved ones they've lost.

Over the last year, more than 175,000 long-term care residents and workers, including 130,000 living and working in federally certified nursing homes, have died of this terrible disease. They were at the center of a collision of mismanagement. In too many nursing homes—even before the pandemic—there was chronic understaffing, slipshod plans for infection control, and abuse and neglect of vulnerable residents. When COVID–19 arrived, the Trump administration came up small by withholding data, failing to distribute PPE, and issuing guidance that put seniors in harm's way. This was a systemic, nationwide failure, and it will be challenging to fix. Members can start by agreeing on basic facts.

First, what's true of the overall population is true in our nursing homes too— blacks, Latinos, and Native Americans are suffering the worst of COVID–19. A recent study authored by Professor Konetzka, one of the witnesses joining the committee today, found that the loss of life was more than three times higher in nursing homes with the highest proportions of black and Latino residents than in facilities with mostly white residents.

Black Americans and immigrants also make up a disproportionate share of nursing home staff. Often they're paid low wages. More than half a million of them have had confirmed cases of COVID–19, and thousands have died. There's also real concern that COVID–19 will continue to circulate among these communities where vaccines aren't as readily available, or where uptake is lower.

These disparities in COVID–19 deaths are the result of generations of inequity in society and in health care. Undoing it is going to take a lot of hard work by this committee and others.

Second, the previous administration actively impeded efforts to address long-running problems in nursing homes. You could fill a library with the watchdog reports calling public attention to these issues: incidents of abuse and neglect, chronic under-staffing, squalid living conditions, inadequate emergency preparedness, and industry-wide failure when it comes to infection control.

Instead of addressing these issues, the Trump administration dramatically reduced the penalties for failing to meet basic Federal protective standards. They went out of their way to undermine any chance at real accountability. When States rushed to develop COVID policies, some followed Trump administration guidance that encouraged nursing homes to accept patients regardless of whether they had tested positive for the disease.

When the pandemic was spreading and nursing homes desperately needed PPE, the Trump administration sent out shipments that reportedly included loose, unusable gloves, hospital gowns that resembled trash bags, and defective masks.

The Trump administration did not want people to know about what was going on in nursing homes. Senator Casey and I spent months pressuring and pleading with them to release comprehensive data. The Trump administration stonewalled and dithered and delayed before they finally began to relent. To this date, there is no reliable data on COVID in nursing homes before May 1st of last year because of the Trump administration's stonewalling.

I'll close on one final point. The terrible impact of COVID–19 on seniors in long-term care isn't a red State or a blue State issue. It is a nationwide tragedy. If you look at the 10 States where nursing homes have been hit the hardest, it's five Republican-led States and five Democratic-led States.

So the reality is, long-term care residents in all 50 States were incredibly vulnerable to a pandemic like COVID–19 for longstanding reasons, but the Trump administration worked harder to protect their unscrupulous friends in management than to improve the safety of residents themselves.

The Biden administration is already working to turn things around, starting with ramping up vaccinations and creating strike teams of highly trained workers who will go into nursing homes and identify safety risks to keep residents safe.

This hearing isn't the first time or the last time that the committee will examine nursing home safety. I want to continue working with members of this committee, because looking after the well-being of America's seniors is right at the heart of our jurisdiction.

Communications

Alzheimer's Association and Alzheimer's Impact Movement

The Alzheimer's Association and Alzheimer's Impact Movement (AIM) appreciate the opportunity to submit this statement for the record for the Senate Finance Committee hearing entitled "A National Tragedy: COVID–19 in the Nation's Nursing Homes." The Association and AIM thank the Committee for its continued leadership on issues important to the millions of people living with Alzheimer's and other dementia and their caregivers. This statement provides an overview on the long-term care policy recommendations released by the Association and the impact COVID–19 has had on persons living with dementia living in long-term care facilities.

Founded in 1980, the Alzheimer's Association is the world's leading voluntary health organization in Alzheimer's care, support, and research. Our mission is to eliminate Alzheimer's and other dementia through the advancement of research; to provide and enhance care and support for all affected; and to reduce the risk of dementia through the promotion of brain health. AIM is the Association's sister organization, working in strategic partnership to make Alzheimer's a national priority. Together, the Alzheimer's Association and AIM advocate for policies to fight Alzheimer's disease, including increased investment in research, improved care and support, and development of approaches to reduce the risk of developing dementia.

The COVID–19 pandemic continues to create additional challenges for people living with dementia, their families, and caregivers including compounding the negative consequences of social isolation that many older adults already experience. Social isolation is an issue within the aging community as a whole, exacerbated due to the current public health crisis, and felt particularly hard in the Alzheimer's and dementia community.

Long-term Care, Dementia, and COVID–19

An estimated 6.2 million Americans age 65 and older are living with Alzheimer's dementia in 2021. Total payments for all individuals with Alzheimer's or other dementias are estimated at $355 billion (not including unpaid caregiving) in 2021. Medicare and Medicaid are expected to cover $239 billion or 67 percent of the total health care and long-term care payments for people with Alzheimer's or other dementias. Total payments for health care, long-term care, and hospice care for people with Alzheimer's and other dementias are projected to increase to more than $1.1 trillion in 2050. These mounting costs threaten to bankrupt families, businesses, and our health care system.

At age 80, approximately 75 percent of people with Alzheimer's dementia live in a nursing home compared with only 4 percent of the general population at age 80. In all, an estimated two-thirds of those who die of dementia do so in nursing homes, compared with 20 percent of people with cancer and 28 percent of people dying from all other conditions. It is critical that all residents of nursing homes, including those in skilled nursing facilities and Medicaid nursing facilities, receive consistent, high-quality care, especially as people can live for many years in these settings.

At least 163,000 residents and employees of nursing homes and other long-term care settings have died from COVID–19, representing over 30 percent of the total death toll in the United States. These communities are on the frontlines of the COVID–19 crisis, where 48 percent of nursing home residents are living with dementia, and 42 percent of residents in residential care facilities have Alzheimer's or another dementia. Residents with dementia are particularly susceptible to COVID–19 due to their typical age, their significantly increased likelihood of coexisting chronic conditions, and the community nature of long-term care settings. Across the country these communities, their staff, and their residents are experiencing a crisis due to a lack of transparency, an inability to access the necessary testing and personal protective equipment, incomplete reporting, and more.

To best support individuals living with Alzheimer's and dementia during the pandemic, the Alzheimer's Association released a comprehensive set of long-term care policy recommendations for federal and state lawmakers, *Improving the State and Federal Response to COVID–19 in Long-Term Care Settings.*[236] These recommendations focus on four areas: (1) rapid point-of-care testing, (2) reporting, (3) surge activation, and (4) providing support.

These policies are designed to create a strong and decisive response to the COVID–19 crisis in all long-term care settings and we were heartened to see them in the American Rescue Plan Act of 2021. We thank you for including these important provisions and strongly believe these provisions are critical to our populations and represent a significant step forward in improving their care during this pandemic and beyond.

Long-term Care Recommendation Specifics

We support the inclusion of dedicated funding for testing and tracing in nursing homes and assisted living communities. All cases of COVID–19 in these settings need to be reported immediately and accurately. These reports should be updated upon remission, death, transfer, or other appropriate status update. With all appropriate privacy safeguards for individuals, this reported data should be freely and immediately accessible to all down to the facility level. It is crucial that data on race and ethnicity are included in this reporting, which will be especially important in ensuring targeted support for the entirety of the COVID–19 pandemic, and preparedness for potential future pandemics.

As "hot spots" occur, they must be dealt with urgently and effectively. Any reported COVID–19 cases should trigger careful, ongoing monitoring and, if conditions warrant, well-trained and equipped strike teams should be deployed to the facility to provide needed support until the outbreak is contained and eliminated. All nursing homes and assisted living communities must have full access to all needed personal protective equipment, testing equipment, training and external support to keep them COVID–19-free. We also strongly support policies to increase access to televisitation technologies to address social isolation in long-term care settings, which can have a devastating impact, to ensure people with dementia are able to communicate with designated family and friends.

Furthermore, now that the first safe and effective vaccines are approved, we urge the continued prioritization of access for Americans over the age of 65, particularly those in long-term care settings. This is consistent with the Centers for Disease Control and Prevention's

---

[236] *https://www.alz.org/media/HomeOffice/Downloads/Alz-LTC-Policy-Rec_1.pdf.*

recommendation that long-term care residents be prioritized for access to vaccines, as well as the health care workers caring for some of the most vulnerable in our country and who provide an enormous service to society as a whole.

Finally, we ask that dedicated funding for home- and community-based services continues. People living with dementia make up a large proportion of all elderly people who use these important benefits. In fact, 31 percent of individuals using adult day services have dementia. Access to these services can help people with dementia live in their homes longer and improve quality of life for both themselves and their caregivers. For example, in-home care services, such as personal care services, companion services, or skilled care can allow those living with dementia to stay in familiar environments and be of considerable assistance to caregivers. Adult day services can provide social engagement and assistance with daily activities. Given the demands on and responsibilities of caregivers, respite services are also critical to their health and well-being, and may allow people with dementia to remain in their homes longer.

Nursing Home Legislation

The Alzheimer's Association and AIM have endorsed the Nursing Home Reform Modernization Act which would help ensure high-quality care by establishing an Advisory Council on Skilled Nursing Facility Rankings under Medicare and Nursing Facility Rankings under Medicaid at the Department of Health and Human Services (HHS). This new Advisory Council would provide HHS with recommendations on how to rank high-rated and low-rated facilities, with information on those rankings posted publicly to the Nursing Home Compare website. Importantly, the Special Focus Facility Program would transition to the low-rated facility program and Quality Improvement Organizations would work with those low-rated facilities to improve their quality of care through on-site consultation and educational programming. When choosing a facility for themselves or their loved ones, families deserve to have all the information available in a clear, easily digestible way. We appreciate that this bipartisan bill also directs HHS to utilize focus groups and consumer testing to ensure these ratings are easily understood by older adults, individuals with disabilities, and family caregivers.

Conclusion

The Alzheimer's Association and AIM appreciate the steadfast support of the Committee and its continued commitment to advancing policies important to the millions of families affected by Alzheimer's and other dementia. Thank you, Chairman Wyden and Ranking Member Crapo, for your continued commitment to supporting individuals living in nursing homes including persons living with Alzheimer's disease and other dementia. We look forward to working with the Committee in a bipartisan way to advance policies that would help this vulnerable population during the COVID–19 pandemic and beyond.

American Geriatrics Society

40 Fulton St., 18th Floor
New York, NY 10038

The American Geriatrics Society (AGS) would like to thank Chairman Wyden, Ranking Member Crapo, and the Senate Finance Committee for their attention to addressing the devastating impact of COVID–19 on nursing homes and for your ongoing efforts to improve nursing home safety now and in the future. The AGS greatly appreciates the opportunity to submit this statement and be part of this important conversation. We are a national non-profit organization of geriatrics healthcare professionals dedicated to improving the health, independence, and quality of life of all older Americans. Our 6,000+ members include geriatricians, geriatrics nurse practitioners and advanced practice nurses, social workers, family practitioners, physician assistants, pharmacists, and internists who are pioneers in advanced-illness care for older individuals, with a focus on championing interprofessional teams, eliciting personal care goals, and treating older people as whole persons. All of our clinician members have been on the frontlines of caring for medically complex older adults during the COVID–19 crisis and teaching others to do the same and more for us all as we age. That work remains critical to ensuring we all have access to high-quality, person-centered, affordable, and age-friendly care as we grow older.

The ongoing public health emergency (PHE) has had a disproportionate physical and emotional toll on older people, including nursing home and other long-term care residents, and the frontline health workers who care for them. Older adults and nursing home and long-term care residents have been at substantially higher risk for serious complications and death compared with other population groups.[237,238] As we move forward from the COVID–19 pandemic, we must address the healthcare workforce shortages and improve the public health system to address care needs for the whole of our population.

The AGS urges the Committee to focus on three critical areas where attention can help achieve our vision for a United States where we are all able to contribute to our communities and maintain our health, safety, and independence as we age; and older people have access to high-quality, person-centered care informed by geriatrics principles. These areas include:

A. Investing in the direct care workforce, which is the backbone of our health and long-term care system.
B. Expanding support for the geriatrics health professions programs under Title VII: Increasing funding for the geriatrics health professions programs and ensuring that these programs are included in public health planning efforts.
C. Investing in public health: Preparing for future pandemics, PHEs, and disasters and ensuring public health planning involve subject matter experts and stakeholders.

Investing in the Direct Care Workforce

The COVID–19 pandemic significantly exacerbated existing gaps in expertise and systemic weaknesses in health care service delivery for older Americans particularly for the direct care workforce.[239] Congress must enact federal and state policies that support the largely female and women of color direct care workforce by increasing compensation and benefits, strengthening training requirements and opportunities, and creating advanced roles. Congress must also

---

[237] Centers for Disease Control and Prevention. (2021). People at Increased Risk: Older Adults. Available at *https://www.cdc.gov/coronavirus/2019-ncov/need-extra-precautions/older-adults. html.*

[238] Centers for Disease Control and Prevention. (2020). People at Increased Risk: People Who Live in a Nursing Home or Long-Term Care Facility. Available at *https://www.cdc.gov/coronavirus/2019-ncov/need-extra-precautions/people-in-nursing-homes.html.*

[239] American Geriatrics Society. American Geriatrics Society (AGS) Policy Brief: COVID–19 and Assisted Living Facilities. *J Am Geriatr Soc.* 2020;68(6):1131–1135. *https://doi.org/10.1111/jgs.16510.*

ensure that all health professionals and direct care workers on the frontlines have access to paid family, medical, and sick leave.

Direct care workers are vital to supporting older adults and their caregivers at home and in congregate living settings (e.g., long-term care and assisted living). They provide hands-on care at the bedside that is physically and emotionally demanding to millions of older Americans. At present, women account for nearly 90 percent of the direct care workforce[240] and women of color account for 48 percent of this workforce in the United States.[241] Hourly rates are low (often $12 or less per hour),[242] and direct care workers often lack paid family leave, and other benefits.[243] Currently, the demand for direct care workers exceeds the supply and this gap is only expected to grow. Investing in building the direct care workforce should be a priority for the United States as a part of investments in the infrastructure that is needed to care for us all as we age.

Expanding Support for the Geriatrics Health Professions Programs

Increasing Funding for the Geriatrics Health Professions Programs

Currently, too few health workers receive adequate, if any, training in providing the highly skilled and complex services that make care different for older people. Furthermore, staff recruitment and retention is particularly difficult due to the medically complex nature of care for us all as we age. The Geriatrics Workforce Enhancement Programs (GWEPs) and the Geriatrics Academic Career Awards (GACAs) are the only federal mechanism for supporting geriatrics health professions education and training. The GWEPs educate and engage the broader frontline workforce, including family caregivers and direct care workers, and focus on opportunities to improve the quality of care delivered to older adults. The GACA program develops the next generation of innovators to improve care outcomes and care delivery

Most recently, the GWEPs and GACAs have been on the frontlines of the COVID– 19 PHE, ensuring clinical and educational training can enhance their communities' response to the pandemic and its impacts on older adults. The GWEPs and the GACAs are the only federal programs that focus on training the workforce to care for older Americans and investing in these programs is imperative to maintaining the health and quality of life for us all as we age. At minimum, Congress should increase annual appropriations to $51 million given the essential role awardees play in their states.

Ensuring that Planning Bodies Include the GWEPs and GACAs in Public Health Planning Efforts

These programs are also playing a key role in public health planning efforts. The GWEPs and GACAs have been an asset for states especially as many states and localities grapple with the

[240] PHI National. (2020). Direct Care Workers in the United States: Key Facts. Available at *https://phinational.org/wp-content/uploads/2020/09/Direct-Care-Workers-in-the-United-States-2020-PHI.pdf.*

[241] PHI National. (2017). Issue Brief: Racial and Gender Disparities Within the Direct Care Workforce: Five Key Findings. Available at *https://phinational.org/wp-content/uploads/2017/11/Racial-and-Gender-Disparities-in-DCW-PHI-2017.pdf.*

[242] Raghu, M. and Tucker, J. National Women's Law Center. (2020). Low-paid Women Workers on the Front Lines of COVID–19. Available at *https://nwlc.org/blog/the-wage-gap-has-made-things-worse-for-women-on-the-front-lines-of-covid-19/.*

[243] PHI National. (2021). Caring for the Future: The Power and Potential of America's Direct Care Workforce. Available at *https://phinational.org/wp-content/uploads/2021/01/Caring-for-the-Future-2021-PHI.pdf.*

rollout of the COVID–19 vaccine and address vaccine hesitancy. GWEPs have been staffing call lines to assist older adults to register for the vaccine, advising local authorities on making the sign-up websites age-friendly, and working with health systems in the rollout of vaccines and outreach to vulnerable and hard-to-reach populations (e.g., homebound older Americans and Americans with disabilities). Through Project ECHO, a telelearning and telementoring program, they have been working with nursing homes to train staff on how to use personal protective equipment (PPE) and on infection prevention protocols. This effort is consistent with CMS's overall priority to reduce COVID–19 infections in nursing homes and keep residents and staff safe during the pandemic. Looking ahead, these programs will be critical in providing assistance for proactive public health planning with their geriatrics expertise and knowledge of long-term care and can help ensure states and local governments have improved plans for older adults in disaster preparedness for future pandemics and natural disasters. To assume these roles, there would need to be additional investments by Congress in both programs to ensure that states have access to the expertise of GWEPs and GACAs. One avenue for ensuring that access is for the Health Resources and Services Administration (HRSA) to include attention to expertise in geriatrics and gerontology in its planning for rebuilding the public health workforce as called for in the American Rescue Plan Act of 2021. One way to accomplish that objective is to increase funding to the GWEP and GACA programs with the specific goal of ensuring that all states have access to the geriatrics education and training that these programs provide to the healthcare workforce.

The reality is that our current healthcare workforce is ill-prepared to care for older adults given the paucity of required training in geriatrics across disciplines. Although AGS does not specifically track the public health workforce, we believe it is critical that investments be made in ensuring that this workforce understand the needs of older Americans so that we can ensure that agencies and organizations focused on the health of the public are meeting the needs of this large and growing demographic group. With funding from the John A. Hartford Foundation, Inc., the Trust for America's Health is exploring the public health needs of older Americans with the goal of ensuring that we are developing age-friendly public health systems.[244] Given their focus on developing age-friendly health systems, focus on transforming primary care, and partnerships with community-based organizations, the GWEPs are well-positioned to assume a greater role ensuring that as we build up our public health workforce we are doing so in a way that supports an age-friendly public health system.

Investing in Public Health

Preparing for Future Pandemics, PHEs, and Disasters

A critical area of focus should be to ensure we have plans for how to protect the health and safety of all Americans in the event of a future pandemic, PHE, or natural disaster. This should include assurance that Crisis Standards of Care that dictate allocation of scarce resources do not include discriminatory policies that are based on age alone.[245] The current COVID–19 PHE underscored the gaps in our planning specific to older adults which, as in natural disasters like

---

[244] Trust for America's Health. (2018). Creating an Age-Friendly Public Health System: Challenges, Opportunities, and Next Steps. Available at *https://www.tfah.org/wp-content/uploads/2018/09/Age_Friendly_Public_Health_Convening_Report_FINAL 1 1_.pdf.*

[245] Farrell T.W., et al. AGS position statement: Resource allocation strategies in the COVID– 19 era and beyond. *J Am Geriatr Soc.* 2020;68(6):1143–1149. *https://doi.org/10.1111/jgs.16537.*

Hurricane Katrina, resulted in the pandemic having a disproportionate impact on older Americans, particularly older Americans of color. It is critically important that the federal government review and revise PHE and disaster guidance related to this population to provide guidance for state and local planning.

Ensuring Public Health Planning Involves Subject Matter Experts and Stakeholders
Public health planning will necessitate coordination with several important stakeholders and across several different priorities.[246] We recommend that public health planning involve subject matter experts and stakeholders including:

a. *Geriatrics health professionals* should be recruited to serve on pandemic and disaster response and planning teams, given their expertise in caring for older people with medical complexity or advanced illness, leading interprofessional collaboration, implementing knowledge of long-term care across settings and sites, and leading advance care planning. This unique skillset is essential for community-level planning.
b. *Nursing homes and other long-term care settings leadership teams* (e.g., administrators, medical directors, and directors of nursing) are vital for planning how resources can be best deployed during a pandemic. These teams have expertise in allocating resources within their own facilities; developing community-wide plans in collaboration with acute care hospitals and other post-acute care institutions in their communities; and building understanding of staffing needs, as well as federal and state regulations.
c. *Hospice and palliative care experts* should be recruited to serve as members of pandemic planning teams, given the need to ensure hospitals and other facilities have access to expertise in advance care planning, symptom management, and end-of-life care, where available.

We encourage you to consider focusing on the three critical areas while examining COVID–19 in the nation's nursing homes.

Thank you again for the opportunity to submit this statement and for your attention to these concerns. The AGS looks forward to continuing to work closely with the Committee as you work to improve the lives of all Americans.

Letter Submitted by Dan Arbeeny

The Honorable Ron Wyden Chair
The Honorable Mike Crapo Ranking Member
U.S. Senate Committee on Finance
Washington, DC 20510–6200

RE: March 17th Hearing "A National Tragedy: COVID–19 in the Nation's Nursing Homes"

---

[246] American Geriatrics Society. American Geriatrics Society (AGS) Policy Brief: COVID–19 and Nursing Homes. *J Am Geriatr Soc.* 2020;68(5):908–911. *https://doi.org/10.1111/jgs.16477.*

Chairman Wyden and Ranking Member Crapo:

My name is Dan Arbeeny and I live in Brooklyn, NY. In one week in April 2020, we had four family members die of COVID: my father, my uncle and two close cousins. Of the four, only one was counted as a COVID death.

Thank you very much for scheduling this hearing on the impact of COVID–19 on nursing homes and continuing the Committee's commendable policy of allowing members of the public to supplement the hearing record with additional and, in our case, personal family experience.

The scope of this nursing home debacle has already been well described in the hearing testimony of the Government Accountability Office (GAO) which pointed out that while "the nation's 1.4 million nursing home residents are a small share of the total U.S. population (less than 1 percent), they comprise nearly 30 percent of COVID–19 deaths reported by the Centers for Disease Control and Prevention (CDC)." In actual numbers, this amounts to more than 174,000 individuals with the numbers still rising.

Our experience in New York, for which I claim no official role but that of a person who has been outspoken and willing to respond to press inquiries about how the situation in our State was made so much worse than it had to be due to the actions of Governor Cuomo and virtually all other aspects of the state government. I refer primarily to the Governor's Directive of March 25, 2020 compelling the State's nursing homes to accept COVID–19 patients.

By no means do I intend to imply that the State of New York's nursing homes were innocent parties in this series of reckless and wrongful actions contributing to the death of my father, other members of our family and thousands of other New Yorkers with whom I have been in close contact now for over a year in time. We have reluctantly become the 100,000 New York State COVID–19 nursing home orphans.

My family has lived on the same block in Brooklyn, New York for five generations. It is a wonderful heritage we were given, but more importantly, it is where my family has deep community roots. My father was a vivacious man of 88 years, still working and driving with a very sharp mind and quick smile. He sat on the stoop of the house always offering a smile, a greeting and keeping an eye-out for neighborhood happenings.

Right after Christmas my father took ill and recovered, but a series of illnesses, non-life threatening, happened that required he be in and out of the hospital and then to a nursing home in our immediate neighborhood called the Cobble Hill Health Center (CHHC). In short, my Dad was doing as best he could and was COVID-free up until the time of the Governor's disastrous March 25th Directive.

It was the CHHC which told us about the Directive and that they were trying to persuade governor's office not to force them to take COVID patients. Unfortunately, Governor Cuomo and the State Health commissioner ignored their pleas. It then took us many days to move him back home and it was during that time in CHHC that he got a low-grade fever. Despite 24-hour care, a week later he developed congestion and his doctor ordered a COVID test. We tested him on Monday, April 20, 2020 at 1:00pm and 12 hours later he was dead and the COVID test came back positive afterwards.

Even as non-medical personnel, we knew it was senseless for the State government to exercise the fullness of its powers to compel contagious patients to the residences where the weakest and most vulnerable were confined. What could they possibly have been thinking and why were there not more nursing homes and their professional associations speaking out against this ill-considered action? Instead, the response of the State Legislature was to roll over at the Governor's request and grant purported immunity to all the players in this dereliction of duty.

Five days after the governor signed his March 25th Directive, the USS Comfort and the Javits Center hospital came online giving NYC and the surrounding area an additional 2,000 hospital beds. The Governor did not use those facilities for patients and the general utilization was minimal. The governor also added more regulations with regard to the use of the Javits Center making it almost impossible to send an elderly patient there.

Six days after the governor signed his March 25th order, the Samaritans Purse field hospital in Central Park opened with 68 beds. Again, for reasons which remain inexplicable, the Governor refused to use this facility for COVID patients.

At this point we had two choices before us, give in to the grief and anger or focus on reaching out to others in order to bring the truth to life. We started by organizing similarly situated individuals and doing fundraising events for Personal Protective Equipment for CHHC and other front-line workers as well as our local police precinct.

At the same time, the media, to its credit, began to focus on CHHC because it was reporting so many COVID deaths as part of the State collection process. As it turned out, the reason for this was that CHHC was the *only* nursing home that properly reported the number of possible covid deaths. To the best we understood it, every other one of the 627 nursing homes significantly underreported and, of course, it was subsequently admitted that the State itself was once again the prime mover in this well-orchestrated cover-up.

Being so closely involved with CHHC, I spoke with many of these reporters covering this story and it was across the full spectrum of news outlets including News1, CNN, CBS, ABC, WSJ, Fox, AP, and many others. There were so many that my brother Peter and I had to divide them up in order to get out the truth of what was really happening. We took hours to explain that CHHC was not a party at fault but that it was the system at large and Governor Cuomo in particular who was understating the New York death toll by midsummer at 6,500 while we had been saying since April 2020 in over 50+ interviews including one with Jake Tapper on CNN that the true number is more like 12,000 to 15,000 deaths.

When the news subsequently came out that the governor was writing a book about his "leadership" during the COVID pandemic we knew it was time to step up our efforts to get the actual truth out to all the aggrieving families and other residents of New York State so they could safeguard themselves against the March 25th Directive. We were also hoping that the appointed and elected officials in New York as well as the federal government would begin to take note.

On October, 18, 2020, our growing but still informal organization hosted a Mock Funeral for Governor Cuomo's so-called "Leadership and Integrity" which focused on two simple points. We asked for an apology and that there be full admission of the true number of our loved ones who had died in nursing homes. There was abundant press coverage which we again appreciated in terms of trying to keep our cause alive.

We watched aghast as the Governor received an Emmy Award for what we now know was a disastrous policy, a cynical effort to cloak it through state-granted immunity and then a program of lying to cover it up as long as possible. Based on what we now know, every statistic the government used was misleading; rather than using facts to point us to the truth, the "guardians of the public interest" used their offices to point us away from the truth.

Finally, on January 28, 2021 the New York State Attorney General belatedly announced what was considered a "bombshell" report confirming that there had been a significant undercount of the number of COVID deaths in New York nursing homes. That was followed very quickly by the governor and State Department of Health losing in its legal effort over reporting the COVID death data to the Empire Center for Public Policy, an independent, non-partisan, non-profit think tank based in Albany, NY. We likewise want to commend Judge Kimberly O'Connor for her fortitude in that case.

Most recently and inevitably, the Secretary (Chief of Staff) to the Governor, Mellisa DeRosa admitted at a private meeting what we had been saying for almost a year, that the State hid the true number of deaths. That meeting soon became public as did the next stage of the Governor's campaign to blame everyone else.

At this point, speaking for myself and I believe almost every other family in this situation, we have accomplished the goal of getting out the truth. But no one in the public or private sector is admitting their culpability for the death, distress, pain, and suffering they have caused and concealed. We respectfully request the assistance of this Committee in continuing its oversight and investigation of New York State and every other state which pursued a similar program of confining the COVID-ill to the most susceptible of the still healthy elderly residing in Medicaid-funded nursing homes.

Conclusion

These are the facts as we see them from the ground:

- The Governor forced 9,000 COVID-positive patients into nursing homes in New York State;
- There are 627 nursing homes in the State of New York but only one spoke the truth;
- The Governor and State Legislature wrongly sought to immunize the medical community, hospitals, nursing homes and their associated trade groups, management consultants, and other service providers that assisted these companies in partnership with Governor Cuomo, the State Department of Health and other State offices and employees;
- The Governor and other State officials and private parties knowingly and now admittedly lied to the public and impugned the character of persons seeking to tell the truth.

Crown Publishing Group has just announced that it has ceased promotions of the Governor's book entitled "American Crisis: Leadership Lessons from the COVID–19 Pandemic," and that there were no plans to reprint the book or to reissue it in paperback. This is an important first step but wholly inadequate still as the proper remedy is for the publisher to disgorge all past and future proceeds and to rescind the advances and any other payments made to the Cuomo in connection with a publishing enterprise built entirely on false pretenses. These funds should then be directed to a charitable fund in order to help defray the burial expenses of the victims of this series of unconscionable activities.

In addition, the Academy of Television Arts and Sciences needs to withdraw the 2020 International Emmy Founders Award which it inappropriately awarded to Governor Cuomo last November.

Thank you for the opportunity to submit these views.

cc: The Hon. Charles Schumer The Hon. Kirsten Gillibrand

Statement Submitted by Marla Carter

Green River Area Development District (GRADD) Ombudsman Advisory Council, Consumer Member

Faithful Friends Nursing Home Ministry leader, Pleasant Valley Community Church

Daughter-in-law of, friend to, advocate for residents in long-term care (LTC)

After watching the full committee hearing on March 17th, I felt compelled to respond; first of all, with my deepest gratitude for the issues that were discussed and the concerns that were raised, and secondly to share my direct experiences that confirm much of what was discussed. Having been volunteering in LTC for almost 3 years now, I will tell you that every harrowing story and every shocking fact shared with your committee is consistent with what I have witnessed. The long-term care system in this country has been broken for quite some time, and the pandemic has simply forced us to look in the mirror and finally see the way we are caring for the elderly and disabled residents of LTC.

My mother-in-law is a resident of a Genesis owned facility here in Owensboro, Kentucky. Before the pandemic, our church had adopted this facility and we were inside the facility weekly; we held Sunday school classes, did crafts with residents, sang with residents, prayed with them, visited with them, and often advocated for them. 60–80% of nursing home residents never receive a single visitor; therefore, for many residents, we became their family.

Before the pandemic, it was not unusual for us to hear residents say, with regards to their care, "I pushed my call button but no one came," or "I keep telling them I need to go to the doctor but they won't make me an appointment," or "they lost my favorite blanket even though it had my name on it," or "I'm out of pull-ups in my size so they told me I have to wear a different size."

Since the pandemic, communication has become very difficult. The facility does not have in-room land line phones, and only a handful of residents have personal cell phones. Most residents must go to the nurses station to use the phone, which is hardly private and very discouraged during the pandemic due to infection control. Even still, here are the kinds of phone calls we've gotten now:

- "There's no one to do the laundry, and I'm out of underwear, so they put me in pull-ups."
- "It's so hot in my room but they won't let me have a fan because it will blow the virus around."
- "We can't have showers because the steam makes the virus more contagious. I haven't had a shower or bed bath in weeks and I smell myself, so I know other people smell me too. I'm embarrassed."
- "I asked for a drink and they told me to get it myself."
- "Help! I'm on the toilet and I pushed the call button but no one has come and I've been sitting here for an hour."
- "Help! They're killing me! No one will help me. Please call my priest and tell him I'm sorry for every sin I ever committed."

- "I had an accident . . . I couldn't get to the toilet in time so I have diarrhea all over myself. I asked for help cleaning up but the staff told me they didn't have time because they were passing out trays."
- "I haven't had my medicine in five days. They ordered the refill but it hasn't come in yet."
- "I like giving my friends snacks but the staff yells at me and says I have to stay in my room all the time. I feel like I'm in a communist country."
- "The staff told me I'm a troublemaker. Do you think I'm a troublemaker?"
- "The traveling nurse gave me the wrong medicine and I had a really upset stomach. She told me not to tell you."
- "I told the staff that my roommate had a fever and was sick but they told me to mind my own business."

Keep in mind that we have an excellent relationship with this facility. The administrator has been very supportive and tries very hard to ensure residents are cared for with compassion and dignity. But she can only work with what she's given by corporate—low wages and the inability to hire more staff—and she can't be there all the time.

Even in the midst of the pandemic, when they were receiving more federal and state funds, I did not see an impact on patient care. For example, this facility received nearly the maximum amount of civil monetary penalty funds for improving virtual communication in the summer of 2020. It's unclear to me exactly what that money was spent on, though presumably it was spent on new iPads. My experience, though, was that staff didn't know how to set up the iPads/Facetime and even when they figured it out, there were only 4 for the building and they had to be shared; residents had to wait for a staff person to bring them an iPad and help them with it. Some residents used them to watch religious services online, and a few virtual "visits" were scheduled for Mother's Day and birthdays.

A few cell phones were purchased so that each unit would have a phone that could be taken to resident rooms instead of them having to use the phone at the nurses station. However, those phones quickly got lost.

The activities director went above and beyond to try to keep residents entertained, though she was limited with her resources as well. Here are all the things our church donated to the facility because they couldn't buy them:

- Shepherd's hooks (to hang bird feeders outside residents' windows);
- 5 CD players (because each wing had to have its own because they weren't allowed to carry their one CD player wing to wing due to infection control);
- Craft supplies: construction paper, glue, markers, crayons, old magazines, paint, cereal boxes, buttons, wrapping paper, note cards, pumpkins; and
- Misc items: 10 sets of drum sticks, 10 large stability balls, 10 laundry baskets, printable games, puzzles, activity pages, Scripture hand outs, Bibles, devotionals, library books, CDs, DVDs, VHS tapes, television

Other items we have donated:

- Clothing, shoes, socks;

- Gift bags for all residents containing snacks, puzzle books, markers, tumblers, lotion, shampoo, hairbrush, tissues, soft candy, pens, notepads (twice yearly); and
- In the past year, our church spent $5,000 on things for this facility—some of that money went for treats for the staff to encourage them. This figure would be much higher if we factored in what folks from our church donated—hundreds of dollars in Christmas gifts and toiletries.

While you would expect that a facility that charges nearly $8,000/month could supply the most basic of things, we are constantly amazed at how many residents are impoverished and needy. We have brought clothing to residents who had only one change of clothes and pajamas to residents who only had a hospital gown. Residents often run out of tissues, pull ups, and personal hygiene items. (Most residents are on Medicaid and thus only receive a $30 allowance each month. Their $30 is all they have for things like haircuts, snacks, clothing, anything "extra.")

You would also expect that such a facility would have a doctor on site at all times; after all, this is a skilled nursing facility that cares for some very acutely ill residents. However, there is only a nurse practitioner on site Monday-Friday. The "medical director" is a local physician who works on the side to "oversee" the medical care the nurse practitioner is providing. He checks in periodically and comes in a few times a month to check over the charts. He is listed as my mother-in-law's primary care physician, yet when I have a question regarding her care, I cannot call him on the phone to discuss her care.

Another thing you might expect from such a facility is that they would provide transportation for residents to and from doctor's appointments or even for "fun" outings. No. This facility does not have a vehicle/bus/van. When residents leave to go to a medical appointment, they must ride on the local GRITS bus (Green River Intra-County Transit System), which is a free or low-cost public transportation service-free for persons receiving Medicaid and low cost to the general public.

One terrible example of facilities relying on this service involved a 92 year-old ward of the state who was being transferred from one skilled nursing facility to another in mid-July. She was transferred on the GRITS bus, wearing a black sweat suit and no shoes (socks only) with none of her belongings except her Bible. It was weeks before she had any of her belongings delivered to her because each facility claimed not to know which one was responsible for transporting her things, and both used the excuse that they did not have a facility vehicle. Additionally, during the pandemic, facilities are still relying on this public transportation—residents that had to leave regularly for dialysis or other regular appointments were not allowed to ride in a family member's car—they had to use the GRITS bus, though their family member was allowed to meet them at the appointment. Illogical!

We have gotten creative during the pandemic to find ways to continue to help the residents and the facility, but we dearly miss the residents and they miss us. I have asked corporate repeatedly to allow us to continue to volunteer, even outdoors if preferable. This facility, like so many others, has struggled to maintain its staff.

They've had a great deal of turnover and are always in need of more staff. They did hire some emergency "unit aide" people, who were untrained but came in for a few months to help with basic, non-medical tasks. These are things we could have been doing for free! Before the pandemic, we were in many ways, "staff extenders."

Here are some things we did:

- Wheeled residents to the dining hall;
- Sat with residents and encouraged them eat;
- Helped them get a different food choice if they didn't like what was served;
- Got them water/drinks (with staff direction- we knew who had fluid restrictions, etc);
- Helped locate lost items in the laundry room;
- Helped write names in/on resident belongings;
- Helped locate lost items in rooms (glasses, dentures, remote controls, etc);
- Helped fix TVs, phones, radios, etc.;
- Went to the store for residents;
- Assisted with holiday parties and crafts;
- Scheduled extra fun activities for residents (for example we had a sweet girl from our church who has no arms come in and paint for the residents with her feet—they loved her!!);
- Held weekly Sunday school classes for residents;
- Helped residents make phone calls;
- Helped re-direct residents who were wandering; and
- Sat with residents who were upset, talked with them.

These are all very important tasks that the staff simply does not have time to do because they are stretched too thin. This summer, when outdoor visits began to be allowed, we offered to come assist with screenings at the door and supervising the visits outside, but were told no. As of today, we are still not allowed inside. Our ministry team of volunteers has been vaccinated and so have over 90% of the residents, while only 50% of staff have been vaccinated. We would like to come inside and help!! If untrained employees could be hired for extra help in the middle of the pandemic, why can't we now enter and help. We can go through the same screenings as staff and be trained in infection control practices. Our services are free and contribute greatly to residents' quality of life! So why would corporate not allow us inside to help at a time when they cannot keep staff?

When we first started visiting my mother-in-law and other residents in the nursing home, I was shocked by the conditions. Since then, I've done much reading about Medicare certified facilities, the care they provide, and the great expense they are to the taxpayer and the government. For example:

- "The vast majority of nursing homes reap substantial funding from Medicare and Medicaid in exchange for the promise of providing quality care to their patients. In fact, a 2015 CMS report found that, in 2014, of the 15.634 nursing homes across the US, 92.2% (14,407) were dually certified to receive both Medicare and Medicaid payments. In other words, federal government taxpayer funding pays for most nursing home care. And the truth is that these nursing home corporations rely upon this steady course of income—government payments—to generate profit. Many, in fact, generate very substantial profits from it."
- In 2009 alone, one out of every four claims submitted by the US nursing home industry was erroneous, resulting in $1.5 billion worth of unjustified payments from Medicare.

- A 2015 article entitled "Nursing Home Care Industry Is a Solid Investment," pointed out the virtues of investing in the nursing home industry: "Profits are staggering, and the nursing home companies have a long time of add-on sales for supplemental services through subsidiaries they control." (Dr. Harold Goldmier, investment strategist, 2015)
- The modern American nursing home grew out of the 19th-century almshouse, a kind of public, charitable organization that was set up to help the "worthy poor" (originally, widows of good social standing who had fallen into destitution). The almshouse system expanded until the 1930s, when officials at the United States Social Security Board began to worry about the "increasing dependency" of "the aged"; they feared that old people would bankrupt the country with their expensive infirmities. They made efforts to shut the facilities down, and they proposed that the government start a small pension, what would become Social Security benefits.

  In place of the almshouses came pay-to-stay "rest homes" and, later, more medically staffed nursing homes, all competing in a private marketplace for elder care. By 2000, nursing homes were a $100 billion business, and the little mom and pop shops that had once dominated the industry were being fused together and swallowed up into larger entities. For a time, it seemed like nothing could stop the growth. It didn't matter when, in the early 2000s, five of the country's top-ten nursing-home chains entered into Chapter 11 bankruptcy proceedings after undertaking a string of heavily debt-financed mergers and acquisitions. The companies were restructured, and sometimes rebranded, and then continued on their way. Today, around 70 percent of nursing homes are for-profit, and more than half are affiliated with corporate chains.

  All the while, nursing-home chains continued to get bigger, until just five companies owned more than 10 percent of the country's 1.7 million licensed nursing home beds. Private equity also entered the sector, buying up four of the ten largest for-profit nursing homes. "There's essentially unlimited consumer demand as the baby boomers age," Ronald E. Silva, president of Fillmore Capital Partners, told *The New York Times* in 2007, after paying $1.8 billion to purchase a large nursing-home chain called Beverly Enterprises Inc. "I've never seen a surer bet." These new ownership groups changed things in ways that people who lived in them could feel. Earlier this year, a Wharton School—New York University—University of Chicago research team found "robust evidence" that private-equity buyouts lead to "declines in patient health and compliance with care standards." When nursing homes are bought by private-equity groups, the team concluded, frontline nursing staff are cut, and residents are more likely to be hospitalized.

  But the most consequential change may have happened within the for-profit companies themselves. It all started, most undramatically, with a 2003 academic article in *The Journal of Health Law.* In "Protecting Nursing Home Companies: Limiting Liability Through Corporate Restructuring," its authors—two health-care lawyers—made note of two financial threats to nursing-home operators: lawsuits by nursing-home residents (for, say, negligence) and efforts by the government to recoup overpayments (for, say, false claims on Medicare billings). The solution, the authors suggested, was in restructuring. Specifically, nursing homes should split up into separate limited-liability corporations, one for real estate and one for operations. This new structure, they wrote, would keep assets safe from litigious family members and retributive bureaucrats. It would also attract money from real-estate investors who were keen on nursing homes but wary of the liability risks. By 2008, the top-ten companies had all split themselves into real estate and operations LLCs.

Then many companies went further, creating networks of sub-companies called "related parties" that could trade and transact with one another. What had once been a nursing home became a corporate cluster, including separate entities for real estate, insurance, management, consulting, medical supplies, hospice, therapy, private ambulances, and pharmacy services. By 2017, three-quarters of nursing homes did business with related parties, according to a study by Kaiser Health News. There was nothing inherently wrong, and certainly nothing illegal, about these increasingly complex formulations. The owners said that they were only creating a vertical supply chain for eldercare. By 2015, nursing homes were spending $11 billion a year on contracts with related parties.

But the structure had an additional benefit that the authors of the article had not pointed out: It allowed companies to siphon profits out of their nursing homes through sometimes exorbitantly overpriced transactions with their sister companies. Instead of hiring salaried managers to oversee a facility, a nursing home could now contract with expensive related-party management corporations and consultancies. Instead of owning the land around a nursing home, a company could lease it from a related-party real-estate business, sometimes at a higher-than-market rate. In this way, a nursing home could appear, on its accounting sheets, to be operating on slim margins, or even at a loss, but only because that loss was offsetting gains within the same company.

"No one begrudges a company for making profits," Dr. Michael Wasserman, president of the California Association of Long-Term Care Medicine, told me. "This is capitalism. This is America." The issue, he said, is that doctors and nurses are pressed to cut costs while related parties are getting rich. "If the real-estate entity is making significant profits and the operation is break-even, then there's a problem. I would compare today's nursing-home real-estate owners to slumlords." This excerpt is from an article that appeared here: *https://story.californiasunday.com/covid-life-care-center-kirkland-washington?fbclid=IwAR24x0cPBI-v3I37CIJpKr0R729Ew9OZ_AfOGUnjE7wHrB-4pLd18r00YIQ*.

- A 2014 report by the Office of the Inspector General of the Department of Health and Human Services about adverse events in skilled nursing facilities found that one in three patients who stay in a nursing home will suffer harm or injury within the first 35 days as a result of the care they receive. The report also found that most of these incidents are "clearly or likely preventable," and attributed much of the preventable harm to "substandard treatment, inadequate resident monitoring, and failure or delay of necessary care."—Levinson, Office of Inspector General, 2014.

  In the above report, 66% of these harmful events were due to preventable medication errors. The report further found an estimated 7,203 hospitalizations for medication events, which on average, cost an estimated $8,372. The estimated total spending related to hospitalizations for medication events was an estimated $57,729,935—just for the month of August 2011. (That is NOT a typo!)
- The nursing home setting is a significant risk factor for sexual abuse. A study of elder sexual abuse in Virginia from 1996 through 2001 which researched sexual abuse in both institutional and residential settings found that nearly three-quarters of all sexual

abuse occurred in nursing homes. (Teaster and Roberto, 2005) In other words, an elderly person is in more danger in a nursing home than on the streets of a typical U.S. city.

- Pressure sores have long been established as an indicator or substandard care. CMS identifies stages III and IV pressure sores as being one of eight preventable conditions. In 2004, more than one in ten nursing home residents had a pressure sore (NCHS, Park-Lee & Caffrey). The total annual cost for treating pressure sores in the US is $11 billion (Institute for Healthcare Improvement, 2007).
- No doubt, the patients and their families are the primary victims, but clearly, lower-level nursing home staff are victimized by the industry's obsession with profits as well. As if being stressed, overworked, and forced by circumstances to mistreat patients weren't enough, the median annual wage of nursing aides and orderlies working in nursing homes is $24,7000 and $19,950 to $22,580 respectively (U.S. Bureau of Labor Statistics, 2016–2017). Effectively, the working poor, who are themselves among the most vulnerable in our society, are the ones taking care of elderly, vulnerable patients. Each is being taken advantage of by the nursing home industry.—Abuses and Excuses: How to Hold Bad Nursing Homes Accountable, by Jeffrey Powless.

In my humble opinion, not only are many nursing homes committing Medicare/Medicaid fraud by failing to provide the services for which they are receiving federal funds, but also by then receiving more money from the government and the taxpayers to take care of the additional health problems that their negligence has created. It's akin to double billing!

It is my firm belief that most all of the issues within the nation's nursing homes can be boiled down to staffing. They don't hire enough and they don't pay enough. However, providers are going to tell you they can't find employees, or that they need more Medicare/Medicaid reimbursements in order to hire more and pay more. I just don't believe that's true. I think the way they have been allowed to structure their corporations with private equity firms controlling the various intertwined entities of real estate, vendors, and goods is the real problem. I have seen non-profit facilities and the difference in care they provide is remarkable.

Statement Submitted by Eilon Caspi, Ph.D.

On June 13, 2019, the GAO released the report: Nursing Homes: Improved Oversight Needed to Better Protect Residents From Abuse. The GAO's investigation reported that CMS does not track "abuse perpetrator type" (such as staff or residents) in over 15,000 nursing homes nationwide. It urged CMS to bridge this major gap in oversight of nursing homes.

Two years prior to the GAO 2019 report, I published an extensive article in the *Journal of Elder Abuse and Neglect* identifying this gap including 20 reasons why it needs to be addressed by CMS.

Caspi, E. (2017). A federal survey deficiency citation is needed for resident-to-resident aggression in U.S. nursing homes. *Journal of Elder Abuse and Neglect,* 29(4), 193–212.

In addition, the MDS 3.0, which is the largest federally-mandated clinical dataset in nursing homes also doesn't track resident-to-resident incidents:

Caspi, E. (2013). M.D.S. 3.0—A giant step forward but what about items on resident-to-resident aggression? *Journal of the American Medical Directors Association,* 14(8), 624–625.

When this public health problem is not being tracked, for all practical purposes, it does not exist and CMS is not in a position to learn from these incidents to inform nationwide prevention. These injurious and deadly incidents remain invisible.

I've been focusing on the prevention of this prevalent and disturbing phenomenon of injurious and deadly neglect for over 13 years. For example, I published the first study in the U.S. on fatal resident-to-resident incidents:

Caspi, E. (2018). The circumstances surrounding the death of 105 elders as a result of resident-to-resident incidents in dementia in long-term care homes. *Journal of Elder Abuse and Neglect,* 30(4), 284–308.

An early Harvard study showed that injurious resident-to-resident incidents are prevalent in U.S. nursing homes:

Shinoda-Tagawa et al. (2004). Resident-to-resident violent incidents in nursing homes. *JAMA,* 291(5), 591–598.

I've also co-directed the first documentary film on this phenomenon. The film is entitled *Fighting for Dignity* and it was produced by Terra Nova Films (released in early 2020).

My book, the first on the prevention of these incidents, will be published by *Health Professions Press* this summer.

Over the years, I've reviewed several hundred injurious and deadly resident-to-resident incidents and came to learn that the vast majority of these incidents, especially in the context of resident with a serious brain disease such as Alzheimer's disease, are a form of neglect such as the neglect of meeting residents psychological and medical needs and neglect of supervision.

When I saw the GAO 2019 report and the aforementioned recommendation in it, I was hoping that CMS will finally require all 50 State Survey Agencies to track "abuse perpetrator type" (staff-to-resident abuse *and* resident-to-resident incidents).

However, nearly 20 months after the GAO report was released, CMS has yet to bridge this major gap in its oversight and enforcement activities of nursing homes. This, despite the fact that HHS concurred with the GAO recommendation.

Residents continue to be injured and die due to these resident-to-resident incidents—even during the pandemic. It is important to point out that the majority of these incidents are preventable.

Would your committee consider urging CMS to implement the GAO 2019 recommendation?

Specifically, this was GAO's "priority" recommendation:

> The administrator of CMS should require that abuse and perpetrator type be submitted by state survey agencies in CMS's databases for deficiency, complaint, and facility-reported incident data, and that CMS systematically assess trends in these data. (Recommendation 1)

This was CMS response to the GAO recommendation:

> HHS concurred with this recommendation. In February 2020, HHS said CMS is developing the ability to review survey trends related to alleged perpetrator and alleged abuse types and aims to implement this recommendation by December 2020.

The son of 87-year-old resident who had Alzheimer's disease and died four days after a resident with dementia pushed him and caused him to hit his head on the floor and sustain a blunt head trauma (determined in autopsy as the cause of death) said:

> We want to see a solution. We do not want the death of our father to be in vain . . . We are out to find a solution. To make sure that our aging population is taken care of. I want to see something done so this doesn't happen again.

Thanks for your consideration,
Yours sincerely,
Eilon Caspi, Ph.D.
Gerontologist and Dementia Behavior Specialist
Assistant Research Professor
Institute for Collaboration on Health, Intervention, and Policy
University of Connecticut

Adjunct Faculty
School of Nursing
University of Minnesota

Founder and Director
Dementia Behavior Consulting LLC

Founding Member and Board Member
Elder Voice Family Advocates

Board Member
Long-Term Care Community Coalition, NYC

Editorial Board Member
Journal of Elder Abuse and Neglect

Statement of Michael G. Bindner

Center for Fiscal Equity
14448 Parkvale Road, Suite 6
Rockville, MD 20853

Chairman Wyden and Ranking Member Crapo, thank you for the opportunity to submit these comments for the record to the Subcommittee. I will not pull any punches.

This crisis is worse than you think. For whatever reason, the Coronavirus Task Force has ignored the first round of symptoms of this ailment. In my experience, it begins as a cold with heavy mucus. Bad timing made many sufferers believe that they had merely suffering from hay fever. There is then a week of dormancy. If you assume that exposure occurs 2 weeks prior to the first symptoms, there are four weeks, rather than two, before SARS symptoms are manifested, including fever, fatigue from low oxygen levels and fatigue from the manufacture of immunity (which feels like a gut punch over a 2-week period).

Ignoring the early symptoms in CDC guidelines means that, even with the best of care, the pandemic can blow through the nursing population before anyone realizes that COVID is running amok. The continuing denial of this model means that the disease will continue unabated until it runs out of vectors—meaning that vulnerable patients will continue to die until vaccinated.

On the positive side, our experience is that once one has marked symptoms, full immunity is most likely. Young people, who laughed off the early symptoms of the virus or simply did not experience it, are now getting sick. This could lead to another round of reinfection in nursing homes staffed with younger workers. Older workers, who likely have had symptoms, are now safer care givers for the elderly.

One of the developments no one talks about is the shedding of PPE. Healthcare workers see patients when they are after the contagious stage. Heavy PPE frightened people with the virus in the first wave had them avoid care until it was too late. Publicizing this will get people into care faster. Fearing death becomes a self-fulfilling prophecy when care given early will save lives.

Getting nursing home patients into a hospital setting will preserve their lives. Leaving their care to nursing home staff, especially when the disease is first evident, means that residents will get care from rookies. This is not a disease that tolerates mistakes in care.

COVID mortality has hastened death for older victims. Those who would have died of a heart attack within the next five years likely died this past year. We will see how high COVID deaths reach in comparison to heart attack death for the year. I suspect the latter will be down and the former may be second to cancer, if not the number one cause of death this year.

In comments provided to congressional committees last summer, I predicted at least 120 deaths per 100,000 individuals in the population. I had assumed that the nation would have done better than New York, which at the time had 150 deaths per 100,000. If mortality mirrors New York from that period, 500,000 people would have died. We have exceeded the more pessimistic estimate by tens of thousands.

Careful chart review will likely show under-reporting, so true death rates may turn out to approach 1,000,000 deaths. Let this sink in for a moment.

This virus originally did not hurt younger people. The latest variant is now making them very ill, but is less likely to kill them. By the time vaccines are available to them, they will have already been ill.

The science is now showing that children have more robust immune systems. To them, COVID–19 is just another cold virus to fight off. Their immune systems are in high gear. For this reason, vaccinating them will be a mistake. They need to build their immune systems by getting sick and recovering. Robbing them of this experience leaves them vulnerable to the next pandemic. They need to play in the dirt and with each other, even when sick. Colds are not Ebola. Treating it as such is counter-survival for the species.

Why were older people more vulnerable at first? Older citizens are farther away from having colds and being exposed to them. Current precautions also degrade immunity because it is not challenged. This is also why Influenza is so dangerous to nursing home residents. Older citizens who are not in a nursing home, especially those in a multi-generational household, are less likely to become sick, primarily because their immune systems are challenged by their snot-nosed grandchildren.

Any parent will confirm that their younger children are constantly sick and that they share the pain—much to the horror of co-workers—although having sick parents come to work also spreads manageable illness. Being shielded, however, leaves one vulnerable to symptoms. My daughter is with her mother in Knoxville. I got sick. My ex-wife probably will not, especially as she has just had her second shot.

A major problem in getting care is our insurance system. A single-payer system, either through a public option, Medicare for All or cooperative care through employee-owned and provided medicine, including nursing homes, will save lives in the next pandemic.

The attachment presented in 2019 is still as timely as it was then. Even more so, since it covers the public option within the Affordable Care and American Recovery Acts. If pre-existing conditions were repealed, for profit insurance would move more people to the public option each year, which would be their undoing. Single-payer health care as part of a bailout of the industry would be the natural result.

A recent paper by the National Bureau of Economic Research asking "Does Private Equity Investment in Healthcare Benefit Patients? Evidence from Nursing Homes" is essential in addressing this issue. I commend it to your attention.

Thank you for the opportunity to address the committee. We are, of course, available for direct testimony or to answer questions by members and staff.

Attachment—Single-Payer, June 12, 2019

There is no logic in rewarding people with good genes and punishing those who were not so lucky (which, I suspect, is most of us). Nor is there logic in giving health insurance companies a subsidy in finding the healthy and denying coverage for the sick, except the logic of the bottom line. Another term for this is piracy. Insurance companies, on their own, resist community rating and voters resist mandates—especially the young and the lucky. As recent reforms are inadequate (aside from the fact of higher deductibles and the exclusion of undocumented workers), some form of single-payer is inevitable. There are three methods to get to single-payer.

The first to set up a public option and end protections for pre-existing conditions and mandates. The public option would then cover all families who are rejected for either pre-existing conditions or the inability to pay. In essence, this is an expansion of Medicaid to everyone with a pre-existing condition. As such, it would be funded through increased taxation, which will be addressed below. A variation is the expansion of the Uniformed Public Health Service to treat such individuals and their families.

The public option is inherently unstable over the long term. The profit motive will ultimately make the exclusion pool grow until private insurance would no longer be justified, leading again to Single Payer if the race to cut customers leads to no one left in private insurance who is actually sick. This eventually becomes Medicare for All, but with easier passage and sudden adoption as private health plans are either banned or become bankrupt. Single-payer would then be what occurs when

The second option is Medicare for All, which I described in an attachment to yesterday's testimony and previously in hearings held May 8, 2019 (Finance) and May 8, 2018 (Ways and Means). Medicare for All is essentially Medicaid for All without the smell of welfare and with providers reimbursed at Medicare levels, with the difference funded by tax revenue.

Medicare for All is a really good slogan, at least to mobilize the base. One would think it would attract the support of even the Tea Partiers who held up signs saying "Don't let the government touch my Medicare!" Alas, it has not. This has been a conversation on the left and it has not gotten beyond shouting slogans either. We need to decide what we want and whether it really is Medicare for All. If we want to go to any doctor we wish, pay nothing and have no premiums, then that is not Medicare.

There are essentially two Medicare's, a high option and a low one. One option has Part A at no cost (funded by the Hospital Insurance Payroll Tax and part of Obama-care's high unearned income tax as well as the general fund), Medicare Part B, with a 20% copay and a $135 per month premium and Medicare Part D, which has both premiums and copays and is run through private providers. Parts A and B also are contracted out to insurance companies for case management. Much of this is now managed care, as is Medicare Advantage (Part C).

Obamacare has premiums with income-based supports and copays. It may have a high option, like the Federal Employee Health Benefits Program (which also covers Congress) on which it is modeled, a standard option that puts you into an HMO. The HMO drug copays for Obamacare are higher than for Medicare Part C, but the office visit prices are exactly the same.

What does it mean, then, to want Medicare for All? If it means we want everyone who can afford it to get Medicare Advantage Coverage, we already have that. It is Obamacare. The reality is that Senator Sanders wants to reduce Medicare copays and premiums to Medicaid levels and then slowly reduce eligibility levels until everyone is covered. Of course, this will still likely give us HMO coverage for everyone except the very rich, unless he adds a high-option PPO or reimbursable plan.

Either Medicare for All or a real single payer would require a very large payroll tax (and would eliminate the HI tax) or an employer paid subtraction value added tax (so it would not appear on receipts nor would it be zero rated at the border, since there would be no evading it), which we discuss below, because the Health Care Reform debate is ultimately a tax reform debate. Too much money is at stake for it to be otherwise, although we may do just as well to call Obamacare Medicare for All.

The third option is an exclusion for employers, especially employee-owned and cooperative firms, who provide medical care directly to their employees without third party insurance, with the employer making HMO-like arrangements with local hospitals and medical practices for inpatient and specialist care.

Employer-based taxes, such as a subtraction VAT or payroll tax, will provide an incentive to avoid these taxes by providing such care. Employers who fund catastrophic care or operate nursing care facilities would get an even higher benefit, with the proviso that any care so provided be superior to the care available through Medicaid or Medicare for All. Making employers responsible for most costs and for all cost savings allows them to use some market power to get lower rates.

This proposal is probably the most promising way to arrest health care costs from their current upward spiral—as employers who would be financially responsible for this care through taxes would have a real incentive to limit spending in a way that individual taxpayers simply do not have the means or incentive to exercise. The employee-ownership must ultimately expand to most of the economy as an alternative to capitalism, which is also unstable as income concentration becomes obvious to all.

The Key to Any Single-Payer Option Is Securing a Funding Stream

While payroll taxes are the standard suggestion, there are problems with progressivity if such taxes are capped and because profit remains untaxed, which requires the difference be subsidized through higher income taxes. For this reason, funding should come through some form of value-added tax.

Timelines are also concerns. Medicare for All be done gradually by expanding the pool of beneficiaries, regardless of condition. Relying on a Public Option will first serve the poorest and the sickest, but with the expectation that private insurance will enlarge the pool of those not covered until the remainder can safely be incorporated into a single-payer system through legislation or bankruptcy.

Statement of Toby S. Edelman, Senior Policy Attorney

Center for Medicare Advocacy
1025 Connecticut Avenue, NW, Suite 709
Washington, DC 20036

The Center for Medicare Advocacy is a national non-profit law organization founded in 1986. The Center provides legal assistance, education, analysis, and advocacy to advance access to comprehensive Medicare coverage and high quality care for older people and people with disabilities. The Center focuses on the concerns of people with chronic conditions and those in need of long-term care. The organization's positions and actions are based on the experiences of the people we hear from every day.

Thank you for holding this important hearing on COVID–19 in the nation's nursing homes. The experience of COVID–19 is indeed a national tragedy. Although the early days of the coronavirus pandemic were especially chaotic, when little was known about asymptomatic spread of the virus, there is no question that better staffing and infection control practices could have prevented, and, in some facilities, did prevent, many cases and deaths among residents and staff.[247]

The coronavirus pandemic has exacerbated longstanding problems in the nation's nursing homes and brought them all too vividly to national attention. These problems must be corrected to ensure that the next public health crisis does not result, again, in such devastation, overwhelming loss of life, and serious harm to residents' health and quality of life.[248]

---

[247] Cinnamon St. John, "Geography Is Not Destiny: Protecting Nursing Home Residents from the Next Pandemic" (Feb. 2021), *https://medicareadvocacy.org/wp-content/uploads/2021/02/CMA-NH-Report-Geography-is-Not-Dest iny.pdf.*

[248] Michael Levere, Patricia Rowan, Andrea Wysocki, "The adverse events of the COVID–19 pandemic on nursing home resident well-being," *Journal of the American Medical Directors Association* (Journal Pre-proof published Mar. 2021), *https://www.jamda.com/article/S1525-8610(21)00306-6/pdf* (documenting negative consequences of pandemic on Connecticut nursing home residents, including increases in depression, unplanned weight loss, and incontinence and deterioration in cognitive function, resulting from residents' loneliness and isolation).

Longstanding Problems

Inadequate Nurse Staffing Levels, Both Professional and Paraprofessional

The lack of sufficient numbers of nursing staff has been known for decades. In 2000, a federal study mandated by the 1987 Nursing Home Reform Law documented that more than 90 percent of nursing facilities did not have sufficient staff to prevent avoidable harm or to meet standards of care set out in the Reform Law.[249] Staffing levels have not changed in the two decades since the report was issued, despite the increased frailty and acuity of the resident population.

The coronavirus pandemic has continued to highlight the dire consequences of inadequately staffing nursing facilities. Study after study documents that facilities without sufficient nursing staff have both more cases of COVID–19 and more deaths from the virus.[250] A study of nursing facilities in Connecticut found that 20 minutes of additional registered nurse care per resident per day was correlated with 22% fewer COVID–19 cases among residents and 26% fewer deaths.[251]

In January 2021, the New York State Attorney General found "Staffing was more determinative of death rates than 'COVID–19 geography' during the initial wave of the pandemic."[252] Attorney General James found that although the harshest impact of COVID–19 was in New York City and neighboring counties at the beginning of the pandemic, the death rate was half in facilities in this geographic area that had the highest (5-star) ratings in staffing.

The direct care workforce also needs to be strengthened. The paraprofessional workers who provide most of the hands-on care for residents need a living wage[253] and comprehensive benefits, including paid sick leave.[254] Over the past year, the virus has been spread to residents and staff by infected but asymptomatic workers who work in multiple facilities, often because they earn such low wages, minimum wage or just above minimum wage, that they need multiple jobs to try to make ends meet and pay their bills. Direct care workers frequently lack health insurance and paid sick leave, leading them to work when sick.[255]

---

[249] CMS, *Report to Congress: Appropriateness of Minimum Nurse Staffing Ratios* (2001).

[250] CMA Alert, "Studies Find Higher Nurse Staffing Levels in Nursing Facilities Are Correlated With Better Containment of COVID–19" (Aug. 13, 2020), *https://medicareadvocacy.org/studies-find-higher-nurse-staffing-levels-in-nursing-facilities-are-correlated-with-better-containment-of-covid-19/*(citing multiple studies). *See also* Jose F. Figueroa, Rishi K. Wadhera, Irene Papanicolas, et al. "Association of Nursing Home Ratings on Health Inspections, Quality of Care, and Nurse Staffing With COVID–19 Cases," *JAMA Network* (Aug. 10, 2020), *https://jamanetwork.com/journals/jama/fullarticle/2769437?guestAccessKey=258f9d19-b7c2-43e2-9218-55c23d3914bc&utm_source=silverchair&utm_medium=email&utm_campaign=article_alert-jama&utm_content=olf&utm_term=081020.*

[251] Yue Li, H. Temkin-Greener, S. Gao, X. Cai, "COVID–19 infections and deaths among Connecticut nursing home residents: facility correlates," *Journal of American Geriatrics Society* (2020), *https://onlinelibrary.wiley.com/doi/epdf/10.1111/jgs.16689.*

[252] New York State Office of the Attorney General Letitia James, *Nursing Home Response to COVID–19 Pandemic,* p. 30 (revised Jan. 30, 2021), *https://ag.ny.gov/sites/default/files/2021-nursinghomesreport.pdf.*

[253] LeadingAge recently released a report finding that paying a living wage to the direct care workforce could pay for itself, just by improving care for residents. *Making Care Work Pay: How Paying at Least a Living Wage to Direct Care Workers Could Benefit Care Recipients, Workers, and Communities, https://leadingage.org/sites/default/files/Making%20Care%20Work%20Pay%20Report.pdf?_ga=2.118488393.1154178586.1601481977-1021098696.1598989890.*

[254] PHI, *Caring for the Future: The Power and Potential of America's Direct Care Workforce* (Jan. 12, 2021), reached through a link at Caring for the Future: The Power and Potential of America's Direct Care Workforce—PHI *(phinational.org).*

[255] Harold Van Houtven, Nicole DePasquale, Norma B. Coe, "Essential Long-Term Care Workers Commonly Hold Second Jobs and Double- or Triple-Duty Caregiving Roles," *Journal of the American Geriatrics Society,* Vol. 68,

Poor Infection Control Practices

In May 2020, the Government Accountability Office (GAO) reported that infection control was the most frequently cited deficiency in nursing homes in the prepandemic period 2013–2017, with 40 percent of facilities cited each year and 82 percent cited at least once in the 5-year period.[256] The guidance for COVID–19 is no different from the guidance for all infections: staff must wash their hands, properly disinfect medical equipment between residents, properly and consistently use personal protective equipment, and identify, track, and isolate residents who appear to have, or who are confirmed to have, infectious diseases.

Limited Enforcement of Standards of Care

The GAO reports that only one percent of facilities cited with an infection control deficiency between 2013 and 2017 received any kind of financial penalty.[257] Facilities ignore deficiencies when they know deficiencies are unlikely to be cited and, if cited, unlikely to lead to any consequence.

The Trump Administration dramatically rolled back the already-weak federal enforcement system, largely through sub-regulatory guidance documents (survey and certification letters addressed to state survey agencies).[258] The result of the changes has been few and comparatively small per instance financial penalties (rather than per day penalties that the Obama Administration mandated as the default type of civil money penalty). The few reported decisions by Administrative Law Judges that have been issued since the Trump Administration decimated the enforcement system suggest that no financial penalties were imposed for facilities' noncompliance or that penalties were so low that facilities chose not to appeal or both.

Solutions

Require Meaningful Nurse Staffing Levels and Reverse the Dismantling of the Enforcement System

The Senate Finance Committee must require meaningful nurse staffing ratios at all levels and require improved salaries, benefits, and working conditions for the para-professional workforce. The Committee further needs to call on the Centers for Medicare and Medicaid Services to reverse the dismantling of the enforcement system so that meaningful and appropriate sanctions are promptly imposed for non-compliance with federal standards of care.

Issue 8, pp. 1657–1660 (published Apr. 27, 2020), *https://agsjournals.onlinelibrary.wiley.com/doi/10.1111/jgs.16509.*

256 "Infection Control Deficiencies Were Widespread and Persistent in Nursing Homes Prior to COVID–19 Pandemic," GAO–20–576R, p. 4 (May 20, 2020), *https://www.gao.gov/products/GAO-20-576R.*

257 *Id.*

258 See Jordan Rau, "Trump Administration Eases Nursing Home Fines in Victory for Industry," *The New York Times* (Dec. 24, 2017), *https://www.nytimes.com/2017/12/24/business/trump-administration-nursing-home-penalties.html?searchResultPosition=2;* Toby S. Edelman, "Deregulating Nursing Homes," *Bifocal,* Vol. 39, No. 3, p. 31 (Jan.–Feb. 2018), *final-bifocal_39_3.pdf (americanbar.org)*; testimony of Toby S. Edelman at Hearing before House Ways and Means Committee, Subcommittee on Health, "Examining the COVID–19 Nursing Home Crisis (Jun. 25, 2020), *https://waysandmeans.house.gov/sites/democrats.waysandmeans.house.gov/files/documents/Toby%20Edelman_Testimony.pdf.*

In addition, the Committee needs to address changes in the nursing home industry since the 1987 Nursing Home Reform Law was enacted that have reduced accountability for the quality of care that facilities provide and for public spending.

Enact Laws to Prohibit or at Least Restrict/Reduce Provider Self-Dealing

Jordan Rau of Kaiser Health News reported in *The New York Times* 3 years ago that nearly three-quarters of all nursing facilities in the country buy goods and services, such as therapy services, management services, medications, and rent, often at inflated prices, from companies that they own and control.[259] The result of these related-party transactions is that facilities are able to hide profits as the cost of doing business. In 2015, facilities' contracts with related parties accounted for $11 billion, a tenth of facilities' Medicare reimbursement. Rau described two New York owners whose family trusts took $40 million of the $145 million that their facilities received as reimbursement over an 8-year period—a 28 percent profit margin. Rau reported Kaiser Health News's analysis that found facilities engaging in these practices have fewer nurses and aides to provide care to residents, "higher rates of patient injuries and unsafe practices," and twice as many complaints as other facilities.

In December 2020, Debbie Cenziper and colleagues at *The Washington Post* documented the self-dealing of California's largest nursing home operator, Brius Healthcare Services, whose nursing facilities paid $103 million to related companies in 2018 for supplies, administrative services and financial consulting, and rent, among other services.[260] Care at many Brius facilities was so poor that, in 2014, then-California Attorney General Kamala Harris took an unprecedented step of filing an emergency motion in bankruptcy court in an effort to prevent the court from giving Brius additional facilities. Harris's motion called the company a "serial violator of rules within the skilled nursing industry."

The Naples Daily News reported in 2018 that Consulate Health Care, the largest nursing home operator in Florida and sixth largest operator in the country (with 210 facilities and 22,059 beds in 21 states), founded in 2006 and owned by the Atlanta-based private equity firm Formation Capital, designed its facilities "to appear cash-strapped."[261] The article described the chain's individual facilities as "essentially empty shells, they pay rent, management and rehabilitation service fees to Consulate or Formation Capital-affiliated companies." One Consulate facility paid $467,022 in management fees and $294,564 in rent to two companies owned by Consulate and Formation Capital. Forty-eight of Consulate's 77 Florida nursing facilities had one or two stars, the lowest ratings, on the federal website, then called Nursing Home Compare. In "an unprecedented action" in January 2018, the state threatened to close 53 of the corporation's 77 Florida facilities under a state law that authorizes revocation of state licenses for serious violations at facilities under common ownership.[262]

---

[259] Jordan Rau, "Care Suffers as More Nursing Homes Feed Money Into Corporate Webs," *The New York Times* (Jan. 2, 2018), *https://www.nytimes.com/2018/01/02/business/nursing-homes-care-corporate.html?searchResultPosition=9.*

[260] Debbie Cenziper, "Profit and pain: How California's largest nursing home chain amassed millions as scrutiny mounted," *Washington Post* (Dec. 31, 2020), *https://www.washingtonpost.com/business/2020/12/31/brius-nursing-home.*

[261] Ryan Mills and Melanie Payne, "Neglected: Florida's largest nursing home owner represents trend toward corporate control," *Naples Daily News* (May 31, 2018), *https://www.naplesnews.com/story/news/special-reports/2018/05/31/floridas-largest-nursing-home-owner-part-growing-national-trend/581511002/.*

[262] Ryan Mills and Melanie Payne, "Neglected: Florida's largest nursing home chain survives despite legacy of poor patient care," *Naples Daily News* (May 31, 2018), *https://www.naplesnews.com/story/news/special-reports/2018/05/31/neglected-fraud-and-abuse-nursing-homes-florida/542609002/.*

Enact Laws (with Enforceable Consequences for Violations) Limiting the Amount of Public Reimbursement That Can Be Spent on Profits, Administration, and Overhead

A financial issue related to self-dealing is the need for new federal and state rules to require facilities to spend designated portions of their reimbursement on care of residents and to set, and enforce, strict limits on how much can be spent on administrative costs, management fees, and profits. Congress enacted such rules, called medical loss ratios, in the Affordable Care Act for Medicare managed care plans. The state of New Jersey recently enacted legislation for nursing facilities to mandate direct care ratios, which limit the percentage of reimbursement that can be spent on administrative costs and profits.[263]

Congress should enact direct care ratio requirements for the Medicare and Medicaid reimbursement that facilities receive.

Enact Laws (with Enforceable Consequences for Violations) Identifying Who Is Eligible to Own and Manage Nursing Facilities

Nursing facilities are bought and sold and management contracts are signed with virtually no oversight and few limits set by states. Increasingly, multiple limited liability companies take pieces of a nursing home business. With multiple companies, it is difficult, and intentionally so,[264] for government and private parties to hold facilities accountable for poor care.

Secrecy surrounds changes of ownership and management. The example of Skyline Healthcare is illustrative. Beginning in late 2015, the New Jersey-based Skyline Healthcare took over management of more than 100 facilities across the country in little more than year. Almost as quickly as it acquired facilities, Skyline began to default, failing to pay vendors and staff. States across the country went to court to get receiverships in order to be able to pay vendors and staff and provide residents with food and medications.[265] Information about new owners was often kept secret. On April 27, 2018, for example, Pennsylvania installed a temporary manager at nine facilities operated by Skyline, but the state declined to identify the manager.[266] As reported on May 5, Pennsylvania identified as the new operator of the Skyline facility in Lancaster a new for-profit company that had been created just three days earlier, on May 2. The so-called new operator was not actually new. It had at least two of the same owners and shared the address of a company, Priority Healthcare Group, that had actually bought 14 facilities in the state in 2016.[267] Priority's record managing 11 former Golden Living facilities in Pennsylvania was poor. Priority cut staffing levels and reduced other spending at the

---

[263] A4482/S2758, *https://www.njleg.state.nj.us/2020/Bills/A4500/4482_*R2.PDF; "Governor Murphy Signs Legislative Package to Strengthen the Resiliency and Preparedness of New Jersey's Long-Term Care Industry" (News Release, Sep. 16, 2020), *https://www.nj.gov/governor/news/news/562020/approved/20200916b.shtml.*

[264] Joseph E. Casson and Julia McMillen, "Protecting Nursing Home Companies: Limiting Liability Through Corporate Restructuring," *Journal of Health Law,* Fall 2003, Vol. 36, No. 4.

[265] Laura Strickler, Stephanie Gosk, Shelby Hanssen, "A nursing home chain grows too fast and collapses, and elderly and disabled residents pay the price," NBC News (Jul. 19, 2019), *https://www.nbcnews.com/health/aging/nursing-home-chain-grows-too-fast-collapses-elderly-disabled-residents-n1025381.*

[266] Harold Brubaker, "Pa. ousts Skyline Healthcare from nine Pa. nursing homes," *Philadelphia Inquirer* (May 2, 2018), *Pa. ousts Skyline Healthcare from nine Pa. nursing homes (inquirer.com).*

[267] Heather Stauffer, "Lancaster nursing home formerly run by Skyline has a new operator," Lancasteronline (May 26, 2018), *https://lancasteronline.com/news/local/lancaster-nursing-home-formerly-run-by-skyline-has-a-new/article_7df1ad0a-6057-11e8-937b-3393e543dbb7.html.*

facilities.[268] Yet this is the so-called new company that Pennsylvania entrusted with a former Skyline facility.

State licensure rules governing ownership and management are openly flouted. For example, New York purchasers of five nursing facilities in Vermont began operating the facilities in October 2020,[269] before going through a new state review process for nursing home sales that requires consideration of past records at other facilities.[270] The New Yorkers' record includes Priority Healthcare Group, whose Pennsylvania facilities were cited with low staffing levels and poor quality care.[271]

The federal government appears to believe that any facility with a state license is eligible for Medicare and Medicaid certification, no questions asked. The abandonment of state or federal responsibility and actions to ensure that only qualified owners and managers own and operate nursing facilities has led to the growing concentration of nursing facilities in private equity firms, real estate investment trusts, and other private owners that have little apparent knowledge about or interest in providing high quality care, to the detriment of residents and staff. This issue is not new but has only gotten worse over time.

More than 25 years ago, in 1994, Jon Robertson formed Phoenix Health Group and acquired nursing facilities in California. *The Los Angeles Times* reported in 1997, "As the money began to roll in from Medicare and Medi-Cal payments to the more than 300 residents at the facilities, Robertson, who had long displayed a fondness for life's pricier pleasures— from Harley-Davidson motorcycles to diamond rings— began to spend conspicuously."[272] In 1996, Robertson checked into a rehabilitation center in Phoenix to deal with a cocaine addiction. Robertson also "served prison time and owed $150,000 in restitution to the IRS for filing a false tax return as president of another nursing home management company."[273] Robertson's California facilities provided poor care for residents and were cited with numerous deficiencies. The company filed for bankruptcy and abruptly closed its facilities.

Despite this record and sometime after his drug rehabilitation and prison sentence, Robertson formed a new company, Utah-based Deseret Health Group. Multiple states gave licenses to facilities owned by Robertson's new company and the federal government certified the facilities for Medicare and Medicaid reimbursement. In early May 2015, Robertson repeated his pattern from California. Deseret abruptly stopped paying for food, medical supplies, and workers' wages and benefits in nursing facilities owned by the company in Kansas, Minnesota, Nebraska, and Wyoming. States pursued court receiverships or otherwise

---

[268] Daniel Simmons-Ritchie, "Worst nursing homes continue to fail the frail despite lawsuit and promises; Golden Living's homes changed hands, but the care never got better," *PennLive* (Nov. 26, 2018), *https://www.witf.org/2018/11/26/worst-nursing-homes-continue-to-fail-the-frail-despite-lawsuit-and-promises/.*

[269] Katie Jickling, "Three New York-based owners take over management of five Genesis nursing homes," *Vtdigger* (Nov. 13, 2020), *https://vtdigger.org/2020/11/13/three-new-york-based-owners-takes-over-management-of-five-genesis-nursing-homes/.*

[270] Bill No. 125, 2018, establishing Nursing Home Oversight Working Group and (section 3) an Interim Review Process for Transfer of Nursing Home Ownership (effective July 1, 2018), *https://legislature.vermont.gov/Documents/2018/Docs/ACTS/ACT125/ACT125%20As%20En acted.pdf; signed by Governor May 10, 2018, hj180510.pdf (vermont.gov).*

[271] Daniel Simmons-Ritchie, "Worst nursing homes continue to fail the frail despite lawsuit and promises; Golden Living's homes changed hands, but the care never got better," *PennLive* (Nov. 26, 2018), *https://www.witf.org/2018/11/26/worst-nursing-homes-continue-to-fail-the-frail-despite-lawsuit-and-promises/.*

[272] Eric Slater, "Entrepreneur Fades From View as Empire Collapses," *Los Angeles Times* (Oct. 23, 1997), *https://www.latimes.com/archives/la-xpm-1997-oct-23-mn-45876-story.html.*

[273] The Associated Press, "Utah company facing bankruptcy; nursing home residents in limbo," *The Salt Lake Tribune* (May 13, 2015).

took control of the facilities to protect residents and ensure they received food and medications.[274]

Private equity ownership of nursing homes has created special problems. In 2007, *The New York Times* reported "more profit and less nursing" in facilities owned by private equity firms.[275]

A research study looking at nursing home ownership between 2000 and 2017 found that private equity (PE) ownership increased the probability of death during a resident's stay by 1.7 percentage points (meaning that "about 20,150 Medicare lives [were] lost due to PE ownership") while Medicare costs for residents' care increased by 11 percent.[276] Facilities owned by private equity firms reduced staffing and increased, by 50 percent, the use of antipsychotic drugs.

During the coronavirus pandemic, *The Washington Post* reported that Portopiccolo Group, a private equity firm with a record of poor care (nearly 70 percent of Portopiccolo facilities have ratings of one or two (of five) on the federal website), short staffing, and coronavirus outbreaks, bought at least 22 nursing facilities, with "scant scrutiny" from state regulators in Maryland and Virginia.[277] As in the facilities it already owned, Portopiccolo reduced operating expenses (reducing cleaning supplies and personal protective equipment) and reduced workers' benefits. The results were poorer care for residents.

A February 2021 posting in *Health Affairs* made these points in a scathing indictment of the nursing home industry:

> Prior to the pandemic, persistent problems with nursing home care had been documented for years, often because of too few and inadequately trained front-line staff. The harm to frail older adults can be quite severe—abuse and sexual assault, infections, overuse of psychotropic medications, pressure ulcers, falls with injuries, weight loss, dehydration, pain, and medication errors. Infection control violations have also been found repeatedly in a majority of nursing homes.
>
> Quality issues persist as policy makers are unable to oversee how nursing homes spend Medicare and Medicaid payments. The growth in complex nursing-home ownership structures has limited financial transparency by allowing nursing homes to hide public payments and stint on direct resident care. We recommend specific policy changes to make ownership, management, and financing more transparent and accountable to improve U.S. nursing home care.[278]

---

[274] *See*, e.g., H.B. Lawson, "Nursing home faces closure," *The Saratoga Sun* (May 6, 2015), *https://www.saratogasun.com/story/2015/05/06/news/nursing-home-faces-closure/3898.html*.

[275] Charles Duhigg, "At Many Nursing Homes, More Profit and Less Nursing," *The New York Times* (Sep. 23, 2007), *https://www.nytimes.com/2007/09/23/business/23nursing.html*.

[276] Atul Gupta, Sabrina T. Howell, Constantine Yannelis, and Abhinav Gupta, "Does Private Equity Investment in Healthcare Benefit Patients? Evidence from Nursing Homes," Becker Friedman Institute, Working Paper No. 2021–20 (Feb. 2021), *https://bfi.uchicago.edu/wp-content/uploads/2021/02/BFI_WP_2021-20.pdf*.

[277] Rebecca Tan and Rachel Chason, "An investment firm snapped up nursing homes during the pandemic. Employees say care suffered," *The Washington Post* (Dec. 21, 2020), *https://www.washingtonpost.com/local/portopiccolo-nursing-homes-maryland/2020/12/21/a1ffb2a6-292b-11eb-9b14-ad872157ebc9_story.html*.

[278] Charlene Harrington, Anne Montgomery, Terris King, David C. Grabowski, Michael Wasserman, "These Administrative Actions Would Improve Nursing Home Ownership and Financial Transparency in the Post COVID–19 Period," *Health Affairs* (Feb. 11, 2021), *https://www.healthaffairs.org/do/10.1377/hblog20210208.597573/full/*.

The Committee should address the issue of nursing home ownership and management and enact, with appropriate enforcement mechanisms, meaningful statutory standards for state licensure and federal certification.

Conclusion

Staffing is the critical factor that makes good care possible. Unless facilities have sufficient professional and paraprofessional staff and treat all staff well, care will not improve. Improving staffing is absolutely necessary, but it is not sufficient.

In addition, states and the federal government need to limit licensure and certification, respectively, to owners and managers that are knowledgeable about and demonstrate commitment and the financial capacity to provide high quality care to residents. Finally, public reimbursement must be spent on care for residents and not diverted to management fees, overhead, and excessive profits.

Many of these issues have been raised before.[279] The Committee now has the opportunity to dramatically improve care for residents and working conditions for workers by addressing these issues.

Statement Submitted by Elizabeth Hamilton

Thank you, Chairman Wyden, Ranking Member Crapo, and members of the Senate Finance Committee, for allowing additional statements to this hearing. My name is Elizabeth Hamilton. My mother is 96 years old and currently is a resident in a memory care unit in Seattle, Washington.

On March 10, 2021 The Center for Medicaid and Medicare Services (CMS) released updated and expanded guidelines for inside and in person visitation in Nursing Homes. Unfortunately the facility my mother is in has not updated their restrictions to comply with these new guidelines stating they are following state guidelines. The Governor as of this writing has not released any changes to the current restrictions now in place.

Residents of long-term care (LTC) have been languishing in facilities across the nation, in varying degrees of "lockdown" since March 13, 2020. Initially, scores succumbed to a deadly virus we knew little about. Facilities were not prepared; none of us were. Much has changed in a year. It's time for CMS to reinforce adherence to existing guidelines for compassionate care visits, essential caregiver designation, and infection control, and to update its guidance for the safe and strategic reopening of facilities.

LTC facilities now have the capacity to follow proven protocols—masking, social distancing, disinfection, selectively restricted movement. Testing is widely available. Infection and death rates in long-term care have dropped dramatically. Many staff, residents and family members have been (or soon will be) injected and protected with incredibly effective vaccines, far more than they typically are from seasonal flu. A year ago we talked about "protecting the most vulnerable." With proven safety precautions in place, testing available, and vaccinations

---

[279] "Buying and Selling Nursing Homes: Who's Looking Out for the Residents?" (CMA Alert, May 23, 2018), *https://medicareadvocacy.org/buying-and-selling-nursing-homes-whos-looking-out-for-the-residents/.*

given, a year later we are "protecting them to death." At the same time, guidelines allowing for compassionate care visits and essential caregiver designation are being completely ignored by many facilities, and proper infection control is not happening everywhere. You can help eliminate these disparities.

Families have been patient, hunkering down outdoors, even in frigid temperatures, to connect with their loved ones. LTC residents are depressed and despondent, as are staff members. Our loved ones are suffering from increased falls and troubling weight loss. Many have gone nearly a year without a haircut or a thorough teeth cleaning. Some have given up and died quietly, either with no family present or with the requisite one or two family members at their bedsides. The negative physical and emotional toll of these policies on our families far outweighs any benefit.

Some facilities in the nation have begun to open up. But with guidelines from last fall still in place, regardless of vaccine status among residents, an entire facility is still on lockdown for a singular asymptomatic case. This makes no sense. The injury to our loved ones and our families goes on and on.

We need swift delivery of updated, common sense guidelines to safely and strategically open up facilities, balancing vastly decreased risk from the virus with quality of life. You have the ability to end the isolation that has devastated lives in long-term care and reunite our families. We have all suffered long enough. It is time.

Statement Submitted by Tamra Holland

Members of the Senate Finance Committee, thank you for choosing to make the tragedies that occurred residential facilities throughout the United States over the past 13 months a focus of your attention. I write to you as one of thousands of family members painfully familiar with an aspect of this story not well understood by the majority of Americans.

My mother Darlene entered a facility on March 18, 2020 for rehabilitation following a stroke the month before. She had made good physical progress in an acute hospital rehabilitation but needed additional time of daily professional therapies. During the hospital rehabilitation prior the lockdown, family was present with her every day for therapy homework, helping with her personal care and emotional well-being. We knew once transferred to the long-term care rehab facility we would not be able to immediately visit but had faith her care needs would be meet and we would be involved in some manner.

My mother-in-law Joan was also a long-term resident of this facility in the skilled nursing wing. My husband and I visited her regularly and were comfortable with her care.

Having many family members on the front lines of healthcare and a long career in pharmacy myself, I understood the need for a lockdown in March of 2020. The pandemic was a roaring freight train and even the best of facilities needed that sudden stop in visitation. There was not enough known about the virus, there was not enough PPE, residential facilities did not have the infection control policies that the pandemic required. They were not prepared, none of us were.

Having to say goodbye to my Mother as the facility van picked her up at the hospital was heartbreaking. However, at that point I still expected the facility care would be appropriate and she would get the rehabilitation therapy she needed to return to independently living in her apartment. What I found was a facility that suddenly had an overwhelmed phone system and no communication plan for families. I could see through my Mom's window that she was still in bed at noon each day. None of her personal belongings were unpacked or put away. She experienced a fall within the first 48 hours of being in the facility. Mom was confused with the change in environment and no one there to help her acclimate. The staff were used to family helping settle in new residents and personalizing the sterile environment of the room. Staff did not seem aware there was a gap in care because family was not inside the building.

In these early days I expected communication was key to Mom's quality of care and rehabilitation as well as the continued good care of my Mother-in-law Joan. Phone contact was difficult because you could not call directly to the nursing unit to speak to staff. A central operator had difficulty suddenly fielding all communication coming in. Calls then transferred to the nursing unit frequently were never answered. Imagine the anxiety of trying to speak to staff about a loved one's care and listening to the phone ring and ring. This lack of contact, the lack of any direct information lead to an assumption of lack of care. When your mind does not have valid information to deal with it imagines something that can be vastly different than the reality. This was the situation for months as no visiting was allowed. I tried email with the facility director which went unanswered. I left voicemails and phone messages. I left things at the front door for both Darlene and Joan hoping they would know that we still cared about them. Darlene had a cellphone and we sometimes were able to speak to her. However, often the phone was not answered because she could not hear it, could not find it or it wasn't charged. Asking staff to help her with the phone required the same phone contact that I described above. Joan was not able to hold a phone and requesting staff help her was often met with exasperation. I established contact with the facility corporate leadership. At first this seemed it would be productive. I asked for some avenues of communication, establishment of a family council, family newsletter, holiday decorating by family (outside). I offered to help in any or all of these ideas. After a few promises of action by the COO that were left unfulfilled all communications ceased.

I applied for job openings at the facility. I am a pharmacist and have during my career done medication record reviews in skilled nursing facilities. I learned that this required monthly reviewed of each patient's record had been suspended at the beginning of the lockdown. The process had gone virtual but with much of the record only on paper a full review was impossible. I applied to work in the kitchen only to be told by human resources even if I was allowed the job, I would be assigned a hallway away from whatever one Darlene or Joan was on. It was a comment rooted in sear meanness. I continued to apply for an ongoing job opening in the food service for months. I never got a response from anyone at the facility about it.

Darlene had some health needs that required physician visits. Each of these were a struggle to schedule. Even when the facility had no cases of COVID, Darlene's right to medical care was questioned at every turn. As the months of the lockdown continued this only grew more difficult. At a time when a single positive case in a separate hallway from Darlene's, and she herself had tested negative, the facility canceled a medically necessary appointment. They did this prior to even discussing it with me her POA. I was livid. I knew how essential this appointment was. I knew the ADON was wrong to deny it and it was not only within Darlene's rights to go but also critical to her health. I pleaded, I argued, I insisted, I requested help from the state ombudsman. My efforts were responded to by a threat of expelling Darlene from the facility by the ADON. That medical appointment was never allowed.

During these months we did window visits. We celebrated Darlene and Joan's birthdays with a window party. We used the iPad. We did outside visits when neither of them could hear us well and a monitor from the facility sat nearby and eased dropped on every word said. We smiled while there and cried all the way home. Wanting only to offer some happiness, some hope, some dignity to these two women that meant so much to us.

In November Darlene suffered a stroke. Although it was a known medical risk for her, I am certain it was brought on by the isolation and lack of hope. Studies have shown that stroke risk is increased by 32% due to isolation. While in the hospital emergency department I was able to be with her. We spent 26 hours holding hands. The facility assured me that she had just gotten a negative COVID test result. Within hours of her admission to the floor a COVID test was performed due to a slight fever, it was positive. With her physical health compromised by the stroke, she could not overcome the virus. She passed away on November 20, 2020. The last 8 months of her life were the saddest of her 82 years.

Joan also contracted COVID at the facility. Although no family were allowed access, staff of course came and went in their daily lives. One after another they tested positive and passed the virus to residents. Joan endured 2 exceptionally lonely weeks in isolation and seemed recovered. Within weeks staff began reporting Joan was not eating and was increasingly weak. The family had end of life discussions. We did not expect her to see the New Year. My husband and his sister applied for compassionate care. It was allowed. As family helped Joan eat meals each day her condition improved. Now 3 months later it is clear that her declining health in December was in large part malnutrition. Residents were required to eat in their rooms alone. Staff would set a tray in front of her which she could not functionally manage. Certainly, she has a small appetite at 89 years of age, but her primary reason for not eating was that she could not do it independently. There is not enough staff to feed residents in their rooms one at a time. This Is such a clear example of why family is essential to the health of loved ones in facilities.

There must be changes in the system. There are vast opportunities for learning from this pandemic. Please do not let stories like Darlene and Joan's be wasted by inaction. Long-term residential facilities for the elderly and the developmentally disabled of any age, need to be reformed. After over 30 years in acute healthcare, I know that caregivers at every level want to provide quality care to patients. Physicians, nurses, PA, CNA among others all have a role in each patient's care. They each deserve a workplace that recognizes the value they bring, provides them with a safe workplace and has policies and procedure that allow them to do a quality job. They need to be listened to. They need to be part of the change that is needed.

Families as well need to be involved. They are essential. Communication is such an undervalued tool to improvement. Family councils should be in every facility. Quarterly care plans may be sufficient in normal times when families are seeing their loved ones regularly. However, during the lockdown families should have heard from a caregiver weekly or more. I know hospitals that had nurses call families for updates daily. I find no excuses for the unanswered emails I sent to facility administrators. A busy schedule is no rationalization for months of time without response under the circumstances of the pandemic.

Facilities need to adopt principles that have guided acute healthcare institutions. Quality improvement, staff development, patient centered care principles long held by hospital systems need to be adapted by long-term care corporations. Residents and family that entrust them for care deserve no less.

Residential facilities will always be needed. Medical care cannot always be provided within the home. Families may not have the physical, emotional or financial means to care for loved ones at home. However, experiences and memories of the lockdown threaten the future of these facilities. People are renovating their homes, changing life decisions about care in their later years. Many facilities managed by big corporation are going to have to rethink their priorities to appeal to many again. This is the perfect time for change, real meaningful change that is good for residents, families and facilities.

Thank you all for your attention to the unfortunate effects the lockdown has had on residents and families. Please do let Darlene and Joan's stories be forgotten. Allow the lessons learned to lead to better care. Quality care that this vulnerable population deserves.

Statement Submitted by Gay L. Hull

Hi, my name is Gay Hull and my daughter Mandy Hull resides at Shapiro Developmental Center in Kankakee, IL. Mandy's service providers have shown us throughout the pandemic that they truly care about our daughter, but her Shapiro family cannot replace the love, affection, and enrichment that we provide towards her quality of life.

We have always been very involved parents. Prior to COVID we would travel 21⁄2 hours, every other weekend, to spend the afternoon with Mandy. During these visits we would take her out to eat, shopping at the Mall or Wal-Mart or for long walks at local parks. We have always had her home during all holidays so she could spend time with her brother and sister and we have never missed a birthday celebration. We love the time that we spend with all of our children, but we especially cherish our time with Mandy.

Since COVID started in March of 2020, we were prohibited from visiting Mandy on many, many occasions. Mandy has not done well with these restrictions. This past year has been heartbreaking for all of us. She has been quarantined off and on to her room or the building. She has also not been able to leave her room, go outside to walk or to get some fresh air, spend time with her family, enjoy a variety of daily activities such as campus vocational training, or have access to her favorite foods and snacks. Her behavior has worsened because of these unreasonable restrictions. We feel that these restrictions have been cruel, inhumane, and discriminatory!

Over the past year, we have tried to do everything possible to let her know that we have not deserted or abandoned her . . . that we were still in her world, but Face Timing, phone calls, and mailed care packages, could not possibly replace the physical presence of her parents. Fortunately, we have been granted Compassionate Caregiver designation, thanks to the Illinois Caregivers 4 Compromise and Mandy is able to see us weekly, but she has NO other freedoms.

As her parents, we want safe, reasonable practices. The isolation must stop! Can you please help us? Thank you.

Letter Submitted by Kathy James

Dear Senators,

A year ago I spent a quiet afternoon with my then 89 year old mother in her assisted living facility. We watched Jeopardy together and then the 4:00 news. At 5:00 I wheeled her down to dinner, hugged her goodbye, said see you tomorrow and that was the last time I would touch her even until today. Each day, I go to her window at the facility and call her on her phone to stand and talk to her. I want her to have my presence near so she does not feel alone. She had only been a widow for one year at the start of the pandemic after being married for 69 years. The loneliness is extreme. It is also difficult for her to get around as she is crippled from arthritis. She has had to manage without the help I would give her in keeping her room clean, watering her plants, putting things away. The staff can only help so much. So all the little things that family can do to help fall by the wayside. I was able to see her at a half hour visit last week and I can see her fatigue after just ten minutes of talking. Because she hasn't talked to anyone for that long in over a year. I would ask that you would take very seriously passing legislation so this complete lockout of families never has to happen again. A time limit should be allowed to get protocols in place and then facilities need to open to families. We fight not just for them but for my future and yours. I know I would not be able to handle what she has gone through. And many, many did not. They are no longer here to tell their stories.

Sincerely,
Kathy James

Justice in Aging

1444 Eye Street, NW, Suite 1100
Washington, DC 20005

Justice in Aging appreciates the opportunity to submit a written statement for the record. Justice in Aging is an advocacy organization with the mission of improving the lives of low-income older adults. We use the power of law to fight senior poverty by securing access to affordable health care, economic security, and the courts for older adults with limited resources. We have decades of experience with nursing homes and other forms of long-term services and supports, with a focus on the needs of low-income enrollees and populations that have been marginalized and excluded from justice such as women, people of color, people with disabilities, LGBTQ individuals, and people with limited English proficiency.

Focus of This Statement: Breaking through the Persistent Public Policy Impasse

In the past month, Congress has convened two hearings addressing the need for nursing home reform: the Senate Finance Committee hearing (March 17th), and a hearing on Examining Private Equity's Expanded Role in the U.S. Health Care System, convened by the Oversight Subcommittee of the House Ways and Means Committee (March 25). These hearings have highlighted the persistently poor care provided to this country's nursing home residents. Unfortunately, these problems are anything but new.

As testimony in the Finance Committee hearing demonstrated, the COVID–19 pandemic has exacerbated preexisting problems within nursing homes, including, but not limited to, inadequate staffing and slipshod infection prevention and control practices. The results have been horrific, with approximately 175,000 deaths among residents and staff of long-term care facilities,[280] along with residents being isolated from family members and friends for an entire year.

Many observers have suggested that now, finally, is the time for reforming our nursing home system. But reform is far from assured. Change will require that Congress break through the gridlock that has stymied nursing home public policy for several decades.

To a great extent, the public policy impasse on nursing home reform stems from one central dynamic: providers claim that improvement is impossible, due to allegedly insufficient Medicaid rates. Although they may concede (for example) that facility staffing levels are too low, they resist efforts to establish national staffing minimums, based largely on arguments that Medicaid rates do not support adequate staffing levels. As a result, nursing homes continue to staff at dangerously low levels, which in turn leads to resident injuries and death—before, during and after the pandemic.

In an effort to contribute to public policy solutions, this statement focuses on one important aspect of the current problem: service providers both a) claiming that Medicaid rates are inadequate while b) organizing their finances in such a way that makes it virtually impossible to determine appropriate rates. These counter-productive practices are part of the dynamic that has made nursing home reform an oxymoron for many years.

Nursing Home Residents Suffer due to Inadequate Staffing Levels Linked to Low Wages

Short staffing is a longstanding problem in nursing homes. A recent report found that 48.2% of direct-care workers earned less than a living wage, with approximately 56% relying in part on public assistance.[281] Another study found nursing staff turnover rates of 94% (mean) and 128% (median) over the course of a single year.[282]

Not surprisingly, poor staffing has consequences. A study mandated by the federal Nursing Home Reform Law determined appropriate staffing levels based on facility quality measures, with the recommended levels specific to nurse aides and nurses, and short-term and long-term resident stays in the nursing home. That analysis found that 52 percent of nursing homes failed to meet any of the recommended staffing levels, while a full 97 percent of the nursing homes failed to meet at least one of the recommended levels.[283]

Numerous studies have confirmed this common-sense conclusion: low staffing levels lead to poor resident care. Specific study results include findings that low staffing levels are connected to avoidable hospitalizations, more deficiencies, and poorer nurse aide performance.[284]

---

280 The COVID Tracking Project, The Long-Term Care COVID Tracker (reviewed March 31, 2021), *https://covidtracking.com/nursing-homes-long-term-care-facilities.*

281 Christian Weller et al., LeadingAge, Making Care Work Pay: How Paying at Least a Living Wage to Direct Care Workers Could Benefit Care Recipients, Workers, and Communities, at 8, 10 (2020) *https://leadingage.org/sites/default/files/Making%20Care%20Work%20Pay%20 Report.pdf.*

282 Ashvin Gandhi et al., High Nursing Staff Turnover in Nursing Homes Offers Important Quality Information, *Health Affairs,* vol. 40, no. 3 (March 2021), *https://www.healthaffairs.org/doi/10.1377/hlthaff.2020.00957.*

283 CMS, Appropriateness of Minimum Nurse Staffing Ratios in Nursing Homes; Overview of the Phase II Report: Background, Study Approach, Findings, and Conclusion, at 5 (2001) *https://www.justice.gov/sites/default/files/elderjustice/legacy/2015/07/12/Appropriateness_of_Minimum_Nurse_Staffing_Ratios_in_Nursing_Homes.pdf.*

284 *See,* e.g., William Spector et al., Potentially Avoidable Hospitalizations for Elderly Long-Stay Residents in Nursing Homes, *Medical Care,* vol. 51, no. 8, at 673 (Aug. 2013) (low staffing linked to avoidable

In related findings, studies also have shown a relationship between quality and the staffing levels for registered nurses. Current federal law requires only that a nursing home employ a registered nurse for eight hours daily.[285] Studies have shown that higher staffing levels for registered nurses lead to better care for residents.[286]

Not surprisingly, the ongoing pandemic has only made adequate staffing more consequential. Studies in both Connecticut and California found that higher staffing of registered nurses allowed nursing homes to better limit the spread of COVID–19.[287] Also, these quality of care problems have fallen particularly hard on persons of color. The Connecticut study, for example, found greater COVID–19 spread among nursing homes with higher percentages of residents of color.[288] Furthermore, the same principal author studied nationwide data and found that nursing homes with a greater percentages of residents of color were more likely to suffer COVID–19 cases and deaths.[289] *The New York Times* reached similar conclusions, noting a "striking racial divide" in how COVID–19 afflicted those nursing home with high percentages of Black and Latino residents.[290]

Notably, provider associations acknowledge to a certain extent the inadequacy of current staffing practices. In a recent policy proposal, for example, the American Health Care Association (for-profit facilities) and LeadingAge (non-profit facilities) recognized the need for around-the-clock registered nurses.[291] Likewise, LeadingAge published a report arguing in favor of paying a living wage to direct care workers.[292] In each of these instances, however, provider associations declined to commit to actually taking these positive steps, which they claim must be contingent upon increased Medicaid reimbursement rates.

Nursing Homes Create Complicated Corporate Structures to Hide Profits.

---

hospitalizations), *https://pubmed.ncbi.nlm.nih.gov/23703648/;* Nicholas Castle et al., Caregiver Staffing in Nursing Homes and their Influence on Quality of Care: Using Dynamic Panel Estimation Methods, *Medical Care,* vol. 49, no. 6, at 545 (June 2011) (better staffing linked to better quality), *https://pubmed.ncbi.nlm.nih.gov/21577182/;* Nicholas Castle et al., Nursing Home Deficiency Citations for Safety, *J. Aging and Social Policy,* vol. 23, no. 1, at 34 (Jan. 2011) (low staffing correlated to deficiencies cited by survey agency), *https://www.ncbi.nlm.nih.gov/pmc/articles/PMC4878686/;* John Schnelle et al., Relationship of Nursing Home Staffing to Quality of Care?, *Health Serv. Res.,* vol. 39, no. 2, at 225 (April 2004) (higher staffing linked to better performance by nurse aides), *https://pubmed.ncbi.nlm.nih.gov/15032952/.*

[285] 42 U.S.C. §§ 1395i–3(b)(4)(C)(i), 1396r(b)(4)(C)(i); 42 CFR § 483.35(b).

[286] *See,* e.g., Mary Ellen Dellefield et al., The Relationship Between Registered Nurses and Nursing Home Quality: An Integrative Review (2008–2014), *Nurs. Econ.,* vol. 33, no. 2, at 95 (March–April 2015) (literature review), *https://pubmed.ncbi.nlm.nih.gov/26281280/.*

[287] Yue Li et al., COVID–19 Infections and Deaths Among Connecticut Nursing Home Resident: Facility Correlates, *J. Am. Geriatrics Soc'y,* vol. 68, no. 9, at 1899 (Sept. 2020), *https://agsjournals.onlinelibrary.wiley.com/doi/epdf/10.1111/jgs.16689;* Charlene Harrington et al., Nursing Staffing and Coronavirus Infections in California Nursing Homes, *Policy, Politics, and Nursing Practice,* vol. 21, no. 3, at 174 (2020), *https://journals.sagepub.com/doi/pdf/10.1177/1527154420938707.*

[288] Yue Li et al., COVID–19 Infections and Deaths Among Connecticut Nursing Home Resident: Facility Correlates, at 1903, *https://agsjournals.onlinelibrary.wiley.com/doi/epdf/10.1111/jgs.16689.*

[289] Yue Li et al., Racial and Ethnic Disparities in COVID–19 Infections and Deaths Across U.S. Nursing Homes, *J. Am. Geriatrics Soc'y,* vol. 68, no. 11 (Nov. 2020), *https://pubmed. ncbi.nlm.nih.gov/32955105/.*

[290] Robert Gebeloff et al., Striking Racial Divide: How COVID–19 Has Hit Nursing Homes, *N.Y. Times,* Sept. 10, 2020, *https://www.nytimes.com/2020/05/21/us/coronavirus-nursing-homes-racial-disparity.html#:_:text=the%20main%20story-,The%20Striking%20Racial%20Divide%20in%20How%20Covid%2D19%20Has%20Hit,the%20population%20is%20overwhelmingly%20 white.*

[291] American Health Care Ass'n and LeadingAge, Care for our Seniors Act, Improving America's Nursing Homes by Learning from Tragedy and Implementing Bold Solutions for the Future, at 4 (2021), *https://leadingage.org/sites/default/files/Overview%20-%20Care%20for%20 Our%20Seniors%20Act.pdf.*

[292] Christian Weller et al., LeadingAge, Making Care Work Pay: How Paying at Least a Living Wage to Direct Care Workers Could Benefit Care Recipients, Workers, and Communities, at 30 (2020), *https://leadingage.org/sites/default/files/Making%20Care%20Work%20Pay%20Report. pdf.*

The recent congressional hearings shone a light into common nursing home business practices that frustrate sane public policy. In particular, testimony submitted to the Oversight Subcommittee of the House Ways and Means Committee showed how nursing homes use corporate organizational structures to hide profits.[293] Similarly, a recent academic paper demonstrated how private equity investment in nursing homes has led to a deteriorating quality of care, including unnecessary deaths, increased use of dangerous psychotropic medications, declining mobility, and increased expense.[294]

In testimony submitted to the Oversight Subcommittee, Ernest Tosh clearly explained the gaping holes exploited by the nursing home industry. First, nursing home business practices have corrupted the cost reporting required by CMS. As Mr. Tosh reports, "[o]n the surface the financial information appears to be useful, until one realizes the financial picture of a single facility can be highly manipulated if it is within a chain of nursing homes that also contains multiple related corporations."[295]

These cost reports may show, for example, that a nursing home has annual revenues approaching ten million dollars, but nonetheless is losing money and has relatively few assets. At first glance, such a nursing home may appear to be in precarious financial shape, but that first glance does not take into account the nursing home's many "related party" transactions. The "related parties" are other corporations owned by the same persons or entities that own the nursing home. By contracting with the related parties to provide various aspects of the nursing home's operation—the building itself, for example, or management services, nursing services, or therapy services—the nursing home can claim expenses even though it is essentially paying itself. This allows a nursing home with few assets and purported annual losses to continue operating successfully: the overall corporate structure is profitable, even though the entity holding the nursing home license consistently claims losses.[296]

The written testimony of David Kingsley highlighted a related problem: nursing homes' frequent use of real estate investment trusts (REITs). REITs are used in a common type of related party transaction—the nursing home operator transfers the real property into a REIT, and then leases back the property from the REIT, claiming rent payments as expenses. Like all related party structures, the REITs create false expenses that are actually just transfers within a single corporate structure.[297]

Mr. Kinsley aptly characterizes the nursing home business as "a financial engineering industry engaged in trading property as a commodity and tax arbitrage as a core technique."[298] The web of related party transactions has no justification from a health care perspective. Indeed, to a significant extent, the provision of care—and the quality of such care—is a secondary concern in such business models.

---

[293] *See* Written Testimony of Ernest C. Tosh, Statement of Sabrina T. Howell, Ph.D., and Written Testimony of David E. Kingsley, Ph.D. Mr. Tosh and Prof. Howell also testified in person at the hearing.

[294] Atul Gupta et al., Does Private Equity Investment in Healthcare Benefit Patients? Evidence from Nursing Homes, at 3 (Feb. 2021). The findings of this study constitute much of the material presented by Prof. Sabrina Howell (one of the study's co-authors) during the recent hearing in front of the Oversight Subcommittee of the House Ways and Means Committee.

[295] Tosh Written Testimony at 2.

[296] Tosh Written Testimony at 2–6.

[297] Kingsley Written Testimony at 2–4.

[298] Kingsley Written Testimony at 5.

Congress Should Provide Better Access to Medicaid-Funded At-Home Care, and Limit Nursing Homes' Use of Deceptive Corporate Structures

We make two recommendations to improve care for older Americans in need of daily care. First, Congress should improve access to Medicaid-funded home and community-based services, so that no one is forced to live in a nursing home if they would rather receive necessary services at home. Under current federal law, a state Medicaid program must offer nursing home care to every qualifying person, but home and community-based services can be subject to a waiting list or other limit on enrollment.[299] Congress should make home and community-based services available to all persons qualifying under Medicaid rules. Such equal access to home and community-based services would provide the dual benefit of enabling persons to receive necessary services at home, and give nursing homes a greater incentive to offer quality care and a good quality of life, in order to compete with home and community-based services.

Second, as set forth in this statement, Congress should take steps to prohibit the financial machinations that distort the business of providing nursing home care. Under current business structures, many nursing homes are focused not on providing high quality care, but rather on funneling profit out of a nursing home to related parties. These practices penalize both residents and staff members, and inevitably lead to deterioration, injuries and deaths.

Also, as addressed above, these financial structures prevent honest evaluation of the adequacy of Medicare and Medicaid reimbursement rates. From our perspective, an increase in Medicaid rates could almost never be justified under current practices, because nursing home operators are not being forthcoming about their true financial status.

On a closely related matter, we support calls for greater transparency in nursing home finances, but are skeptical as to whether transparency alone can address the current problems. It is not realistic to expect CMS to perform forensic accounting on the incredibly intricate corporate structures in use today.

And, finally, we assert that it is entirely fair to prohibit certain corporate structures as a condition of Medicare or Medicaid certification. Nursing homes rely on public funding for the bulk of their revenue.[300] Given that relationship, along with the importance of setting appropriate Medicare and Medicaid reimbursement rates, it would be eminently reasonable for Congress to prohibit the corporate structures that currently hamper our ability to make meaningful reforms.

Letter Submitted by Lydia Nunez Landry

Chairman Wyden, Ranking Member Crapo, and distinguished Members of the Committee,

My name is Lydia Nunez Landry and I am writing to you today *not* as someone the American Health Care Association and LeadingAge would reduce to the characterization (in

---

[299] 42 U.S.C. §§ 1396d(a)(4)(A) (obligation to provide nursing home services), 1396n(c) (home and community-based services waivers).

[300] *See,* e.g., Medicaid's Share of Nursing Home Revenue, Resident Days Hits Record High as Medicare Drops to Historic Low, *Skilled Nursing News* (Dec. 11, 2019) (Medicaid and Medicare funding constituting over 72% of overall nursing home revenue) *https://skillednursingnews.com/2019/12/medicaids-share-of-nursing-home-revenue-resident-days-hits-record-high-as-medicare-drops-to-historic-low/.*

their "Care for Our Senior's Act")[301] of a "frail [or] elderly adult with underlying health conditions" at risk of dying from COVID "630 times higher than an 18 to 29" year old, that is, someone these lobbyists designate as prone to death.

Rather, despite reductions of people like me—or any other marginalized group—to underlying health conditions or comorbidities or biased stereotypes, I write to you today as an alive and thriving disabled woman, one who lives in and contributes to her community, and as someone who questions the motives of those who attribute grave injustice to exploited or oppressed people's own supposed deficiencies. Without a supportive partner to care for me in our home, I could as easily have died from neglect *or* COVID–19 in the average nursing home. My point here is to show that the long-term care industry is peddling this narrative simply to avoid responsibility for wrongdoing; that is, they want to pretend that people are dying in their facilities not because of the industry's negligence, greed, or malfeasance, but instead because disabled and older people have a particular tendency to die en masse. The narrative in "Care for Our Senior's Act" is yet another example of the industry's connivery and manipulation (I will append a brief example at the end of my testimony to show how they advance this narrative by playing with statistics).

Generally speaking, when *any* group of people are marked as suspect or inferior[302] in some manner, when they are segregated and denied the resources[303] and liberties that others enjoy, their flourishing will indeed be impeded,[304] and they will be at a greater risk of contracting infections or disease. This is evidenced throughout history from the decaying and dank tenement houses of the early 19th century,[305] the horrific conditions of the Warsaw ghetto,[306] to the abuses that occurred in state institutions[307] for people with disabilities. Given a deadly pandemic *combined* with deplorable (or at best unsafe) conditions, where people are segregated and treated as fungible objects from which to extract government benefits[308] (or cheap labor), even AHCA and LeadingAge lobbyists like Mr. Mark Parkinson or Mr. David Gifford might be at a mortality risk 630 times higher than 18 to 29 year olds *not* forced to endure similar circumstances. (The industry's claims are rarely supported by evidence, and with brief examination, can be shown inaccurate. Their act is at best slipshod and indicates an arrogance reinforced by years of overindulgence and a lack of accountability.)

In contrast to those who are key players on K Street or spend most of their time in boardrooms or lobbying in the halls of Congress, I want to emphasize that my perspective is informed by my advocacy work in nursing homes where I have spent a great deal of time. I form bonds with residents. I know many of their spouses and children's names, where they were from, the hobbies they enjoyed, and the kind of work they did. All of this they generously shared with me. I learned what it was like working in a Pennsylvania textile mill in the 1930s, surviving a chemical plant explosion in Texas and the revolution in Cuba, and growing up in Mexico in the 1940s. I have heard stories from war brides from France and Vietnam or the time

---

301 *https://www.ahcancal.org/Advocacy/Documents/Care%20for%20Our%20Seniors%20Act%20-%20Overview.pdf.*

302 *https://press.rebus.community/introductiontocommunitypsychology/chapter/oppre-ssion-and-power/.*

303 *https://www.who.int/disabilities/world_report/2011/accessible_en.pdf.*

304 *https://www.ama-assn.org/delivering-care/patient-support-advocacy/how-racism-segre-gation-drive-health-disparities.*

305 *https://socialwelfare.library.vcu.edu/issues/poverty/tenement-house-reform/.*

306 *https://www.iwm.org.uk/history/daily-life-in-the-warsaw-ghetto.*

307 *https://files.eric.ed.gov/fulltext/EJ844468.pdf#page=6.*

308 *https://prospect.org/familycare/the-corporatization-of-nursing-homes/.*

a woman had to sew thousands of sequins by hand on her daughter's quinceanera dress. I feel myself privileged to be granted the opportunity to listen. And unlike CEOs who earn $1,427,192[309] for lobbying, state ombudsman programs rely on volunteers. I have dedicated my life to this issue and yet rare is the occasion that I am asked to contribute to this topic. I—and other disability justice activists—have not been lavished the same platforms to speak given to long-term care industry CEOs and lobbyists. As a result of this, the voices of significantly disabled people, those at imminent risk of institutionalization or those in institutions, are squelched by the industry narrative. When I initially started out as ombudsman, I applied the principle of charity to the industry's narrative, but with careful appraisal of the incongruity between what residents, families, ombudsmen, advocates, experts, HHS regulators, CNAs, CMS, and the OIG evidenced compared to the industry's slant, it became apparent that industry representatives either have a deficient understanding of the culture and operations their business practices engender, or worse, they are impervious to the suffering of disabled people. Choosing *not* to see injustice or corruption, however, seems contrary to their lofty mission statements and commitments they have made to taxpayers.

On occasion, circumstances force us to confront the ugliness and brutality that inevitably festers where we sequester vulnerable people; stories of abject cruelty rip away the veil of inattention we cultivate to block from our view the relentless mill of everyday abuse, neglect, and hopelessness. In these moments of outrage, we perceive the true nature of institutionalization and perhaps even what we must do, but those flashes of insights quickly fade. Soon those with vested interests haul out the timeworn reform narratives and "bad apple" scapegoats that persuade us to look away again, to participate in systemic neglect from afar.

As an LTC ombudsman I could not simply look away from the toll of daily abuse and neglect residents experience or ignore their justified feelings of abandonment and the despair it begets. My ombudsman work bears out what ought to have long been obvious to any attentive person, namely, that segregating people in institutions can never foster or indeed ever permit equal treatment.[310] Nor—as over a hundred years of disability history attests[311]—can this model be fixed through reform. We cannot fix that which, by its nature, leads to systemic human rights violations. Severing people (like older and disabled people) from their homes and communities necessarily devalues them as persons and citizens. The diminishment is felt immediately. The freedoms they enjoyed vanish as institutional regiments constrict the courses of their lives. These utilitarian routines deprive them of their privacy and autonomy for the sake of efficiency and cost-effectiveness. Confined in these facilities without the projects and relationships that endowed their lives with meaning and shaped their social identities, they experience a kind of social death.[312] And so too their former communities, continuing on without them, lose the connection to them as full persons still deserving of the moral consideration and respect we are obliged to confer on those people in the community. Isolated, powerless, and dehumanized, people institutionalized inevitably suffer grave harms, not only from abuse and neglect, but

---

309 *https://nonprofitlight.com/dc/washington/american-health-care-association.*

310 See, for example, Liat Ben-Moshe, *Decarcerating Disability: Deinstitutionalization and Prison Abolition* (Minneapolis, MN: University of Minnesota Press, 2020).

311 Sara F. Rose, *No Right to Be Idle: the Invention of Disability, 1840s–1930s* (Chapel Hill, NC: The University of North Carolina Press, 2017).

312 3Jana Kra´lova´, "What Is Social Death?" *Contemporary Social Science* 10, no. 3 (2015): pp. 235–248, *https://doi.org/10.1080/21582041.2015.1114407.*

from the very act of banishing them from the moral communities that granted the rights and benefits they are now denied.

To be sure, congregate institutions try to simulate community to hide these realities, but such ersatz contrivances are no substitute for genuine social inclusion and belongingness; the simulations are parodies. Such a model cannot produce "person-centered care" no matter how many CMS regulations we enact *and* enforce. Nor can quarterly congressional hearings[313] and regulatory tweaks[314] — informed by the usual actors[315] they serve to benefit—amount to anything more than theater, political performances that strike those people who must endure the injustice[316] as thoughtless cruelty.

Only a transformative shift in public policy can end these injustices. This shift will require scrutinizing narratives widely considered axiomatic. These include the beliefs that institutionalization is an unavoidable consequence of aging[317] and disability, that institutions provide safer[318] environments (a claim long used to rationalize the barbarity of social removal despite evidence demonstrating the contrary),[319] that uprooting people from the homes, communities, and personal identities they spent lifetimes nurturing is compatible with our most revered social ideals, and finally that we can outsource our humanity—that is, our moral and social obligations to one another, including our disabled parents and children—as a revenue source for corporations and the workers they exploit[320] and expect humane results.

By now, we know these outcomes of the institutional model; it is a model that objectifies deeply human concerns and favors economic values and imperatives such as competitiveness, efficiency, and profit margins, values that tend to attract predatory actors.[321] And yet we persist with it, and one must ask why. Why do we continue to allow neglect, abuse, and dehumanization to go unchecked? Why do we allow those same predatory actors to manufacture and control the narratives[322] that frame these issues, and indeed provide them platforms[323] in the halls of Congress and in the media to influence unwitting advocates? Why do we persist with this cultivated naivety in the face of so much everyday suffering? The poor human rights records of congregate care facilities long predate the COVID–19 crisis, but the crisis has laid bare[324] the preexisting conditions that led to deaths of over 181,000 disabled people in these institutions.[325]

The horrors I witnessed as an LTC ombudsman keep me up at night, but also inform my disability justice work. And both my insomnia and activism partly derive from frustration. In

---

313 *https://www.finance.senate.gov/hearings/a-national-tragedy-covid-19-in-the-nations-nursing-homes.*

314 *https://www.kxan.com/investigations/obscure-program-sends-big-money-to-texas-nursing-homes-amid-pandemic-is-it-protecting-residents/.*

315 *https://www.npr.org/2020/05/21/855821083/ideal-nursing-homes-individual-rooms-better-staffing-more-accountability.*

316 *https://www.cnn.com/interactive/2017/02/health/nursing-home-sex-abuse-investi-gation/.*

317 *https://www.irishtimes.com/opinion/nursing-homes-must-be-made-a-thing-of-the-past-1.4257422?mode=amp&fbclid=IwAR2NDUH2vj4HrwoBbpOG9iF0SYqz5RM2jTAx4BnYqVe5MKBBr--j6Cp6FLY.*

318 *https://oig.hhs.gov/oas/reports/region1/11600509.asp.*

319 *https://www.ncbi.nlm.nih.gov/books/NBK217552/.*

320 *https://www.finance.senate.gov/imo/media/doc/AdelinaRamos_WrittenTestimony%20 March%2017.pdf.*

321 *https://www.nytimes.com/2021/03/13/business/nursing-homes-ratings-medicare-ovid.html.*

322 *https://www.finance.senate.gov/imo/media/doc/FINAL%20Dr.%20Gifford%20SFC%20 Hearing%20Testimony%203.17.2021.pdf.*

323 *https://www.providermagazine.com/Breaking-News/Pages/AHCA,-NCAL-Head-Parkinson-Named-a-Top-Lobbyist-for-2020.aspx.*

324 *https://www.aclu.org/news/disability-rights/covid-19-deaths-in-nursing-homes-are-not-unavoidable-they-are-the-result-of-deadly-discrimination/.*

325 *https://www.kff.org/coronavirus-covid-19/issue-brief/state-covid-19-data-and-policy-actions/.*

deference to the industry, the system defangs oversight. I have fought countless nursing home attempts to involuntarily discharge residents only to have found that those residents, some with severe dementia, had disappeared the following week—to where, the nursing home curiously had (or at least offered) no clue. Sitting at their bedsides, I have held residents' hands as they recounted instances of rape and abuse, often by staff. Residents have had limbs amputated due to a lack of wound care, understaffing, and poor training. I have seen residents gasp for air as nursing home staff rationed oxygen to save money. I have called Health and Human Services on multiple occasions for residents due to cruel instances of retaliation, only to leave the residents open for more of the same because they sought assistance from a deliberately debilitated regulatory system. Finally, I, myself, have been threatened on multiple occasions by staff and operators. Despite my notifying HHS regulatory and the Ombudsman Program, nothing of substance was done. To the industry, ombudsmen are gnats to swat away; they well know consequences will not be forthcoming. After all, there are few if any consequences for the negligent deaths of residents.

Culture change is impossible within the institutional habitus, particularly so when professional and agency advancement, corporate profit,[326] race, age, and ableism are added to the brew. From the institutional point of view, the dehumanizing model is working as intended. Hence, pumping in ever more money to fund the same solutions and reforms will not bring about different results. As we have seen during the COVID–19 pandemic, nursing homes made record profits[327] from taxpayer funded COVID subsidies,[328] yet COVID cases and deaths, along with non COVID deaths resulting from inadequate infection control practices and severe understaffing,[329] continued to rise.

There will be no substantive change until we end the Medicaid institutional bias by diverting taxpayer funds away from institutions and to programs that maintain or reestablish community integration. As I often explain, nursing homes are the most subsidized[330] industry in the United States and increased monetary rewards[331] serve only to entrench industry malfeasance.[332] Diverting Medicaid dollars to fund HCBS not only reaffirms our commitments to the Americans with Disabilities Act (ADA), the Supreme Court's *Olmstead* decision, and our professed democratic principles, it will also do more to soften the resolve of a recalcitrant industry (and similar nonprofits) than years of congressional hearings. In the long run, we will waste fewer resources on researching deficient industry practices and developing complex strategies to instigate change (only to be undone by lobbyists), on Office of Inspector General (OIG) and the U.S. General Accounting Office (GAO) investigations, on Ombudsman programs, on regulatory agencies to maintain the illusion of oversight, on healthcare costs resulting from the industry's negligence, and on subsidizing the industry's cost of doing business.

---

[326] *http://tallgrasseconomics.org/2021/02/1539/.*

[327] *http://tallgrasseconomics.org/2021/02/the-ensign-group-americas-biggest-nursing-home-corporation-had-a-banner-year-in-2020/.*

[328] *https://www.mcknightsseniorliving.com/home/news/assisted-living-eligible-for-20-billion-in-new-relief-funding-for-covid-19-related-losses-expenses/.*

[329] *https://apnews.com/article/nursing-homes-neglect-death-surge-3b74a2202140c5a6b5cf05 cdf0ea4f32.*

[330] *http://tallgrasseconomics.org/2021/01/the-media-is-promoting-a-dangerous-false-narra-tive-by-claiming-that-the-nursing-home-industry-is-struggling-financially/.*

[331] *https://www.mcknightsseniorliving.com/home/news/assisted-living-eligible-for-20-billion-in-new-relief-funding-for-covid-19-related-losses-expenses/.*

[332] https://www.youtube.com/watch?v=ee-rnrbrD1g.

Sincerely,
Lydia Nunez Landry
Certified Volunteer Long-Term Care Ombudsman
Organizer for Gulf Coast Adapt

Appendix

As promised, I want to briefly review a few of the rhetorical and statistical practice employed by the industry and their lobbyists to reframe the human catastrophe exacerbated by the negligent practices in LTC facilities. The author of Care for Our Seniors Act,[333] which aspires to learn from "tragedy" and implement bold solutions, concedes that LTC facilities were the epicenter of the "once-in-a-century" pandemic's ravage. The force-of-nature language distances the 170,000 deaths (now up to 181,286[334] deaths) from any culpable agent. And indeed, no one is to blame for the virus, just as we can blame no one for a major flood. But we can blame them for negligent and habitual substandard practices (such as not maintaining levees) that substantially worsen the toll. The author mentions "independent research" by "leading experts" which shows that "COVID–19 outbreaks in nursing homes are principally driven by the amount of spread in the surrounding community." The only actual research offered[335]—conducted in May, 2020, long before the vast majority of cased occurred—did conclude that size and location of facilities were factors while traditional metrics such as star ratings and prior citation for poor infection control were not. (Most of the citations were articles from industry magazines, one of which mentioned the article just cited.) It's unclear how this exonerates the industry. Moreover, the study, thus interpreted, becomes an outlier, as much more research has found direct links between poor quality ratings and significantly higher numbers of COVID cases and deaths (see here[336] and here[337]).

Instead of dueling studies, we might focus on statistics. The author notes another force of nature behind the deaths, namely time: aging and the fragility of bodies. The virus just happens to target the frail and elderly adults with underlying health concerns that live in their facilities. The author incorrectly asserted that the average age of nursing home residents is 85, but correctly asserted that most residents have underlying conditions, as indeed most people over 65 years old have multiple chronic conditions, in and out of LTC facilities. First some number:

The U.S. has approximately 52 million citizens aged 65 or greater. Of them, 430,000 have died from complications of COVID–19 infections. Of those, 130,000 died in nursing homes—the author mention 170,000 deaths, but that includes congregate facilities the data from which is sparse, so I shall stick with the 130,000 in nursing homes (NHs). Thus, 300,000 died elsewhere than a NH. NHs warehouse approximately 1.4 million residents, ~90% of whom are 65+ years old. The total number of cases in NHs is, at the moment, 643,314, and, for non-NH people in the same age group, 2,666,625. Looking at the bare infection and death numbers, one might think that nursing homes did well—too well, in fact, for the author's contentions.

---

333 *https://www.ahcancal.org/Advocacy/Documents/Care%20for%20Our%20Seniors%20Act%20-%20Overview.pdf.*

334 *https://www.kff.org/coronavirus-covid-19/issue-brief/state-covid-19-data-and-policy-actions/.*

335 *https://agsjournals.onlinelibrary.wiley.com/doi/full/10.1111/jgs.16661.*

336 *https://www.sciencedirect.com/science/article/abs/pii/S0195670121000086.*

337 *https://www.sciencedirect.com/science/article/pii/S1525861020305211.*

But consider again that most people over 65 years old have chronic conditions and most people, even with their bleach wipes, have rudimentary infection controls in their homes. Now, 9.28% of the 1.4 million people in NHs have died from COVID; we can round that up to 1 in every 10. But if non-NH people in the same fragile age group died at that rate, we would have an incredible 4,342,857 more deaths than we do, as only 1 in 167 non-NH elderly people died from COVID. Indeed, examining only those infected, you are nearly twice as likely to die (20% vs. 11%) if you're in a NH than not. Indeed, the infection rate in NHs is 46% vs. 5.3% for non-NHs fragile people.

Now, ultimately, industry spokespeople will claim that the deaths occurred because all these people are interacting in close quarters, and so on. But this is not something that can be fixed, and so it underscores why we need to turn back to community integration instead of warehousing people in admitted death traps.

LeadingAge

2519 Connecticut Avenue, NW
Washington, DC
20008–1520

Thank you for the opportunity to comment on the above hearing. Our members and the older adults they serve have been irrevocably affected by this pandemic. We appreciate the concern that this Committee has expressed over the past year and its efforts to address the significant challenges posed by both public and private responses to the public health emergency.

LeadingAge is a tax-exempt national organization focused on education, advocacy, and applied research. The mission of LeadingAge is to be the trusted voice for aging. Our 5,000+ not-for-profit members include the entire field of aging services providers—nursing homes, home care and hospice, affordable housing, life plan/continuing care communities and assisted living.

We begin our statement by asking the most difficult question, what happened?

If only it were easy—if only there was an answer to the question, what happened? Why did so many people die in nursing homes? What magic bullet could we have fired to prevent this? What magic bullet can or should we look to in the future?

As Dr. Tamara Konetzka testified, based on her rigorous, highly respected research, "the two strongest and most consistent predictors of worse COVID–19 outcomes are nursing home size, with larger facilities being more at risk, and COVID–19 prevalence in the surrounding community," as opposed to star rating, staffing, access to PPE, etc.[338] The greater the presence of the disease in the community, the greater the impact on residents and staff. The second condition is something that we have tolerated for many years—large poorly funded nursing homes with many residents, many of the long-stay residents poor and racial minorities, again, at greater risk for this disease for all the reasons that we know as we attempt to address the

[338] We appreciate that there is research showing that nonprofit nursing homes and nursing homes with higher rankings, many of whom are our members, fared better. However, they too faced all the public health challenges we discuss, herein, and without addressing those challenges, we consign all nursing homes, even the best performers, to an intolerable situation.

impact of centuries of discrimination. In those communities with the highest spread, where staff are as affected as residents, the disease was at its deadliest.

When Dr. Kontezka was asked, what could have been done to reduce this tragedy, she responded, better use of public health to control spread in the community We needed a fast, all of government public health response to contain and control the disease and that did not happen.

This pandemic was a failure of our public health infrastructure, and that failure trickled down to infect all the public and private health care and housing entities that supported at risk populations, both residents and staff.[339]

The underlying challenge to this disease—its very newness—was faced by all our members. It is called the novel coronavirus for a reason. Each day brought new knowledge about the disease, but that means that the day before, we were operating on old and not necessarily accurate information. For example, during the early days when the pandemic was new—March and April 2020—a lack of understanding of how the disease spread resulted in inconsistent and often changing advice (e.g., when to use masks; testing limited to symptomatic staff and residents, before we realized it was spread asymptomatically and was not contained; inconsistent directives from state, local and federal public health authorities).

In addition, the entire health care system was left to fight it out for essential supplies rather than having a centralized source (indeed, even FEMA couldn't adequately fulfill the White House's April directive to send 2 weeks of supplies to nursing homes months into the pandemic.)

Failure of public leadership to understand the disease led to new problems placed at the feet of nursing homes trying to follow the ever-changing directives—e.g., closing down nursing homes to visitors saved lives (because of asymptomatic carriers, speed with which older persons died from infection) but because we had NO idea how long the crisis would last, created its own secondary health crisis, isolation.

Why is it so important to stress the public health failures? Because we must learn the right lessons if we are not going to repeat this disaster as this public health emergency continues and we also examine how to avoid future disasters.

To fix public health infrastructure in the future we must have:

- *Transparency and honesty;* credibility of public and private systems can only be built on a foundation of transparency and open communication, even but perhaps most importantly when we do not have answers.
- *National public reporting system* to ensure accuracy and consistency, including reporting of race, ethnicity, gender and age.[340]
- *National testing strategy* to eliminate duplicative, contradictory policies; and public financing to ensure that private entities are adequately compensated for mandatory requirements.[341]

---

[339] We note that the negative impact of the pandemic on older persons and persons living in nursing homes and other congregate settings, along with public and private response, is not limited to the United States. A survey conducted by Global Ageing Network, representing aging services providers throughout the world, revealed eerily similar experiences. *https://globalageing.org/gan-covid-report/.*

[340] *See,* e.g., LeadingAge's letter to Sec. Azar asking for a uniform reporting system. *file:///C:/Users/Marsha/Documents/CDC%20reporting%20letter%20final.pdf.*

[341] *See,* e.g., LeadingAge's letter to Congressional leadership, *file:///C:/Users/Marsha/Downloads/Testing%20letter.pdf.*

- *Public access to PPE,* to eliminate the "hunger games" scenario where providers are mandated to use PPE but PPE is in short supply globally, leaving providers to find PPE by themselves, hoping their standard supplier has access or they can find some other supplier who is reliable and honest. Public access would also reduce the problem of price gouging, where the cost of a disposable gown increases from 25 cents pre-pandemic to $4.00 during the pandemic. It truly is the federal government's responsibility to manage access to and distribution of rare but life-saving essential products.
- *Emergency preparedness infrastructure* must include aging services. Examples include retaining the strike teams that some states created earlier in the pandemic (and now funded though CMS); and effective use of the public health workforce to supplement workers who are in quarantine or sick leave. This is essential not only for nursing homes but all congregate and senior housing, including HUD housing where low-income seniors at highest risk live in the "community" but with little access to necessary services (e.g., Wi-Fi, access to testing and vaccines). Aging services providers must be at the table at all levels. This is the lesson we thought was learned from Katrina, but it is not clear we did.
- *Telehealth/technology/broadband* issues of fairness and access remain. We clearly need to improve broadband access in rural areas; provide access to reduced rates for rural home health providers as we do for nursing homes; reimburse telehealth capabilities in non-rural nursing homes and other care settings; and address access and availability in community settings, for example by allowing HUD housing providers to wire their apartment buildings for Wi-Fi for tenants.
- *Effective public/private partnerships.* The long-term care pharmacy partnership to deliver vaccines to almost every nursing home is a good example of the federal approach that has been sorely missing. While not perfect, with improvements it could be a model for addressing specific needs in future emergencies.

The second cause identified by Dr. Konetzka—large poorly funded nursing homes—embodies long-standing challenges to the way we deliver long-term services and supports. To address these issues, we must:

- *Focus on long-stay residents*—financed through Medicaid and to a much smaller extent, private pay—and rebuild our communities to address the social and health needs of these residents.
- *Rethink how nursing homes are conceived and structured,* moving to a smaller setting, with single rooms, again focusing on the needs of long-stay residents;
- *Address workforce issues;* the continual shortage of qualified staff at all levels and the serious underpayment especially at the direct care worker level must be addressed; LeadingAge's Center for Workforce Solutions[342] and the LeadingAge LTSS Center@UMass[343] are both dedicated to identifying solutions to these issues.
- *Address critical financing* issues associated with under-payment from Medicaid and the negative impact that underpayment has on quality and services. LeadingAge

[342] *https://leadingage.org/workforce.*
[343] *https://www.ltsscenter.org/.*

members regularly report that they must raise millions of dollars annually through charitable donations to provide high quality care because of underfunding from Medicaid.

- *Recognize that nursing homes are part of a continuum* of services primarily financed by public programs. We critically need a non-means tested public long-term care insurance program to ensure that all persons have an affordable means of paying for long-term care, are able to age or live with disability in the setting of their choice for as long as they can, with both quality of life and quality of care.

In addition, witnesses at this hearing and at other hearings before this committee and the Special Committee on Aging have raised concerns about how to ensure nursing homes provide high quality care, and how to respond to nursing homes that are poor performers.

Care for Seniors, the 8 point program LeadingAge and AHCA have put forward, addresses many of the concerns raised during this hearing, and identifies public and private financing mechanisms to implement these policies.[344]

1. *To enhance quality of care:*
   a. *Enhanced Infection Control:* we strongly agree that infection control is critical and have proposed updating the current guidelines to address some of the challenges around workforce and training to make it possible to employ infection control specialists in each nursing home.
   b. *RN 24/7:* many of our members already employ registered nurses on a round-the-clock basis. In many parts of the country, however, there is a shortage of qualified nursing staff, and Medicaid, the primary payer for long-stay nursing home residents, is not funded in a way that covers current costs, much less the addition of, in effect, 6 full time nurses just to have one nurse on staff all the time. We provide a number of recommendations on how to implement expanded staffing.
   c. *Maintaining a minimum 30-day supply of PPE,* to address current and future infectious diseases and other conditions that require extensive protective equipment. Again, this will require not just action by nursing homes but also a commitment from the public sector to ensure that adequate supplies are available continually.
2. *Recruit and Retain a Long Term Care Workforce Strategy:*
   a. For decades the nursing home field has been plagued by shortages in staff, whether because it is easier and more lucrative to work in settings like hospitals, as Ms. Ramos so accurately testified, or because there simply are not sufficient numbers of persons interested in this field. As mentioned above, LeadingAge's Center for Workforce Solutions and LTSS Center have been working on attracting workers for many years, culminating in the ground-breaking work, *Making Care Work Pay,* which addresses the economic benefits and necessity of providing a living wage, along with the challenges of implementing this policy.
   b. Care for Seniors recommends a multi-phase tiered approach to supply, attract and retain the long term care workforce, including leveraging federal, state, and academic entities to provide loan forgiveness for new graduates who work in long

---

[344] *https://leadingage.org/care-our-seniors-act.*

term care, tax credits for licensed long term care professionals, programs for affordable housing and childcare assistance, and increased subsidies to professionals' schools whose graduates work in nursing homes for at least 5 years.

3. *Improve Systems to be More Resident-Driven*
   a. *Survey Improvements for Better Resident Care:* Over many years, numerous studies by private and public entities have documented failures in the survey system, from inconsistent results to failure to identify and fix significant deficiencies. This over 30-year old system needs to be re-vamped to reflect modern thinking on addressing medical errors (e.g., using the elements in the patient safety model) and the significant changes in nursing homes and the residents we serve since this system was inaugurated in 1987. LeadingAge strongly supports the study currently undertaken by the National Academies of Science, Engineering and Medicine (NASEM) reexamining the current way we identify, measure and enforce quality of care and quality of life in nursing homes.[345] Additionally, Care for Seniors makes recommendations that support development of an effective oversight system and processes that support improved care and protect residents.
   b. *Chronic Poor Performing Nursing Facilities and Change of Ownership:* A corollary of the failure of the current survey and certification system is the continued and seemingly intractable problem of chronic poor performers. LeadingAge supports the Nursing Home Reform Modernization Act (S. 782) introduced by Senators Casey and Toomey as an excellent example of a creative way to address improving care by creating a separate program within CMS to provide mandatory counseling, education and assistance for poor performers. In Care for Our Seniors, we propose a detailed process for working with poor performers: (1) Identify chronic poor performing facilities; (2) Conduct an analysis to determine the reason for chronic poor performance; (3) Develop a turn-around plan; (4) Monitor progress; and (5) Determine if the plan of correction goals have been met or the need for plan revisions. Finally, we "bite the bullet" and state, "If milestones are not met within six to 24 months (median time of one year), a temporary manager, change in management/ownership or the closure of the facility may be required."
   c. *Customer Satisfaction:* As we note in this last recommendation, nursing homes are the only Medicare health care provider that does not include customer satisfaction in the data collected and reported by CMS. Hospitals, hospice, and home health collect customer satisfaction, which is part of their publicly reported data. We recommend adding a customer satisfaction measure to the 5-star rating system, to help consumers and family members monitor the quality of nursing homes.

Finally, we should use this crisis as an opportunity to think more broadly about how we want to age, what services we will need in the future, how we will want to live, and how we expect to finance the aging services ecosystem. While we understand the importance of addressing care in nursing homes during the pandemic, we would note that more older adults

345 *https://www.nationalacademies.org/our-work/the-quality-of-care-in-nursing-homes.*

live in the broader community than in nursing homes. We have very little data on the impact of COVID on older adults who receive LTSS in the community.

We must, therefore, also address loss of community-based services. Closure of adult day programs, PACE, senior centers, loss of access to HCBS and home care workers all had a negative impact on seniors now and will in the future. LeadingAge members who provide home-based care, whether through Medicare, Medicaid or private pay, had trouble accessing PPE, testing, and vaccines, which would be essential to their being able to serve their clients. The adults we serve as well have had difficulty being prioritized for testing and access to vaccines, especially home-bound clients. In this respect, a more robust public health infrastructure, with community mobile clinics, is critical, as well as addressing the needs of individuals in HUD-supported housing.

In conclusion, we thank you for the opportunity to engage in this very critical endeavor, improving the care and services our provide to the most vulnerable and frail in our society. This pandemic has been devastating to the people we serve, our staff, and our leadership. We must learn the right lessons so that we are able to come out of this crisis stronger and able to provide older adults with true quality of life and services.

Letter Submitted by Carrie Leljedal

A National Tragedy: COVID–19 in the Nation's Nursing Homes
Wednesday, March 17, 2021
To: Senate Committee on Finance

Thank you for allowing me to submit a statement in regard to the COVID–19 crisis in Skilled Nursing Facilities (SNF) in the United States. My name is Carrie Leljedal, and I have a 33-year-old son who resides in an Intermediate Care Facility for adults with Developmental Disabilities (ICFDD), Skilled Nursing.

I am also the leader for Illinois Caregivers for Compromise, we advocate for residents and families in all kinds of residential long-term care facilities (LTCF) in Illinois, and with our National Chapter. Recently, I started volunteering with the Illinois Ombudsman office.

When most families must deal with long-term care it is for less than 5 years. I am in this for the long haul, my son will always require skilled nursing he has resided in his facility for seven and half years and could easily be there another 40–50 years.

My Lynn, was born with a rare seizure disorder, called Sturge-Weber Syndrome (SWS) and a host of other serious health conditions. Lynn has had over 100 surgeries in his life, and close to 45 hospital stays. Lynn is currently followed by three different kind of neurologist, three different eye doctors, two endocrinologist, one GI doctor along with both physical and psychologist therapist. One of the biggest issues we face early on into the pandemic was we had to cancel all of Lynn's doctor's appointment.

Lynn has lived in his ICFDD in Southern, Illinois. On March 9, 2020, I received a call from the Executive Director telling me that the county health department was restricting all visitors to the facility. Five days later, CMS issued guidance on March 13, 2020 to shut down all facilities to anyone who was not employed at the facility.

I had seen Lynn on March 9th and was unable to see him again until late June, I do not consider virtual, or window visit a visit to see my son. When I finally was able to see my son, it was only at doctors' appointments and I was required to stay 6 feet away, socially distanced. When I met him at his ICFDD, for his first post quarantine doctor's appointment the ED came outside and informed me that I was not allowed to hug or kiss my son, I was an inch shy of fully hyperventilating while driving to follow them to the doctor's appointment. Explaining to my son, why I could not hug or kiss him was exceedingly difficult for both of us.

In a years' time, my son has been able to come home for three different long weekends, when returning to the ICFDD, he was required to quarantine for 14 days. I have been told, that would continue even though he is fully vaccinated and so are my husband and myself.

Residents of LTCF, have suffered in ways that will take us years to fully understand. The fear of the unknown might have been one of the hardest parts of this. My son is verbally high functioning and understands things well, as much as he understood why he had to be quarantined it still affected him mentally and physically. Early on as COVID first entered the building, my son would ask me if I knew which of his friends had tested positive and if anyone had died. Never did I think this would be a regular question from my son. Explaining all of this to an adult who functions at around a 10–12-year-old level was quite difficult.

CMS issued some visitor guidance on September 17th, the guidance was extremely limited, but it was a start, until the states got their hand on it. As the leader of the Illinois Caregivers for Compromise, I heard from members all over Illinois and with leader of the other states. CMS guidance did little to nothing to assist residents with being able to see their family members. Many states would only allow for compassionate care visit, at end of life and still required family members to remain socially distanced from their loved ones. The number of people that have died alone in the US over the past year, because hospitals and long-term care facilities would not allow family members to remain until the end is unfathomable.

September 17th guidance allowed for outside visits for residents and family members. This was set up to fail on day one. By the time you require 6 ft social distance and barrier and masks between the resident and the visitor, most residents could not hear the visitor and or recognize them.

The director of Nursing Homes Division for CMS, Evan Shulman, has publicly stated multiple times that he has heard from residents that they would rather die from COVID–19 than go another year without seeing family.

The effects the isolation has caused on residents of all kinds of long-term care facilities in the United States is cruel and unusual punishment. Why are we punishing some of our most fragile residents in the United States, who need extra care to live.

Are you aware that long term care effects every age? There are children who can spend years in long term care because they require more medical care than a parent can provide at home, but not enough to keep them in a true hospital setting. Adults with developmental disabilities (DD) usually enter long-term care in their late teens or early twenties and remain there the rest of their lives. Even residents of adult DD community living arrangements have been isolated from their families this last year.

Early in the pandemic, the mandated quarantine of residents on any kind of long-term care facility made sense. One we were past the first few months and had reliable testing and PPE the residents should have had as many of their rights restored as possible. Residents of long-term care are entitled to the same freedom and right to make their own choice as any other resident of the United States. There could have been many ways to restore some of the resident's rights to allow some visitors, using common sense and core safety protocol, while treating residents and family members with respect and not like guilty criminals.

A year later, with new visitation guidance in place that does allow for visitation and physical contact, most facilities and quite a few States are making their own rules and in turn they continue to violate the resident's rights. If I had to guess over 50% of residents in long-term care have not seen a family member or friend in over a year without a window between them and a supervised visit as if they were in prison.

There are so many things that have gone wrong over the past year in long term care, we all know that the entire system from pediatrics to geriatrics needs a complete overhaul. To do this and to do it right, you need all stake holders at the table. *The fact that there was not a single resident or family members asked to give testimony during the public hearings speaks volumes as to where they stand.*

In Missouri and Illinois, CMS issued penalties to 258 nursing homes during 2020 and earlier this year for infection control deficiencies. Of those, 220 also received incentive payments for low COVID–19 transmission rates.

The largest infection control-related penalty for any nursing home across the two states in 2020 went to Life Care Center of St. Louis. CMS issued a penalty of almost $500,000 in May for issues that inspectors said "placed all residents in the facility in immediate jeopardy."[346]

So far, Life Care Center has reported eight residents' deaths due to COVID–19 to CMS.

In October, the facility received nearly $60,000 in incentive payments.

At Crystal Creek Health and Rehab Center in Florissant, 13 residents died of COVID–19. For infection control deficiencies in February and September 2020, CMS issued a $153,842 penalty. The next month, Crystal Creek received an incentive payment from HHS. By December, the incentive payments totaled $146,088, almost completely wiping out the penalty.

Across Missouri and Illinois, almost 200 nursing homes received incentive payments that were greater than their infection control-related penalties from 2020 or 2021.

A statement from the Health Resources and Services Administration, which administers the incentive program, said that there are two criteria for an actively certified nursing home to receive an incentive payment: "First, a facility must demonstrate a rate of COVID–19 infections that is below the rate of infection in the county in which they are located. Second, facilities must also have a COVID–19 death rate that falls below a nationally established performance threshold for mortality among nursing home residents infected with COVID–19."

However, the calculations for the incentive payments do not take into account[347] whether a facility has a previous or ongoing deficiency from a CMS inspection.

Instead of giving bonus payments to the nursing homes, they could have used those monies to require more staff to be hired and people given jobs and the residents would be safe.

An HRSA statement said the incentive money must be spent in certain ways: "Nursing home QIP recipients must utilize the resources they receive to continue to protect their residents and staff against this devastating pandemic and they must at-test to the terms and conditions outlined in the program for payment. For example, quality incentive payments may be used for costs associated with administering COVID–19 testing for both staff and residents; reporting COVID–19 test results to local, state, or federal governments; hiring staff to provide patient

[346] *https://www.medicare.gov/care-compare/inspections/pdf/nursing-home/265610/health/infection-control?date=2020-05-18.*

[347] *https://www.hrsa.gov/sites/default/files/hrsa/provider-relief/nursing-home-qip-metho-dology.pdf.*

care or administrative support; efforts to improve infection control, including activities such as implementing infection control 'mentorship' programs with subject matter experts, or changes made to physical facilities; and providing additional services to residents, such as technology that permits residents to connect with their families if the families are not able to visit in person."

We need a complete overhaul of the long-term care system in the United States. The priority must be quality of life for the residents. The fact that we have lost over 150,00 residents in Long-Term Care due to COVID–19 proves we can not protect than from COVID. The number of people who died from Isolation, Failure to Thrive, Neglect and Abuse might never been know, but by protecting them to death we took away any quality of life that they might of had.

I am begging all of you, put yourself in my shoes, imagine knowing your child will live in long-term care for another 40–50 years, would you want them to go through another year like 2020. If we can find a way to bring the right people to the table, we can find a way to better the system to prevent anyone from having to relive 2020.

Sincerely,
Carrie Leljedal

Statement Submitted by Ja'Nisa Mimbs

My Mother is in Eastview Nursing Center in and we've not been allowed to touch or spend any valuable time with her since February 19, 2020. We've visited at her window, which they refuse to even crack for her to hear us. Then they started these outdoor visits for 30 minutes. Keep in mind, it was on Tuesdays and Thursdays from 9:00 a.m.–10:00 a.m. and 4:00 p.m.–5:00 p.m. That's eight visits a week for the entire nursing home, you had to make a reservation and pray you got a spot. The visits were outside with a table between us and an aid watching our every move to ensure we didn't touch her. They stopped those visits in September and just started them back on March 1, 2021.

My Mother was walking with a walker, dressing herself, using the restroom, feeding herself and needed little assistance with her daily activities. In October she started to decline, she had a severe UTI that had gone unnoticed by the staff and as we weren't allowed to spend anytime with her, we couldn't alert them that something was wrong. By the time it was caught, it was severe! She was very confused, was incontinent and in a diaper. Something she'd never been before. They gave her the antibiotic Vancomycin intravenously and it was so strong it almost killed her. She was so weak and she's never come back from it. This was the start of her decline in October, we were never allowed Compassionate Care Visits to try to boost her spirits and entice her to improve. Yet they tell us she's depressed, not eating and they're putting her on an antidepressant. At this point she was not walking, any longer and was placed in a wheelchair. She was moving herself around in her chair with her feet and was still getting up every day. Then it got to where they were leaving her in her wheelchair all day while she's complaining that her bottom hurt and we now have a bedsore on her bottom. Thanksgiving Day we visited at her window and they allowed me to give her a plate of banana pudding, she sat and fed herself the entire plate. Many visits at her window in the cold with my 78-year-old stepfather is all we had. Christmas Day, again, a plate of food, she fed herself and by mid-January she was bed ridden, she's now in the bed being turned every 2 hours from side to side to help the bedsore, she's 90 pounds, now on pureed foods, being fed and can do nothing for herself not even hold a cup of water. We've signed the paperwork as last week (March 8, 2021) to put her on Hospice, at the advice of the nursing home physician and we're still not being allowed Compassionate Care Visits.

We can do the 30-minute visits which they make her get in a geriatric chair while she complains that it hurts her bottom. We've asked the administrator about Compassionate Care Visits and were told, they will do them on Mon., Wed., Thurs., Fri. between the hours of 11:00 a.m. and 4:00 p.m. We must allow the staff to administer a rapid antigen COVID test, be dressed in full PPE gear (head to toe) and can't touch her, only sit 6 feet from her in her room, but these have not been arranged yet. While the staff come and go as they please with nothing but a mask on.

Also, she's in a room by herself, she's basically quarantined already and we still can't see her, touch her or speak to her without the staff monitoring us.

My Mother deserves so much more, all the residents do. Without family, what quality of life do they have? They've lived their lives and their only comfort is family and that has been snatched away as they're treated like hostages and I never thought this world would come to me having to beg for permission to hug my Mother, care for her, sit by he side and hold her hand while she leaves this cruel world!

National Consumer Voice for Quality Long-Term Care et al.

Jonathan Evans, President Lori Smetanka, Executive Director

March 29, 2021

U.S. Senate Committee on Finance

Dirksen Senate Office Bldg. Washington, DC 20510-6200

RE: Statement for the Record: A National Tragedy: COVID–19 in the Nation's Nursing Homes; Hearing before the U.S. Senate Committee on Finance March 17, 2021

Dear Chairman Wyden, Ranking Member Crapo, and Members of the Committee:

The National Consumer Voice for Quality Long-Term Care, Community Legal Services of Philadelphia, and the Michigan Elder Justice Initiative would like to thank Chairman Wyden and Ranking Member Crapo for holding this hearing on the devastating impact of the COVID–19 pandemic on nursing home residents

Our organizations advocate for quality care, quality of life, and the rights of nursing home residents and other long-term care consumers. We appreciate the opportunity to share our input on this critical issue with the Committee.

No group of Americans has suffered from COVID–19 more than nursing home residents. Over 130,000[348] residents have died from COVID–19, while over 1.1 million residents and staff have been infected.[349] At the same time, countless others have suffered from isolation and

---

[348] *https://data.cms.gov/stories/s/COVID-19-Nursing-Home-Data/bkwz-xpvg/.*

[349] Both numbers are an undercount. CMS did not require nursing homes to start reporting data regarding COVID–19 cases and deaths until May 8, 2020 and did not require facilities to report COVID–19 data back to the beginning of the pandemic. Other totals, such as *The New York Times,* are much higher. However, the *Times* total includes all long-term care facilities, for instance, assisted living facilities, and not just nursing homes.

neglect. An Associated Press article[350] from November 2020 estimated that there had been over 40,000 excess deaths in 2020 compared to 2019 that were not attributable to COVID–19. That number is likely much higher now. Adding to the suffering, one year after nursing homes were locked down, tens of thousands of nursing home residents continue to have extremely limited, if any, in-person contact with their families and loved ones.

These numbers are even more tragic because much of this suffering and death could have been prevented. Years of insufficient staffing and the nursing home industry's focus on profits over residents, combined with the slow and inadequate federal response to the pandemic in long-term care facilities created a perfect storm resulting in tragedy. COVID–19 has also exposed the failures of nursing homes to care for and protect residents adequately. Without significant policy changes, long-standing problems will continue, future pandemics will be equally devastating, and residents will be the ones who suffer and die.

We urge Congress to:

- Initiate an investigation into the devastating impact of COVID–19 on nursing home residents.
- Support nursing home staff by requiring minimum staffing standards, training, and increased wages and benefits.
- Require the rescission of all waivers of nursing home regulations established during the Public Health Emergency.
- Ensure access to COVID–19 vaccines for all residents and staff who choose to be vaccinated.
- Ensure protection from COVID–19 for residents and staff by ensuring ongoing access to PPE and testing.
- Fully restore visitation in nursing homes.
- Reinstate standard and complaint surveys and strengthen regulations and enforcement.
- Require transparency and accountability around nursing home ownership and finances.
- Address disparities in care for racial and ethnic minorities.
- Expand choice through the expansion of Medicaid Home and Community Based Services.

Many of these recommendations will have the immediate effect of preventing further harm from COVID–19 while also having the long-term benefit of increasing the overall quality of care and preventing a recurrence of the devastation wrought by COVID–19 in the future.

Investigate the Full Impact of the COVID–19 Pandemic on Residents of Long-Term Care Facilities, Including the Disproportionate Impact on People of Color

Before the pandemic, 82% of nursing homes in the United States had been cited for an infection control violation, with 50% of those homes having repeated problems.[351] The deadly impact on nursing home residents from infections has long been known. Infections have been a leading

---

[350] *https://apnews.com/article/nursing-homes-neglect-death-surge-3b74a2202140c5a6b5cf05cdf0 ea4f32.*
[351] *https://www.gao.gov/products/gao-20-576r.*

cause of morbidity and mortality among nursing home residents, with 1.6 million to 3.8 million infections per year before the pandemic.[352] Yet, many nursing homes were utterly unprepared to prevent the spread of infectious disease among residents. In August 2020, five months into the pandemic, former CMS Administrator Seema Verma noted that nursing home inspections continued to find widespread failures in basic infection control procedures, such as handwashing.[353]

From the outset, the industry has asserted that since COVID–19 rates in the community heightened the risk of spread in the facility, there was little it could do to protect residents. This claim has been proven inaccurate by numerous studies that show that similarly situated nursing homes that invested in staffing and care quality did better than homes that did not.[354] Recently, the New York Attorney General released a report[355] finding that a facility's prior history of inadequate staffing was more predictive of outcomes than other factors, including its geographic location.

COVID–19 has had a disparate impact on nursing home residents of color. Data shows that homes with large populations of Black and Latinx residents were disproportionately affected compared to other homes.[356] Congress must ensure that the causes of these disparities are investigated and addressed.

CMS was slow to require transparency of conditions in nursing homes as a result of the pandemic. It was not until May 2020 that CMS required all facilities to report data to the CDC about COVID infections, deaths, etc., and it failed to require the reporting retroactively. As a result, there is little data from the months before May, when tens of thousands of residents contracted COVID–19 and died.

At the same time, CMS waived facility reporting of staffing data to the Payroll-Based Journal and delayed reporting assessment data. Complete reporting is essential to establish an accurate and complete picture of what occurred during this time. It is vital to have this information to learn from early failures and help ensure they do not recur. We urge Congress to investigate the effect of COVID–19 on nursing home residents thoroughly. Any investigation should include recommendations to improve care quality and prevent a recurrence of the nursing homes crisis.

---

[352] Richards, C. Infections in residents of long-term care facilities: An agenda for research. Report of an Expert Panel. 50 *JAGS.* 570–576 (2002).

[353] *https://skillednursingnews.com/2020/08/cms-targets-infection-control-in-new-nursing-home-training-program/.*

[354] Figueroa, J.F., Wadhere, R.K., Papanicolas, I., Riley, K., Zheng, J., Orav, E.J. and Jha, A.K.. Association of nursing home ratings on health inspections, quality of care, and nurse staffing with COVID–19 Cases. *JAMA:* (2020): August 10, E1–E2; He, M., Li, Y., and Fang, F. Is there a link between nursing home reported quality and COVID–19 cases? Evidence from California skilled nursing facilities. *JAMDA.* 2020: 905–908; Li, Y., Tempkin-Greener, H., Shan, G. and Cai, X. COVID–19 infections and deaths among Connecticut nursing home residents: facility correlates. *JAGS:* June 18, 2020.

[355] *https://ag.ny.gov/sites/default/files/2021-nursinghomesreport.pdf.*

[356] Li, Y., et, al, Racial and Ethnic Disparities in COVID–19 Infections and Deaths Across U.S. Nursing Homes, *Journal of American Geriatric Society,* 2020 Nov., 68(11):2454–2461; *NY Times, https://www.nytimes.com/article/coronavirus-nursing-homes-racial-disparity.html?action=click&module=Well&pgtype=Homepage&section=US%20News.*

Support the Long-Term Care Workforce Through Minimum Staffing Standards, Training, and Increased Wages and Benefits

Staffing

Since CMS began releasing weekly data in May 2020, on average, 19% of nursing homes have reported a shortage of nurse aides, while 16% reported a shortage in nurses.[357] Over 554,000 nursing home staff have been infected with COVID–19, and at least 1,625 have died.[358] Many workers have resigned due to fear of contracting COVID, family and caregiving responsibilities that have increased during the pandemic, or frustration due to untenable working conditions. These factors exacerbated insufficient staffing levels that pre-dated the pandemic and placed workers in impossible situations and residents at risk of harm.

The federal government does not require minimum staffing levels, and as a result, inadequate staffing has long been a problem in nursing facilities. Numerous studies have linked higher staffing levels to better care.[359] CMS's own study on appropriate staffing found a clear association between nurse staffing levels and quality care.[360] Insufficient staffing proved deadly during the pandemic, with studies showing that facilities with higher staffing levels and ratings fared better on controlling COVID– 19 spread and resident outcomes than poorly staffed homes.[361]

Before the pandemic, RN presence was directly related to quality care and better outcomes for residents.[362] It also proved to be predictive of outcomes during the pandemic, as homes with total RN staffing levels under the recommended minimum standard (.75 hours per resident day) had a two times greater probability of having COVID–19 infections.[363] Yet, nursing homes are only required to have an RN present 8 hours daily.

Training

Early in the pandemic, the previous administration waived the requirement that nurse aides meet training and certification requirements[364] during the Public Health Emergency. CMS claimed that the waiver was necessary to address staff shortages. In reality, the waiver resulted in Temporary Nurse Aides (TNAs) who were ill-equipped to provide necessary care and services to residents and put the workers and residents at increased risk of injury. TNAs who

---

[357] *https://data.cms.gov/stories/s/bkwz-xpvg.*

[358] *Id.*

[359] Castle, N.G., Wagner, L.M., Ferguson, J.C., and Handler, S.M. Nursing home deficiency citations for safety. *J. Aging and Social Policy,* 2011; 23 (1):34–57; Castle, N.G. and Anderson, R.A. Caregiver staffing in nursing homes and their influence on quality of care. *Medical Care,* 2011:49(6):545–552; Schnelle, J.F., Simmons, S.F., Harrington, C., Cadogan, M., Garcia, E., and Bates-Jensen, B. Relationship of nursing home staffing to quality of care? *Health Serv Res.,* 2004: 39 (2):225–250; Spector, W.D., Limcangco, R., Williams, C., Rhodes, W. and Hurd, D. Potentially avoidable hospitalizations for elderly long-stay residents in nursing homes. *Med Care,* 2013: 51 (8):673–81.

[360] Centers for Medicare and Medicaid Services, Abt Associates Inc. Appropriateness of Minimum Nurse Staffing Ratios in Nursing Homes. Report to Congress: Phase II Final. Volumes I–III. Baltimore, MD.

[361] Li, et al. 2020, "COVID–19 Infections and Deaths Among Connecticut Nursing Home Resident: Facility Correlates;" *Journal of the American Geriatrics Society,* Vol. 68, Issue 10, 2153– 2162.

[362] Dellefield, M.E., Castle, N.G., McGilton, K.S., and Spilsbury, K. The relationship between registered nurses and nursing home quality: An integrative review (2008–2014). *Nurs Econ.,* 2015; 33(2):95–108, 116.b.

[363] Harrington, et al. 2020, Nursing Staffing and Coronavirus Infections in California Nursing Homes; *Policy Politics and Nursing Practice,* 2020, Vol. 21(3) 174–86.

[364] *https://www.cms.gov/files/document/summary-covid-19-emergency-declaration-waivers.pdf.*

had not been trained in proper infection control entered a medical setting where protecting residents from infectious disease was paramount.

To date, this waiver is still in place, and proposals exist at the state and federal levels for waving the training and certification requirements for these workers permanently. If the pandemic has taught us anything, it is that more training is needed, not less.

It is also unclear how many untrained and uncertified workers have fallen under this waiver and how much training and supervision they have had. In fact, it is doubtful whether CMS will be able to determine the total number. It would be highly irresponsible to waive these requirements without knowing how many staff, and in turn, residents will be affected.

The current training requirements for CNAs are inadequate as well. CNAs have more contact with residents than any other staff members. However, federal training requirements for CNA certification are only 75 hours. Increasing acuity and complexity of residents' needs, including higher incidences of dementia, warrant a need for increased training standards. In its report on the adequacy of the healthcare workforce for older Americans (*Retooling for an Aging America,* 2008), the National Academy of Medicine (formerly the Institute of Medicine) recommends that "federal requirements for the minimum training of certified nursing assistants (CNAs) and home health aides should be raised to at least 120 hours and should include demonstration of competence in the care of older adults as a criterion for certification" (Recommendation 5–1).

Increased Wages and Benefits

A report[365] released by LeadingAge, an organization representing non-profit nursing homes, documented that almost half of nursing home care workers earned less than a living wage, with nearly 57% relying on public assistance. One study[366] documented that nursing homes' nursing staff turnover rate was roughly 100% annually, even before the pandemic. The LeadingAge report states that increasing wages for nursing home workers would reduce this turnover and significantly improve residents' health outcomes. Increased wages are necessary to attract and retain highly experienced and well-trained workers. On the one hand, we cannot call our nursing home workers heroes, while on the other, paying them wages that require them to rely on government assistance.

Further contributing to unsafe conditions for staff and residents, too many facilities do not have a qualified infection preventionist to support and implement infection prevention and control protocols necessary to sufficiently address the spread of COVID–19.

Lastly, understaffing is made worse by the failures of CMS to enforce adequate staffing levels. A recent report[367] by the Office of Inspector General found that CMS should do more to strengthen oversight of nursing home staffing.

To better support the facility's staff and attract and retain experienced and qualified workers that can increase positive health outcomes, Congress should urge CMS to:

- End the Trump Administration's waiver of training requirements for nurse aides and feeding assistants enacted in March 2020. Require temporary nurse aides hired under this waiver to complete full training and certification within a designated timeframe to

---

[365] *https://leadingage.org/sites/default/files/Making%20Care%20Work%20Pay%20Report.pdf.*

[366] Gandhi, A., Yu, G., Grabowski, D. High Nursing Staff Turnover in Nursing Homes Offers Important Quality Information, *Health Affairs,* 2021, Vol. 40, No, 3.

[367] *https://oig.hhs.gov/oei/reports/OEI-04-18-00451.pdf.*

continue working and require nursing homes to identify and publicly report numbers of Temporary Nurse Aides currently employed.

- Increase initial nurse aide certification training requirements from the current 75 hours to adequately prepare frontline aides for the complex needs of the people they are hired to assist. Require facilities to cover the cost of training.

In addition, Congress should pass legislation that:

- Strengthens the direct care workforce by (a) increasing compensation, including hazard pay (b) improving access to affordable health insurance, paid family and medical leave, paid sick leave, and affordable childcare.
- Requires a minimum staffing standard of at least 4.1 hours per resident day.
- Requires 24-hour RN presence in all nursing homes.
- Establishes a robust enforcement mechanism to ensure adequate staffing levels.

Require the Rescission of all Waivers of Nursing Home Regulations Established under the Public Health Emergency

In addition to the training and certification waiver, the previous administration issued multiple waivers of standards and requirements for healthcare providers, including nursing homes, through the use of 1135 waivers.[368] These waivers included waiving notice of transfer or discharge and facility reporting requirements, including resident assessment information and staffing information.

The waiver allowing facilities not to report resident assessment information and staffing information has been rescinded. However, CMS has publicly stated that it will not require facilities to provide the staffing information for the period that reporting was waived, even though it is readily accessible to nursing homes. When CMS made this decision, the period for which the reporting waiver applied had been the deadliest for nursing home residents. If we are to understand what happened during the pandemic, facilities must provide this information.

Waivers must not continue indefinitely without evaluation to assess whether they continue to be needed or effective. Many of the waivers referred to in this document remove essential resident rights articulated in law and regulation.

Congress should urge CMS to:

- Rescind the waivers of nursing facility requirements that permit waivers of notice for transfer or discharge due to cohorting and nurse aide training.
- Require facilities to report data on staffing from January 1st–May 2020. All of this data is already in the possession of nursing homes and is critical for analyzing what happened during that time and what we can do to prevent it in the future.

---

[368] *https://www.cms.gov/files/document/summary-covid-19-emergency-declaration-waivers.pdf.*

Ensure Access to COVID–19 Vaccines for All Residents and Staff Who Choose to be Vaccinated

The discovery and release of highly effective and safe COVID–19 vaccines has offered promise to residents and staff. Since residents and staff began receiving vaccinations, COVID–19 case numbers and deaths have plummeted. Yet not all residents have equal access to the vaccine in nursing homes.

In all states but West Virginia, the CDC partnered with outside pharmacies to conduct clinics at nursing homes to have residents and staff vaccinated. These pharmacies have adopted a policy of only visiting nursing homes three times to vaccinate residents. As a result, residents who entered the facility after the second clinic have just received one dose of the vaccination. Others who were admitted after the third clinic have not received a vaccine at all. In some states, plans have not yet been established to ensure continued access to vaccines, and in some cases, facilities are requiring residents to obtain the vaccination themselves. This policy creates an unacceptable burden on residents and families to ensure they become fully vaccinated. For many residents, this task will be impossible and will result in them going without the protection of a vaccine.

New residents and staff continue entering nursing homes and should be offered the vaccine. Currently, there is no policy from the federal government setting forth a plan for ensuring these residents can become fully vaccinated.

Early reports[369] 22 stated nursing home staff were refusing vaccination at a rate as high as 60%. This high refusal rate has been attributed mainly to distrust of the vaccine and a lack of information accessible to staff.[370] CMS and CDC must continue efforts to provide staff with information on vaccines that address staff concerns and help increase vaccination rates among staff.

It is also vitally important for current and future residents and their families to have access to information that shows how many residents and staff have been vaccinated in each facility. This information will be essential for residents to make informed decisions on their care and where they want to reside. Although the CDC is releasing total numbers of staff and residents who have been vaccinated, it is not at the facility level.

To ensure all residents and staff have access to the COVID–19 vaccination, Congress should:

- Require federal, state, and local coordination for ensuring ongoing access to vaccines for all residents and staff of long-term care facilities.
- Require nursing homes to report the number and percentage of their residents and workers who have been vaccinated and disclose that information to residents, families, staff, the LTCOP, the State Survey Agency, CMS and CDC. Vaccination rates in nursing homes should be reported to the CDC and shared publicly on Nursing Home Compare (Care Compare).

---

[369] *https://www.cnbc.com/2021/02/09/covid-vaccine-60percent-of-nursing-home-staff-refused-shots-walgreens-exe c-says.html.*

[370] *https://www.health.harvard.edu/blog/why-wont-some-health-care-workers-get-vacci-nated-2021021721967.*

Ensure Protection from COVID–19 for Residents and Staff by Ensuring Ongoing Access to PPE and Testing

As with many health facilities, nursing homes have struggled to obtain and maintain adequate supplies of high-quality personal protective equipment (PPE). Many nursing homes continue to report less than one-week supplies of masks, gowns, and gloves.[371] Additionally, ensuring facilities have sufficient access to accurate COVID–19 testing will be essential in helping prevent outbreaks. To ensure all facilities have adequate PPE and testing, Congress should:

- Establish an effective supply chain for the distribution of PPE to long-term care facilities, and ensure funding for sufficient, usable PPE to supply nursing home staff, visitors, surveyors, and LTC ombudsmen.
- Require all facilities to have a 30-day supply of PPE on hand.
- Provide funding and hold facilities accountable for paying for accurate point-of-care testing with rapid turnaround of results for staff, residents, and their families who visit.

Fully Restore Visitation in Nursing Homes

On March 13, 2020, CMS issued an order[372] prohibiting anyone other than essential health care workers from entering nursing homes. As a result, residents were isolated from their families and subject to neglect and harm due to inadequate staffing. As time passed, the harm from isolation and neglect began to take a toll on residents' health and well-being.[373] These problems mainly went unseen, as facility surveyors, families, and long-term care ombudsmen were restricted from entering facilities. Residents could no longer rely on their loved ones to draw attention to health declines or inadequate care. As some facilities re-opened their doors to visitation, many family members discovered their loved ones had experienced a devastating decline, including significant weight loss, cognitive decline, emotional distress, and extremely poor hygiene.[374]

On March 10, 2021, CMS issued new visitation guidance[375] that relaxed some of the visitation restrictions. While a step in the right direction, the guidance does not go far enough, however, to protect residents from the effects of isolation and neglect. The guidance language allows facilities significant discretion when determining the length and frequency of visits, including for compassionate care. CMS must require facilities to permit visits based on the needs of each resident and enforce those requirements.

Further, residents continue to need access to telecommunications devices and Internet services in order to communicate with family and friends who are unable to visit in person. Such access is necessary for supporting many residents who suffer from isolation. Despite efforts to increase access during the pandemic, many facilities do not have devices that can be

---

[371] For instance, for the week ending February 14, 2001, 5% of nursing homes reported they had less than a one week supply of N–95 masks, *https://data.cms.gov/stories/s/bkwz-xpvg.*

[372] CMS, QSO–20–14–NH, updated by QSO–20–39–NH (Sept 17, 2020).

[373] *https://apnews.com/article/nursing-homes-neglect-death-surge-3b74a2202140c5a6b5cf05cdf0ea4f32.*

[374] *https://theconsumervoice.org/uploads/files/issues/Devasting_Effect_of_Lockdowns_on_Res idents_of_LTC_Facil ities.pdf.*

[375] CMS, QSO=20–39–NH.

used by residents who do not have their own, and there are facilities that refuse to allow a resident to connect their personal device to the facility's Internet connection.

To help protect residents, Congress should:

- Allow every resident to designate an essential support person (ESP). The ESP must be allowed unrestricted access to residents to provide physical and emotional support and assistance in meeting residents' needs. ESPs should be treated as employees of the facility for infection control purposes, including routine COVID–19 testing and the wearing of PPE (cost to be borne by the facility).
- Urge CMS to modify its visitation guidance to require facilities to permit visits based on the needs of each resident and, until full visitation rights are restored, ensure that visits are no less than one hour weekly.
- Require CMS to enforce visitation guidance.
- Pass legislation that provides access to telecommunications devices and the Internet for all residents.

Reinstate Annual Recertification and Complaint Surveys and Strengthen Regulations and Enforcement

Recertification and Complaint Surveys

At the same time visitation bans were instituted, the previous administration suspended surveys and enforcement except in very limited situations. CMS directed State Survey Agencies to prioritize the most egregious complaints (triaged as immediate jeopardy) and implemented a new type of survey focused on infection prevention and control requirements,[376] to the exclusion of all other issues. As a result, state survey agencies did not conduct complaint investigations (except for immediate jeopardy) or annual surveys for months. Complaints of rights violations, neglect, eviction, and similar serious issues were ignored to the residents' great detriment.

While CMS issued guidance in September 2020 to reinstate survey activities, not all states have. As of the date of this hearing, California, Ohio, and Tennessee, for example, still have not begun completing annual recertification surveys. California is still only investigating IJ-level complaints.

Congress should urge CMS to ensure that all states are conducting annual recertification surveys and investigating all complaints.

Regulations

In 2017 CMS issued final federal rules for nursing homes that rolled back the ban on pre-dispute arbitration and in 2019 issued proposed rules to further roll back the revised nursing home rules published in 2016. These proposed rules would provide fewer protections for residents and less accountability for nursing facilities by, among other things, weakening standards relating to

[376] CMS, QSO–20–20–All.

infection prevention, use of antipsychotic medications, and responding to resident and family grievances.

Congress should:

- Urge CMS to rescind its 2019 proposed rules to ensure that nursing home residents are not stripped of these necessary protections.
- Pass legislation banning forced arbitration agreements in nursing homes.
- Urge CMS to reinstate the regulation banning nursing home arbitration agreements.

Enforcement

Prior to the pandemic, insufficient enforcement of regulations long plagued nursing home care. Deficiencies were under-cited and often did not[377] identify serious problems. Enforcement actions are also not sufficiently meaningful to bring about lasting change, as evidenced by a 2019[378] OIG report that found that 31 percent of nursing homes had a deficiency (violation) cited at least five times during 2013–2017, and[379] a study which determined that 42 percent of deficiencies were given for chronic or repeated deficiencies in a 3-year period.

Enforcement was further weakened by actions taken under the previous administration. In 2017, CMS revised its enforcement policy to change the default method of assessing civil money penalties for past non-compliance from the imposition of "per-day" fines to "per-instance" fines. This change removes any incentive for facilities to identify and correct non-compliance as early as possible, resulting in residents subjected to potentially harmful non-compliance for an extended period. We believe this revision was made in violation of proper administrative procedures.

These failures of enforcement certainly contributed to the crisis in nursing homes during the pandemic. Repeated and long-standing violations are the result of facilities facing little pecuniary punishment. As noted above, 8 out of 10 facilities had infection control violations before the pandemic, with half of those having repeated problems. Until CMS adopts a rigorous and consistent enforcement strategy, the issues that led to the devastation in nursing homes will continue.

Congress should:

- Require CMS to ensure that comprehensive and complaint surveys have been fully restarted in all states.
- Direct CMS to withdraw the proposed rules on nursing facility Requirements of Participation published Federal Register, Vol. 84, No. 138, July 18, 2019, 34737.
- Strengthen federal and state enforcement by requiring pre-established per-day penalties and utilizing denials of payment for resident admissions for non-compliance

---

[377] Office of the Inspector General (OIG). *States continued to fall short in meeting required timeframes for investigating nursing home complaints: 2016–2018.* Data Brief. Washington, DC: OIG OEI–01–19–00421. September 2020.

[378] Office of the Inspector General (OIG). *Trends in deficiencies at nursing homes show that improvements are needed to ensure the health and safety of residents.* HHS Data Brief. April 2019. 09–18–02010.

[379] A Long Term Care Community Coalition. Issue Alert. Chronic deficiencies in care: The persistence of recurring failures to meet minimum safety and dignity standards in U.S. nursing homes. *LTCCC,* February 2017. *http://nursinghome411.org/nursing-homes-with-chronic-deficiencies/.*

with specific requirements, such as staffing, transfer/discharge, life safety, emergency preparedness, and infection control.

- Instruct CMS to rescind the Trump Administration directive, "Revision of Civil Money Penalty (CMP) Policies and CMP Analytic Tool" (S&C 17–37–NH), which instructed State Survey Agency Directors and CMS Regional Offices that "per-instance" CMPs would be imposed for past non-compliance, conflicting with the enforcement provisions in the Social Security Act that provide for the imposition of CMPS for "each day of non-compliance."

Require Transparency and Accountability Around Nursing Home Ownership and Finances

For years, the nursing home industry has been plagued by poor care brought on by the purchase of homes by corporations and Private Equity Investment (PE) firms with little or no experience in healthcare or with a long history of providing sub-standard care. A study released in February 2021 estimated that PE ownership of a nursing home increases the mortality of Medicare residents by 10%, results in declines in many measures of well-being for residents and increases taxpayer spending per resident by 11%.[380] A recent report in the *Washington Post* revealed that even during the pandemic, investment groups with a long track record of owning homes that provide poor quality care were allowed to buy over 20 homes and that care suffered.[381]

Corporate and PE firms have slashed resources, including cutting staff and supplies.[382] It is common practice for them to pay related third parties, such as vendors, management companies, and others, for services as a means of funneling money to themselves.[383] Yet, there is no system to audit the use of federal funds and determine whether they go to profits or resident care.

To improve the quality of care in nursing homes and to ensure the appropriate use of taxpayer money, Congress should pass legislation:

- Mandating audits to determine how facilities spend taxpayer money.
- Setting limits on administrative costs and profits for all payors.
- Requiring CMS to establish federal regulations to specify the minimum criteria for purchasing or managing any nursing home.

Address Disparities in Care for Racial and Ethnic Minorities

All residents are entitled to quality care and services, access to justice, and protection from discrimination. Black and Latinx nursing home residents have been disproportionately affected

---

[380] *https://www.nber.org/system/files/working_papers/w28474/w28474.pdf.*

[381] *https://www.washingtonpost.com/local/portopiccolo-nursing-homes-maryland/2020/12/21/a1ffb2a6-292b-11eb-9b14-ad872157ebc9_story.html.*

[382] Harrington, C., Olney, B., Carrillo, H., Kang, T. Nurse staffing and deficiencies in the largest for-profit chains and chains owned by private equity companies. *Health Serv Res.*, 2012; 47(1 pt. I):106–128.

[383] Harrington, C., Ross, L., Kang, T. Hidden ownership, hidden profits, and poor quality of nursing home care: A case study. *International Journal of Health Services,* 2015;45 (4): 779–800.

by COVID–19.[384] Research has shown the disparities in care experienced by individuals based on race, ethnicity, and socioeconomic status have become pronounced during the COVID pandemic.[385] This research points to long-standing racial inequities that pre-date COVID–19. Due to discriminatory lending policies, housing segregation, greater reliance on Medicaid, and inequitable healthcare access, marginalized populations are more likely to reside in racially and ethnically identifiable nursing homes that provide poorer care. Data gathering practices and targeted interventions must be developed to ensure that residents' care needs are met.

CMS policies make addressing disparities in care difficult. Although CMS collects data on race and ethnicity, it does not release this data to the public, which has created a gap in knowledge regarding how minority groups are treated in nursing homes. However, COVID–19 has laid bare that residents of color receive inferior quality of care when compared with others.

We urge Congress to:

- Require CMS to collect and report nursing home resident demographic data specific to race and ethnicity, source of payment, and ownership.
- Require CMS to require facilities to report racial demographic data as part of the weekly data facilities report to the CDC.
- Make CMS race and ethnicity data publicly available dating back to the beginning of the pandemic. Policymakers, government agencies, advocates, providers, and researchers need this information to identify disparities in care and to develop enforceable public policies to ensure equitable care for all residents.
- Investigate and address the disparities in care and access to services for racial and ethnic minorities, including disparate care and outcomes in nursing homes under common ownership and operation, Medicare and Medicaid policies that allow or promote discrimination based source of payment, and other factors that result in disparate placement in poor-performing, racially identifiable nursing homes, such as hospital discharges.

Expand Choice Through Expansion of Medicaid Home and Community Based Services

For many older adults with limited income and resources, needing assistance with activities of daily living means going to a nursing home. However, during the pandemic, many older adults chose to remain home without sufficient supports to avoid the risk of being infected with COVID–19 in a nursing home. While the implementation of Medicaid waivers has improved access to home and community-based services (HCBS) for these individuals, HCBS is not a required benefit under Medicaid, and for those states where waivers exist, there often are limits on coverage, limited availability of service providers and affordable housing, and long waiting lists. The devastating effect of COVID–19 on people living in congregate settings has only

[384] Li, Y., Cen, X., Cai, X., and Temkin-Greener, H. Racial and ethnic disparities in COVID– 19 infections and deaths across U.S. Nursing Homes. *JAGS,* 2020:1–8 DPO:10:1111/jgs.16847.

[385] Gebeloff, R., Ivory, D., Richtel, M., Smith M, Yourish K., Dance, S., Fortie´r, J., Yu, E., and Parker, M. (2020). Striking racial divide: How COVID–19 has hit nursing homes. *The New York Times,* May 21, *https://www.nytimes.com/article/coronavirus-nursing-homes-racialdisparity.html?action=click&module=Well &pgtype=Home-page&section=US%20News.*

highlighted the need to make HCBS a required benefit. Increased access to HCBS would likely have saved lives during the pandemic.

To allow individuals who could successfully remain in or transition back to their homes or community-based settings instead of entering or staying in a nursing home, we urge Congress to:

- Make HCBS a required benefit under Medicaid and allow coverage of housing-related services and retroactive coverage for HCBS services.
- Permanently reauthorize the Money Follows the Person program, which has helped older adults and persons with disabilities transition from institutions into the community.
- Direct resources for more low-income housing and residential care.

The pandemic's tragic impact on residents and staff of nursing home residents was years in the making. Many of the recommendations in this statement have been made by advocates for years, in part because it was foreseeable that a virus like COVID–19 would devastate nursing homes. We call on Congress to act now and take decisive steps to not only prevent the next crisis, but to increases the quality of care in nursing homes for current and future generations.

Sincerely,
The National Consumer Voice for Quality Long-Term Care
Community Legal Services of Philadelphia
Michigan Elder Justice Initiative

Statement Submitted by Mary Nichols, Texas Caregivers for Compromise

March 13, 2021 was one year since families were declared non-essential and prevented from freely visiting loved ones in long-term care facilities. CMS issued new guidance on March 10, 2021 that allows expanded visitation but not only are most nursing homes still not in compliance, but the guidelines do not apply to assisted living facilities, group homes, intermediate care facilities and group homes that do not received Medicaid and Medicare funding so those facilities are still largely autonomous when it comes to regulating visitation. Families must learn complex guidelines in order to argue to be admitted to facilities or obtain assistance from an ombudsmen. This is disproportionately skewed against lower income populations who work multiple jobs and lack the luxury of being full-time advocates, populations with language barriers, and those populations without higher levels of education who struggle to decipher technical legalese and analyze these complicated regulations against the restrictions being given to them by their loved one's facility.

The severe weight loss, rapid cognitive decline, and extreme despondency in residents from COVID–19 protocols continue to result in loss of both life and quality of life. The mental health crisis taking place among residents, families, and long-term care staff members cannot be overstated as the intense pressures on people affected by guideline enforcement increase daily. For a full year, residents have felt abandoned and forgotten, life-long spouses have been separated, adult children with cognitive disorders have not seen a parent or sibling, dementia and Alzheimer's residents have lost memory of their loved ones, people have died alone, and families have lost what time remained with their loved ones who passed away in this last year.

CMS Guidance Is Misused

Guidance put in place by CMS on September 17, 2020 and March 20, 2021 is widely misunderstood by facilities and the visitation provisions within them have neither been acknowledged nor implemented in a great many facilities in a majority of states. Commonly, facilities point to CMS guidelines as the reason they cannot allow any form of visitation. This is false. Meanwhile, recourse by state health authorities is absent and there is no reason to anticipate that facilities who ignore current visitation standards will follow future or amended rules.

Essential Caregivers Are Not a Permanent Solution

Many states are adopting essential caregiver provisions that allow one or two family members access to care for a resident for a few minutes or an hour or two a week. Essential caregivers are a temporary solution for visitation as they only allow a small increment of restoration of resident rights. As we see many states beginning to adopt programs similar to the Texas and Florida programs, our concern is that the perception by our lawmakers will be that this is an acceptable permanent alternative to visitation in long-term care facilities when, instead, it is an emergency answer to be used as a last resort.

ADA Violations

Current prohibition of visitation has resulted in widespread and readily accepted violation of the Americans with Disabilities Act.

Unequal Family Access. Those residents who are cognizantly healthy enough to use telephones, virtual visits and talk through closed windows have far more access to family than those bed-bound, deaf, blind, and intellectually disabled residents as well as residents with advanced dementia and Alzheimer's who are incapable of seeing virtual technology as anything other than white noise, are bed-bound and unable to go to a window, or become agitated and harm themselves when they don't understand why a relative remains on the other side of glass. Blind adults who depend on tactile communication are eliminated from these visits, deaf adults are restricted by small screens and windows are often not even wheelchair accessible.

Unequal Protection from Abuse and Neglect. Intellectually disabled adults and residents with dementia or Alzheimer's have unequal protection from abuse and neglect as those residents who are able to push a call-button or phone a relative. Outside visitors, clergy, family, powers of attorney, hospice workers, ombudsmen, and legal guardians are the extra eyes that assess a resident's environment and welfare and affect change should there be an issue or deficiency. The absence of those eyes removes that protection from people incapable of calling for a tray because the lunch cart missed their room, asking for a shower, reporting a bedsore, or complaining about soiled clothing. They have also lost those eyes that are familiar enough to notice the subtle differences in the health or behavior of the resident that staff members—frequently temporary substitutes—might miss. This was one of the major purposes of the 1987 Nursing Home Reform Act.

Results of Facility Autonomy

Facilities have had twelve months of authority over decisions related to and rights of residents in long-term care facilities. While they must have ability to make administrative choices that best suit their facility's needs, these choices have crossed over into decisions that:

- Deny rights of residents guaranteed in state and federal law;
- Make care decisions without resident and/or family input;
- Circumvent guidelines put in place by Texas Health and Human Services;
- Circumvent Centers for Medicaid and Medicare Services guidelines; and
- Ignore recommendations of the CDC regarding discontinuation of transmission based precautions for patients recovering from COVID–19

Facilities will not release this authority without argument and resistance as the involvement of family members is often no longer welcome but considered interference. While CMS guidelines do not apply to all facilities, the ones that they do apply to often either do not know the guidelines, do not understand the guidelines, or simply choose not to follow the guidelines. The issues rising from those facilities are many and egregious:

- Refusing essential caregivers in states that allow them;
- Not allowing hospice workers for a year;
- Denying end-of-life visits;
- Denying compassionate care visits;
- Not following CDC recommendations re: discontinuation of transmission-based precautions when a resident has recovered from COVID–19 and isolating asymptomatic residents 24 to 35 days instead of 10;
- Denying closed window visits;
- Not allowing a resident to use his/her own property;
- Making residents remain in their room, refusing communal dining, and not allowing outdoor recreation, walks, or fresh air;
- Prohibiting residents from opening or receiving mail;
- Requiring a family to use the hospice company of the facility's choice;
- Refusing indoor plexiglass visitation;
- Making resident care decisions without consulting legal guardians, family, or Medical POAs;
- Not allowing resident to participate in religious activity;
- Not holding required care plan meetings with family members;
- Denying resident a right to refuse a treatment; and
- Denying ability to report abuse or neglect by refusing to allow use of facility telephones

One Year Is the Remainder of a Lifetime

The life expectancy of a resident once he or she moves into long-term care is six months to two years depending on which statistics you believe, the health of the resident and the type of care required. The restrictions will have been in place a year on March 13, 2021. That is the remainder of many people's lifetimes.

Post-Vaccine Visitation

New CMS guidance discriminates residents based on whether they choose or decline the vaccine. There is much vaccine reluctance at this time among many minority populations and this regulation makes visitation rights disproportionately skewed against those minorities. Residents in a county with 10% or more positivity who have not received the vaccine are denied visitation. Not only is this a disguised mandate of an emergency use vaccine but it makes a resident's rights dependent on the choices of everyone else in the county to mask, social distance, practice infection control, or receive the vaccine. Nobody's statutory and federal rights should be dependent on the choice somebody else makes.

Dangerous Precedent

COVID–19 was an unprecedented crisis in our country. But the unprecedented has now become precedented and we have set a dangerous one. Imagine a war, emergency, crisis, or pandemic in the future that disproportionately affects children under a certain age or people of a certain genetic background or race. Would this country stand for stripping them of their rights for their own good for over a year? As ridiculous as that sounds, could we have imagined eighteen months ago that residents in long-term care facilities would be restricted from visitation and all those rights in the 1987 Nursing Home Reform Act for a year? It's time that we agree that in the United States of America the rights of no population should ever again end the moment a pandemic begins.

Statement of Dr. Emily Morgan, Assistant Professor of Internal Medicine and Geriatrics, Oregon Health and Science University; Medical Director, Mirabella Skilled and Long Term Care

Oregon Health and Science University
3181 S.W. Sam Jackson Park Rd.
Portland, OR 97239

Chairman Wyden, Ranking Member Crapo, and Members of the Committee:

We are pleased to submit this statement for the record to offer feedback on the Department of Health and Human Services Centers for Medicare & Medicaid Services' (CMS) memorandum on Nursing Home Visitation during the COVID–19 Public Health Emergency published on March 10, 2021. We greatly appreciate the continued efforts of CMS to ensure the health and safety of our vulnerable nursing home population and we wholeheartedly agree with CMS' commitment to ending the social isolation faced by many nursing home residents during this pandemic. However, we feel it is important that we voice our concern regarding how these changes are implemented, with the shared goals of reducing the burden of isolation and keeping our most vulnerable population protected.

We are concerned that the emphasis placed on allowing indoor visitation "at all times and for all residents" will unduly place residents and facility staff at increased risk without additional limitations in place. We ask that CMS consider adding an exception that clearly states that indoor visitation will not be permitted when a facility cannot safely ensure appropriate physical distancing and oversight during visitation. We are concerned that facilities overwhelmed with visitors will not have the available staffing needed to ensure safety protocols are being appropriately followed, while at the same time delivering adequate care to residents.

We would also like CMS to consider changing the use of 10% county test positivity rate as an exception scenario for allowing un-restricted indoor visitation. Test positivity is a crude measure of transmission risk, but most would consider a rate of >10% as indicative of widespread and un-controlled transmission in the community. Happily, many counties in Oregon as well as other states have not seen positivity rates this high even during the peak of the pandemic. We believe that protecting the safety of residents and staff would best be served by continued limits on visitation unless the local risk of disease is low, for example, <5%. Also, since test positivity rates may be highly dependent on access to testing, consideration should be given to including other metrics, such as the rate of new cases/per 100, 000 population over the preceding 14 days (incidence rate) to determine restrictions on visitation. (See *https://coronavirus.oregon.gov/Pages/living-with-covid-19.aspx#current risklevelbycountyma* for an example of how incidence rates and test positivity may be combined as indicators of COVID–19 spread in the community). In our opinion, restriction of indoor visitation should be allowed unless local disease transmission has been minimized.

Lastly, we are concerned about the CDC's Updated Healthcare Infection Prevention and Control Recommendations in Response to COVID–19 Vaccination, published March 10, 2021 which states "quarantine is no longer recommended for residents who are being admitted to a post-acute care facility if they are fully vaccinated and have not had prolonged close contact with someone with SARS–coV–2 infection in the prior 14 days. The potential for recent SARS–CoV–2 exposure of patients who are being newly admitted to nursing homes cannot always be accurately determined, whether they are being admitted from an acute care hospital or the community. Risk of exposure may be highly variable depending on community rates and/or the quality of infection control practices at the referring care facility. In addition, we know that vaccination is not 100% effective in preventing SARS–CoV–2 infections, and the level of protection provided against emerging virulent and highly communicable genetic variants of concern is still uncertain. Although the risk of COVID– 19 disease among fully vaccinated patients may be relatively low, the consequences of transmission within a nursing home can be devastating. Quarantine of newly admitted nursing home residents remains an important tool in outbreak prevention. While quarantine is isolating, perhaps the best way to address this would be to recommend quarantine for 7 days accompanied by testing to shorten the quarantine period while maintaining this important safeguard.

We are thankful for the continued efforts of CMS and the CDC to prioritize the health and wellness of our nursing home residents and staff. It is with much excitement that we look forward to increased visitation and decreased isolation for our residents that have suffered so much in this last year. We appreciate the Committee's interest in this issue and CMS' willingness to consider the feedback we offer here and move to implement safe visitation and transitions of care policies that continue to offer the highest degree of protection to our nursing home communities.

With Many Kind Regards,

Emily Morgan, M.D.

Cc: Liz Richter, Acting Administrator, Centers for Medicare and Medicaid Services

Letter Submitted by Carolyn Piper

Thank you for the opportunity to add my statement to the record of this hearing. I am a 70 year old daughter, living in NV, of parents residing in long-term care in PA. Unfortunately they are in two separate "facilities" in a continuing care conglomerate, since they need different levels of care. My mother requires skilled care, on the second floor of her building. My father requires assisted living care, residing on the ground floor of the same building. Thus their dwellings are under separate licenses, making my father the dreaded "Visitor" this past year.

From the time of my mother's stroke almost 4 years ago, I was traveling to PA every month for the first year, then every 6–8 weeks after that until Feb 2020. My mother has no language and no mobility, totally helpless and dependent on others. Every single communication is done by the same hand wave, and we spent hours trying to determine what she wanted or needed. The frequency of my visits was to ensure that my parents' needs were being met, to participate in planning meetings, and to advocate for unmet needs. I was also able to provide extra direct care and stimulation to my mother for participation in some activities (she declined everything that staff offered), general stimulation and conversation, *long* walks outside in her wheel-chair (which staff never had time to do and which was the *only* recreation that was meaningful to her in any way) and eating assistance because we discovered through diligent trial and error what she liked to eat and how it could be prepared on her tray to help her to be the most independent in feeding herself as possible. I was her voice, because she no longer had one. Prior to COVID, I worried about the long hours that she was languishing alone in her bed for 20 hours every day. But I knew that between my visits, my 2 brothers and sister, and my nephew were visiting sometimes multiple times a week. They provided all of these same things.

And then with no warning, no one was allowed back in. My mother, who does not read a newspaper, and does not watch TV, and whose brain is severely damaged from her massive stroke, only knew that no one was coming anymore to take her outside, or wheelchair walks through the building, or fix her meal tray, or brush her hair, or brush her teeth, or clean her dirty face, or wipe the scum and smell from between her clenched fingers, or make sure staff saw the crust and redness on her inner elbow or under her breast or on her elbow, and then treated it properly. She surely must have felt abandoned, alone, depressed, despondent. She had no concept of virus, or mitigation, or pandemic. Not even my father was allowed back in. And what we thought would be a two week separation turned into a year. My brother and nephew got a couple "window visits," but my hard of hearing mother could not hear them through the glass door and masks. She did not comprehend why they did not come in. Then there were Facetime calls, which she did not even understand before her stroke, and with no communication on her part, all we could do was to "eyeball" her and try to explain in words she probably did not remotely comprehend why we were no longer coming. My sister had one compassionate visit with her in her room during the year, but could not go at lunch to provide feeding help, could not walk her anywhere (not allowed out of the room), could not go on the weekend (not enough staff) and was allowed two visits and *done*. Just an arbitrary rule from what we could understand. I was "not allowed" in for a year, because the PA governor issued a prolonged 14 quarantine stipulation for out of state travelers into PA, and my finances did not allow for two weeks in PA and *then* two visits with my parents.

In addition to my own personal story, I am a member of a national Facebook group called Caregivers for Compromise-Because Isolation Kills too. There are over 14,000 members. The

PA chapter that I belong to has over 600 members. So, over the last several months, I have read *hundreds* of tragic stories about long term care residents and their families suffering through this often *total* and prolonged isolation, as they lived and too often died *alone*.

Here is what I have learned this past year, and what I would like to share about my perspective on this tragedy.

I shudder to think what would have happened to my mother without family there to support her and encourage her and advocate for her and sometimes even fight for her 4 years ago when she first entered the nursing home. Her care was standard, but I know without any doubt that her family was the critical element to her living. We supplemented direct care and our presence was her medicine. We saw things that staff missed and interpreted her hand waves because in their busy every day work life, there was not time to spend hours to figure out what she wanted or needed. We helped to relieve her anxiety because she no longer spoke but we knew she was aware and afraid and helpless. We were there to help her match cards, and copy letters, and try to speak, and exercise her arms and legs. Having lost all mobility on her own, we walked her miles in her wheelchair. We were her lifeline and her connection to the world outside of her 12 by 12 room.

How many thousands of new residents have entered long-term care facilities this past year with *no one* to support them or encourage them or advocate for them, or report neglect that they saw? How many were unnecessarily medicated because they seem depressed, or anxious, or starting having "behaviors"? How much was all of this due singularly to isolation? How many died with no one by their side, and no good byes? Have you seen all the pictures that have been posted of accelerated decline? The "unintended consequence" to the lockdown? Or as residents would say, the lock-up? Residents suffered and families suffered and there will never be closure for them.

We learned that facilities earned "rewards" from the federal government for reducing COVID cases. On the surface, that mitigation success seems to be a very good thing. But how did this very monetary award incentivize keeping families out? How were those funds used to enhance ongoing and meaningful connections with

In May 2020, the Centers for Medicare and Medicaid Services (CMS) issued some visitation guidelines but I don't think families ever grasped very well that these existed and how to get them enforced. By the time of the new guidelines in Sept. 2020, we were more educated and sharing information with each other. Still, the guidelines were vague and up for much interpretation.

Just to summarize the great disparity, and with all other things being equal related to outbreak status and county positivity rate:

- Some facilities arranged compassionate care visits. Others absolutely did *not*.
- Some facilities eventually worked with families to a compromise. Others stood with a firm *no*.
- Some facilities told families, well if we let you in, we will have to let others in. So they still said *no*. And yet *every single* resident should have been entitled to a compassionate visit after 10 months of being confined to their room and many times not even understanding why their family had abandoned them to be left alone.
- Some allowed daily up to two hours. Even twice daily. Some allowed twice a week, because they said CMS said that these visits should "not be routine."

- Some allowed these visits at meal times (so the family member could actually support a need.) Others said absolutely not at meal time (even in a resident's private room) because the resident would have their mask off. But really, families could wear masks while they helped with a meal, just like staff could.
- Some required the family find their own COVID test. Others (a very few) would provide the test on site prior to the visit. Where were all the tests that the Governors had received? Wasn't finding ways to *safely* reunite families a priority?
- Some required testing every three days, some twice a week, even when staff were tested weekly or monthly. That was a monumental challenge and hardship for family members who were trying to stretch the truth so they could schedule free tests at CVS. Or it's out of pocket at a private lab, up to $125.
- Some continued Compassionate visits with county positivity over 10%. Others shut down all but perhaps a single end of life visit when positivity exceeded 10%. Some even restricted *all* Compassionate visits for up to 4 weeks based on this positivity rate, when there had been only one or two ("reported") asymptomatic positive non-resident cases and no one in the building was in isolation. The PA Division of Nursing Facilities told me, and the CMS document from Sept 17 stated, that CC visits are to supersede county positivity. My correspondence to a CMS Triage email verified this. But who are we to argue with facilities when we have no backing because there was just enough vagueness in the guidance that they could "twist it," or perhaps merely misunderstand it?

What was most frustrating to us as family members, was that all these facilities say they are following "The Guidelines." The Sept. CMS guidelines were vague, ambiguous, and contained too many gaps. And there has been no one for us to ask, unless a formal complaint is made. Family members have feared further reprisals for complaining to their State Nursing Division more than anything. Many are even reluctant to call the State Ombudsman office for compassionate visitation help, out of fear of what the facility will do going forward in disguised retaliation.

Now CMS has new "guidance," issued in March, and residents and families have been deluded to think this will answer our prayers and our grass roots advocacy goals. Families in many locations are still begging for Compassionate visits. *But what does a Compassionate Visit mean?* In recent interviews Evan Shulman, the Director of the CMS Division of Nursing Home Quality and Safety, has said that they cannot possibly define all examples of a Compassionate visit. So after a year of lock-up, some facilities around the country are *still* denying these, because "mom has not declined enough." "Dad's problems are not acute enough." "Your sister is not depressed enough." What? A year without a family visit is not in and of itself reason enough to allow a compassionate visit? Or families plead for an end of life visit, which is sometimes denied until the *very end*. "Grandma is not close enough to death to allow you in." Have you seen any broad news coverage about people who try to visit a dying loved one in a nursing home and the police are called to escort them out, as their loved one is actively dying? Probably not. It has been hard to get media attention to this tragedy. But it is happening. And we see it up close and personal on our Facebook page.

Mr. Shulman also says these compassionate visits should not "be routine." *What does "Not Routine" mean?* Some families are allowed a 15 minute visit once per week. Weekdays only.

No children. Sometimes only one visitor, maximum is two. CMS says that they "understand." I do not believe they do. They say these guidelines are what facilities "should follow" since they are not federal "regulations." In PA, where my parents live, the Governor and Acting Health Secretary say facilities "should" follow these new guidelines, and that they "encourage" it. So, please help me to understand. If states say that facilities "should" follow the guidelines that CMS says that they "should" follow, then how is *any* of this enforceable? Some state Nursing Division agencies have been very helpful when people do take the leap to make a complaint. Others side with any arbitrary restrictions that the facility imposes. Some State Long Term Care Ombudsman offices have been very helpful when people do take the leap to make a request for advocacy. Others say there is nothing they can do, placing them precisely in concert with any arbitrary restrictions that the facility imposes. And from the family vantage point, CMS and State regulators are doing *nothing* to ensure this is being understood and universally implemented in facilities across our nation. That has left us fighting individual battles all over the country, because they tell us they will "investigate" our "complaints" but they have not been *proactive* to clarify guidance or issue clear expectations that it is being adhered to.

Mr. Shulman says these compassionate visits should be "person-centered." Facilities do not understand what this means on a normal day. So, what does person-centered even mean when every right is being taken from individuals residing in long-term care facilities? And what gives the facility administrator the right to measure and to determine the value and worth and necessity of a resident being "allowed" to see a family member?

This is an injustice to loved ones who are seniors, adults and children who are living in long term care. Their rights have been stripped, not for 2 weeks which we could have probably lived with, but for a year. How have we allowed this to happen? Where is the outrage? This is a humanitarian crisis going on for thousands across our own country. Right here, in the USA. People have stated this week that the disparity of the NCAA men's and women's locker rooms and food is "disgusting." The NCAA has "apologized" to the women. Where is the outcry over long term care residents locked up for over a year? Who has apologized to them? Who has given them an ounce of attention for months? Who has cared about them? Why are people in isolation no less a disgraceful situation than the fact that locker rooms have different equipment? Where are our priorities?

This can *never* happen again, and we apparently need Regulations to make sure that it does not happen again. I beg you to respond to this crisis by having a Committee that will legislate humanity and compassion for all of these residents, current and future. Because it is clear that compassion and humanity are optional in our current world. On any given day, I could be the next person locked up in long term care without access to my family. Any one of you could be as well. Or your spouse or parent or your child.

Believe me, I do not for one minute dismiss the severity of this pandemic, nor do I have any disregard for the tremendous loss of life it has caused. But with no one seeming to be paying any attention for the last year, there has been an equally devastating loss of life, or devastating loss of physical and cognitive capacity to those have suffered alone on the inside. They have lost their will, and their spirit, and their mental health, and their emotional health as well. And yet facilities would deny that those individuals "qualify" for a compassionate visit from a loved one? And CMS would condone the inconsistencies in the implementation of their so-called guidelines through their own very stance of *inaction* to ensure this is properly interpreted and happening? CMS "shoulds" are inadequate. Our State-based "shoulds" are meaningless. We need federal laws that will mandate that Essential Caregivers are allowed for long term care residents, even in a pandemic, and even when other regular visitation might have to be limited for safety reasons. And I would propose that we need another federal mandate that says that the Resident Rights, as guaranteed and protected by the federal Nursing Home Reform Act established in 1987, can *never again* be violated to the extent that we have just witnessed. Even in a pandemic, residents should be entitled to the "quality of care that will result in their achieving or maintaining their 'highest practicable' physical, mental and psychosocial well-being." Any thing less is unjust, immoral, and inhumane. Just as this very *tragedy* has been for a full year.

Respectfully submitted
Carolyn Piper
Daughter of parents residing in Long Term Care
Member of National and PA chapters of Caregivers for Compromise—Because Isolation Kills Too

* * *

Statement of Premier Inc.

444 N. Capitol Street NW #625
Washington, DC 20001

The Premier healthcare alliance appreciates the opportunity to submit a statement for the record on the Senate Finance Committee hearing titled "A National Tragedy: COVID–19 in the Nation's Nursing Homes." We applaud the leadership of Chairman Wyden, Ranking Member Crapo and members of the Committee for examining the factors that contributed to the nursing home response during the pandemic and assessing necessary improvements going forward.

Premier Inc. is a leading healthcare improvement company, uniting an alliance of more than 4,100 U.S. hospitals and health systems and approximately 200,000 non-acute providers, including 28,000 nursing homes around the country, to transform healthcare. With integrated data and analytics, collaboratives, supply chain solutions, and consulting and other services, Premier enables better care and outcomes at a lower cost.

It is indisputable that COVID–19 has had devastating consequences for the nation's nursing homes. Deaths among senior-care center staff and residents appear to represent at least 25 percent of the overall count of more than 500,000 U.S. fatalities related to COVID–19, as compiled by the Centers for Medicare & Medicaid Services (CMS).[386] Since the COVID–19 outbreak, a key focus area of Premier has been ensuring nursing homes, which were wholly unprepared to deal with the magnitude of the pandemic, have personal protective equipment (PPE), supplies and equipment at their sites so they can continue to deliver high-quality care to residents.

Through two comprehensive surveys and dozens of individual conversations to understand the needs of senior living providers during the pandemic, Premier developed solutions and recommendations that we shared with the Administration. In addition to supply chain issues,

---

[386] *https://data.cms.gov/stories/s/COVID–19-Nursing-Home-Data/bkwz-xpvg/.*

which require critical thought moving forward, we believe additional funding is necessary to implement technological supports in nursing homes. Specifically, infrastructure is needed to help infection preventionists and clinical pharmacists at facilities detect, manage, control and report infection-related conditions related to COVID–19 and beyond. We urge Congress to address known supply chain and surveillance vulnerabilities for this unique population in the next COVID–19 package.

Congressional Action Is Needed to Address Supply Chain Vulnerabilities

As a supply chain leader, Premier has been at the forefront of COVID–19 response efforts and has been working around the clock to ensure a consistent supply of medical supplies for nursing homes, including PPE. Premier has been actively engaged with the Administration and federal agencies to track developments and offer guidance, providing real-time data on ordering patterns, current consumption rates and future demand forecasts in order to inform our government's understanding of the current state and potential future vulnerabilities.

Premier conducted several surveys[387] to better understand the needs of nearly 2,500 skilled nursing and assisted living facilities during the pandemic response and found that:

- About 43 percent of senior living facilities did not have a consistent ordering history for PPE at the outset of the pandemic, effectively leaving them without a legitimate channel for purchasing supplies that may be necessary to protect workers and elderly residents. Of senior living providers that did have a consistent purchasing history of PPE products, 87 percent were not receiving the full quantity of products ordered at the outset of the COVID–19 pandemic.
- By early April, 24 percent of senior living facilities did not have N95 masks on hand, and the majority had fewer than 2 weeks' supply of surgical masks, isolation gowns and face shields.
- Additional products in high demand for senior living facilities and short supply from manufacturers and distributors included thermometers, exam gloves, shoe covers, bouffant caps, alcohol pads, disinfecting products, hand sanitizer, and disposable paper items. This demonstrated the unique needs of nursing homes from other healthcare settings.
- These supply chain challenges have left nursing homes vulnerable, as 70 percent reported they are not fully prepared to treat an increasing number of COVID–19 cases as the virus surges.

Given these findings and barriers for nursing homes to obtain PPE through traditional distribution channels, Premier created an e-commerce platform, Stockd, to ensure nursing homes were able to access critical medical supplies during the pandemic in a timely manner. Built by providers for providers, Stockd helps solve the issue of gray market sellers and illicit marketeers that were rampant during the pandemic through:

---

[387] *https://www.premierinc.com/newsroom/premier-in-the-news/senior-living-facilities-lack-supply-of-protective-gear-survey-finds and https://www.premierinc.com/news-room/press-releases/as-covid-19-pushes-hospital-patients-to-post-acute-care-settings-supply-and-resource-needs-grow-per-premier-inc-survey.*

- Robust security settings to prevent the selling of "gray market" goods, or those that are sold outside of the brand owner's approved distribution channels.
- Stringent vetting policies that safeguard buyers and ensure that they're purchasing from verified manufacturers and distributors, not third-party sellers who may price gouge or make suspect product claims based on market demand.

Stockd will continue to be a critical resource for nursing homes moving forward as they adjust to the new normal and continue to obtain PPE to protect both healthcare workers and nursing home residents.

To strengthen the supply chain to address future global pandemics, Premier has robust recommendations on how the existing private sector supply chain can be further enabled and augmented. Premier's guiding principles include:

- Augment the existing private sector supply chain to better respond to global pandemics through diversification and transparency. The private sector supply chain is highly functioning and should be further enabled, not disrupted.
- Develop a cohesive and holistic national strategy for addressing global pandemics and stabilizing the US supply chain to respond to surge demand for critical medical supplies and drugs.
- Identify critical medical supplies and drugs needed to treat a global pandemic and associated comorbidities. This identification should occur via a public-private advisory council that includes representatives from manufacturers, group purchasing organizations (GPOs), distributors, physicians, pharmacists, laboratorians, nursing homes, and others. This list must be dynamic and regularly updated as technology advances, best practices are identified, and the practice of medicine evolves.
- Create upstream visibility into the supply chain to understand sources of raw materials and manufacturing facilities. This information is critical to assess vulnerabilities and prioritize what critical medical supplies and drugs should be focused on initially to assure adequate diversification of the supply chain.
- Design stockpiles to create coordination rather than competition between state, local and national stockpiles.
- Invest in a robust, real time HIT infrastructure that will provide an on-call, nimble data collection infrastructure that the nation can call upon in any future major crises. Rather than standing up an inadequate and duplicative system as we experienced during the pandemic, the nation needs a system that can track critical product availability—from the raw materials, to manufacturer, to distribution, to hospital inventory. This system would exist behind the scenes and be ready to be "turned on" in a moment's notice. This information would inform dynamic and appropriate product allocation and distribution strategies, minimize hoarding, and enable powerful and accurate prediction, enabling the nation to manage supplies during the crisis.
- Leverage supply and demand data from GPOs, who serve as neutral, vendor-agnostic, and value-orientated entities to drive transparency in the supply chain and forecast demand needs.
- Advance payment and delivery system reforms that hold providers, including nursing home providers, accountable for the health of a population, budgets and transparent

outcomes. This will incent improving the health of a population, which will both improve patients' comorbidities and attention to care management for sick patients. Acting within a budget helps reduce long-term financial pressure from rising healthcare costs.

- Leverage technology to implement comprehensive infection prevention and antimicrobial stewardship programs in nursing homes to provide meaningful assistance with infection control.

Premier urges Congress to ensure that nursing homes are represented in the development of a cohesive and holistic national strategy for addressing global pandemics. Furthermore, a customized stockpile for nursing homes should be created with appropriate supplies, drugs and other needs.

Funding for Infection Prevention Clinical Surveillance Will Improve Outcomes

COVID–19 has brought to the forefront the specific challenges nursing homes face in containing the spread of infectious disease. The virus has accelerated at nursing homes because residents are generally vulnerable to its complications and more susceptible in the contained space of the facilities. While data about infections in nursing homes is limited, the CDC notes that, even prior to the pandemic, a staggering 1 to 3 million serious infections occur every year in these facilities and as many as 380,000 people die of the infections in nursing homes every year.[388]

Infection prevention oversight and training at nursing homes is a challenge in and of itself with limited staffing and several layers of reporting requirements. This challenge is compounded by limited electronic health record (EHR) functionality at the sites with only an estimated 66 percent of skilled nursing facilities currently using an EHR.[389] Data regarding use of EHRs in other segments of nursing homes such as long-term care facilities and independent living are considered to be much lower. The use of paper records in these care settings inhibit swift data collection and proactive tracking and trending to identify potential infections before they become rampant in the congregate setting. Surveillance, tracking, documenting and reporting of infections is not only necessary for COVID–19 but could be used to better position nursing homes for future outbreaks and other indicators that would result in improved quality of care.

Nursing Homes Now Have Multiple, Expanded Layers of Infection Prevention Requirements and Face Unique Challenges with Oversight and Training without Electronic Surveillance Capabilities

- CMS now requires facilities to:

---

[388] *https://www.cdc.gov/longtermcare/index.html#:_:text=1%20to%203%20million%20serious,infections% 20in%20LTCFs%20every%20year.*

[389] *https://www.healthit.gov/sites/default/files/page/2018-11/Electronic-Health-Record-Adoption-and-Interoperability-among-U.S.-Skilled-Nursing-Facilities-and-Home-Health-Agencies-in-2017.pdf.*

- *Establish and maintain an infection prevention and control program* (IPCP) that includes, at a minimum, a system for preventing, identifying, reporting, investigating and controlling infections and communicable diseases for all residents, staff, volunteers, visitors, and other individuals providing services under a contractual arrangement.
- *Report on at least a weekly basis* confirmed and suspected COVID–19 cases, or face penalties.

- This is on top of infection reporting requirements that vary by state and can often require using phone, fax or mail, as well as reporting requirements within facilities' own organizations.
- Infection prevention oversight and training is challenging, which is compounded by limited technology nursing homes due to:
  - High resident-to-staff ratios which are associated with infection spreads;
  - A lack of on-site specialty services, such as pharmacists for antimicrobial stewardship;
  - Functions that are often outsourced to outside agencies, which then hold the data;
  - Surveillance, tracking and reporting processes lack automation for everyday risks such as multidrug resistant organism (MDRO) and for outbreaks like COVID–19.

Clinical Surveillance Solutions Should Be Implemented to Improve Quality and Decrease Costs

- Clinical analytics technologies are currently widely leveraged in hospitals and acute settings, including 46 Veterans Affairs hospitals, to detect patient care issues through surveillance, interventions and reporting capabilities that are needed to support antimicrobial stewardship programs. These systems utilize data from EHRs and have significantly helped clinicians and pharmacists in acute settings identify overuse of antibiotics and drug-bug mismatches, reduce time-to-appropriate therapy and enhance therapy for difficult-to-treat pathogens. Those health systems already utilizing clinical surveillance technology were well positioned to respond to COVID–19 before the pandemic hit. This technology is ready to optimize for nursing homes, delivering similar results to those below.
  - *Three Veterans Health Administration medical centers (VAMCs)* saved $2.3 million in just two years by changing the way they administer antibiotics, using a clinical surveillance system to ensure appropriate and safe use of antibiotics for the men and women who have served our country.
  - *Hartford Healthcare* in Hartford, CT, streamlined its workflow for identifying high-risk patients, conducting patient reviews, completing documentation, and reporting infection data to CDC's National Healthcare Safety Network (NHSN) across its six hospitals. This saved 10 hours per week per infection preventionist, allowing them to spend more time with clinical staff educating and observing infection prevention processes.

- *Ellis Medicine,* in Schenectady, NY, saved more than $122,000 in a year by implementing clinical surveillance to meet both New York State Department of Health and Joint Commission requirements for stewardship to easily identify bug-drug mismatches, duplication of therapy, and opportunities for de-escalation or discontinuation of therapy.

Incentivizing This Technology Would Help Nursing Home Preparedness beyond the COVID–19 Public Health Emergency

- We urge Congress to designate funds specifically to ensure nursing homes can implement electronic clinical surveillance technology (ECST) that will provide meaningful assistance with infection control.
  - For the purposes of the public health emergency and for 180 days after, Congress should incentivize facilities that already have EHRs to adopt and integrate ECST.
  - For those facilities that do not have existing EHRs, Congress should designate additional resources to implement that foundational technology and to also adopt and integrate ECST.

Unfortunately, clinical analytics technologies are currently not widely used in nursing homes. Nursing homes should have the same access to tools that will help them combat infection spread during any future outbreaks of COVID–19 and during their day-to-day operations, but unfortunately funding remains a significant barrier. Nursing homes are already challenged with meeting their more visible needs, such as testing and securing adequate PPE levels at their sites, but a comprehensive approach is additionally needed to ensure data collection is efficient, non-duplicative and being analyzed in ways that are helpful for facilities. Furthermore, it is critical that lessons learned from meaningful use are applied forward as we develop cohesive solutions to address the lack of EHRs and clinical surveillance technology in nursing homes and create appropriate incentives for adoption.

Premier urges Congress to designate funds to incentivize nursing homes to implement EHRs and electronic clinical surveillance technology that will provide meaningful assistance with infection control.

Conclusion

In closing, the Premier healthcare alliance appreciates the opportunity to submit a statement for the record on the Senate Finance Committee hearing to examine the COVID–19 nursing home crisis. As an established leader in the healthcare supply chain and healthcare data analytics, Premier is available as a resource and looks forward to working with Congress as it considers policy options to continue to address these very important issues.

Statement Submitted by Beth Rister

Hello, I am Beth Rister from Southern Illinois. I am an educator, currently serving as Regional Superintendent of nine counties. I consider myself a very hard worker. While serving in a full-time job, I also look after my mother who has Parkinson's, and is starting down the road of dementia. I will not bore you with all the details, but just know through a very trying year, my mother had to move from an assisted living to a nursing home. I stood at the window of the nursing home from May to October every evening. I tried to comfort my mother by talking to her on a cell phone through a glass. The facility would not allow the screen to be opened, which would have allowed fresh air in, thus helping the ventilation and the communication. I would leave after working all day, and standing an hour or two, crying my eyes out. It was so hard on me, as well as on her. I could see things that needed to be done in her room. I could see personal care that needed to be done for her well-being. One very important thing was walking. She had broken her hip, and she needed to walk more than 10 minutes a day. As an essential part of her care, I would have gone in daily and walked her, to keep her strength up. She was losing the ability to walk right in front of my eyes. She is unable to brush her teeth appropriately due to shaking. I again, would brush her teeth daily for her. I would help her with her supper. Many times the tray was just set down in front of her, and the aide (sometimes a housekeeper) would turn around to walk out of the room. I would be knocking on the window, asking them to open her Jell-O, her crackers, cut her meat, etc. If I had not been at the window, she would have been unable to eat some of the items on her tray. I know at lunch and breakfast, she was not properly cared for, because I was unable to be at the window. There are many situations, where essential caregivers from family are needed. The long-term care facilities are short staffed, many not properly trained. Many residents, like my mother need so much care, and during COVID was unable to get this care. The facility does not always have the capacity to care for the residents like they deserve to be taken care of. These are former hardworking members of our nation, law abiding citizens, taxpayers, being held hostage in their last months of their life. It is a crying shame for anyone to be treated like this, and kept from family members who are willing to help them.

I ended up taking my mother out of the facility on October 11th. I was not about to stand outside all winter to see about my mother. She and my father lived very conservatively, and was able to build a small nest egg. They never made big money, but just new how to manage. The nursing home cost was $5,000 a month, I am now paying over $11,000 a month for 24 hour care at home. We will be running out of money very soon. I want to see a solution to this problem, before my mother has to return to such a facility. I want to be able to go to her room, help her with essential care. I shouldn't have to watch a video, take a quiz, etc. to do so. Some of the facilities are trying to make it so hard, people will give up. This is America, we deserve better treatment than this! My mother was a former nursing home administrator. She ran a fine long term care facility. The residents were like family to all the staff. Boy, how times have changed!

I am asking you, no begging you to pass a bill, like SB 2160 to allow one or two essential family members to enter a facility, go to their loved one's room, to take care of the essential needs of their loved one. There are many physical needs, as well as the social emotional needs. They need to be shown love, not isolation.

Thank you for your time and consideration. I could care less if I inherit a dime. I will spend ever last penny my parents saved over their lifetime to care for my mother. My father passed in 2019, before the pandemic. He was fortunate enough to stay home, with just 6 months of caregivers. The money is running out very quickly. Please help.

Statement Submitted by Nora Toscano

I am 60 years old, and live in Tucson, AZ. I graduated from the University of Connecticut in 1983 with a dual degree in Electrical Engineering and Computer Science. I have been married for 36 years. My husband is also a University of Connecticut graduate with an Electrical Engineering degree. We have no children. I retired from Raytheon Missile Systems as a Senior Manager Systems Engineer. Prior to COVID, I volunteered 1 day a week at a local hospital. Recently I started volunteering at a local AZ COVID vaccine site.

My Mom, Aneita Babicz, passed away at the age of 82 from COVID on July 7, 2020 after living in a Memory Care facility since Jan 2020.

My Mom's Story

My Mom was diagnosed with Dementia and Early Onset Alzheimer's in late Nov 2019 from the University of Arizona Alzheimer's Institute. I learned dementia patients need structure, activities, and socialization; two things my husband and I struggled to provide her during several months that she lived with us. She became a resident of Catalina Springs Memory Care in Oro Valley, AZ in Jan 2020. With the environment at the Memory Care Facility, she really improved and loved being with "new best friends." She enjoyed many daily activities and structure. I would visit her at least 3 times a week just to make sure she was doing well and was happy. It was a great place for her.

On March 13th the Memory Care facility started implementing restrictions due to COVID, which included no longer allowing visitors. The staff started wearing face masks at this point.

Beginning in May residents were also given masks and were asked to wear them when they were in the common area. Residents were also told to sit apart from each other, and they were no longer allowed to hug each other anymore. My Mom struggled because she needed a hug every day. But at the same time my Mom really tried to do as she was told.

Around the end of May new mandates were imposed that all residents must eat all meals in their own rooms by themselves (Mom had a single room). Dementia residents need to be around each other and because of this mandate my Mom started withdrawing and no longer ate her meals like before. I would stop by during lunch to watch her through her closed window, and she would just push food around on her plate. It was hard to get her to eat. She really needed her friends to eat with her. Initially I would call her on her own phone and talk to her during lunch to convince her to eat. She was able to see me standing at her window. However, being in isolation and her seeing me at her window would only upset her more, so eventually I had to stop calling her. I would still visit at her window but I would not let he know I was watching her during lunch. It was so sad to watch.

The situation got worse for my Mom when a revised mandate from the AZ Governor was issued for all Nursing Homes and Long-Term Facilities to mandate all residents to stay in their rooms, alone, all day long. This meant my Mom had to sit in her one chair, without a TV, or radio, and her eyesight was bad so she couldn't read. She had no contact with other residents all day long. This isolation does not work for dementia patients, and it would not even work for individuals without dementia; it is essentially solitary confinement. At times my Mom would call me from her personal phone to complain about being mistreated. Other times she yelled at me, her anxiety was getting worse. She did not want to be in "jail." She was done with the facility and wanted to go home. It was really hard on me too since there was not much I could do to help. We considered moving her to another facility but the state was not releasing COVID test results data for Long Term Facilities so we were unsure if we would be placing her at a greater risk elsewhere.

Being alone also caused my Mom's dementia to quickly worsen. Her anxiety issues and her perception of reality was declining. She feared that a big bad man was coming into her room at night to get her. I later found out the staff would periodically peak in on residents at night, but in the dark and with the staff wearing masks, it scared my Mom. Therefore, my Mom was not getting much sleep at night either.

I could not reach any staff in the Memory Care Facility to help with this matter. I kept hearing they were short staffed. It was impossible for me to reach anyone to ask for help for my Mom or find out what was really going on. There was no feedback for me, nor was there anyone for me to talk to about how she was doing and how we could help her. It was just that she was in a facility with a big wall around it and I could not get any information personally or by phone. Communication was nil.

The facility was also not telling me much about whether a resident had COVID or not. I heard from a friend who was an employee that a new resident was moved into the facility with COVID, but they were isolating that person in their room. However, the same staff that took care of the COVID patient cared for everyone else in the facility. It seems to me that things could have been handled better. I did not expect the facility to admit COVID positive patients and risk my Mom's health.

At the time COVID testing and PPE were hard to come by in AZ.

The facility did test residents for COVID, but between the months of March and July my Mom was only tested twice for COVID, the second time being the week before she was sent to the hospital where she was diagnosed as COVID positive. I never did hear the results of the second test performed by the Memory Care Facility.

On Monday June 29, 2020, my Mom, a Type II Diabetic, was found slumped over in her room on her chair unresponsive. They called for an ambulance which identified her with low blood sugar (12) and took her to the local hospital. There she was diagnosed as COVID positive and they put her in the COVID ICU ward. She was still asymptotic and doing well for a couple days, but by Wed July 1st she took a turn for the worse. The doctor put her on Remdesivir and Dexamethasone but she showed no signs of improving. Since she also had heart valve issues she did not want to be put on a ventilator. I was able to meet her doctor in person at the Hospital on Thursday July 2nd outside the ICU ward to get a briefing on expectations, etc., but to my surprise I was not able to go inside the ICU ward due to lack of proper PPE. Therefore, I could not say good-by to my Mom.

The hospital told me I would get daily updates by phone, but that did not always happen, they were so swamped taking care of patients it was hard for them to find the time to talk to family members on the phone. By Sat July 4th I heard from the doctor that my Mom was not getting any better and there was nothing more they could do for her. I was told I needed to think about Hospice care. On Monday July 6th they transferred her to a nearby Hospice called Casa de la Luz. I had selected them because the assured me that they had PPE I could use to visit her once a day.

Once at the Hospice I found out I could not go inside because they did not have proper PPE to give me, despite what they told me in advance. I was able to see her outside her first story open window, but at this point she just lay in bed with her eyes closed. It was Tucson in July and temperatures reached over 105. I saw several other families gathered outside the windows of their dying COVID loved ones. It was all very sad. However, I don't think my Mom knew I was there. I was able to play her a CD of her Dad singing Irish music through her window which I think she could hear. She passed later that night.

The last time I saw my Mom in person was March 10th. She passed, alone, in a strange room on July 7, 2020.

Issues

While at the Memory Care Facility there were several issues that I believe were Systemic Failures:

- Lack of availability of COVID testing and how it took way too long for the PCR tests to be reported back to the individuals tested (7–10 days).
- Lack of sufficient available PPE for me to visit my dying Mother in the hospital and in Hospice prior to her passing.
- Inadequate staffing at the Memory Care Facility to identify that my Mom was sick with COVID prior to sending her to the hospital, or to identify someone else in the Long Term Facility was asymptotic with COVID before this person was able to pass COVID on to other residents, including my Mom.

Conclusion

I believe there was a Systemic Failure caused by a lack of leadership from the Federal government which flowed down to the state governments, and in the end hurt most Long-Term Memory Care and Dementia Facilities and their residents. If only there was cooperation and synergy among the states and the Federal government, many lives could have been saved.

Dementia patients cannot be treated like those in Nursing Homes and other non-dementia patients.

PPE availability was not well regulated nor distributed, therefore every Long-Term Facility, Hospital, and Hospice seem to be on their own to find available PPE and were competing with each other for whatever limited PPE was available.

COVID testing was also scarce and the few local places that were performing PCR tests at the time were so overloaded with requests that the test results would take 7 to 10 days, or longer. Waiting for results for that long seem unproductive, since a lot could happen in 10 days with this rapid spread of this virus, plus the individual being tested could get worse within these critical 10 days. In addition, asymptomatic individuals ended up spreading the virus to those more susceptible to COVID.

Inadequate staffing for Long Term Facilities resulted in patients who were sick with COVID symptoms being overlooked until they got to the point where they had to be hospitalized. In addition, results from COVID testing on asymptomatic individuals came too late to quarantine those asymptomatic from the rest of the residents in the facility before they spread it to others.

Recommendation

If the message from the Federal Government would have been consistent and more proactive, I believe many more innocent people may have survived 2020. Better management of PPE and COVID testing expectations, along with separate guidance for Dementia patients vs. Nursing Homes from the Federal Government would also have saved lives. It is a shame that mandates like wearing masks became so political, and still is. Individuals no longer act for the best of the national, but for themselves.

The year 2020 was a difficult time for many Americans. Any help you can bring to protect the welfare of our elderly, would be greatly appreciated.

Statement Submitted by Michael R. Wasserman, M.D., CMD

To paraphrase the historian Toynbee, “a society’s quality and durability can best be measured by the respect and care given its older adults.” I am both appreciative and disappointed by today’s testimony by John E. Dicken, “COVID–19 in Nursing Homes: HHS Has Taken Steps in Response to Pandemic, but Several GAO Recommendations Have Not Been Implemented.” With the devastation that nursing home residents and staff have experienced over the past year, the gravity of this issue and the urgency needed to address underlying faults in the long term care system should be apparent. The bottom line is that there is still much that needs to be done to protect the most vulnerable members of our society.

One year ago I said the coronavirus was “the greatest threat to nursing home residents that we have seen,”[390] and that nursing homes could become our “killing fields.”[391] My experience as a clinical and quality expert, in addition to having been the CEO of a large nursing home chain gave me a unique perspective into COVID– 19, and how existing structural weaknesses in the nursing home industry would have tragic outcomes. It is unfortunate, but my predictions have come to pass, with devastating consequences in nursing homes across the country.

I am board certified and fellowship trained in geriatric medicine. In 1989, I opened Kaiser-Permanente’s first outpatient geriatric consult clinic and in 1994 founded Kaiser’s second Continuing Care Department in the country. I subsequently went on to become the president and chief medical officer of GeriMed of America, a geriatrics medical management company, before founding Senior Care of Colorado, which became the largest primary care geriatrics private practice in the country at the time. I was the Executive Director, Care Continuum, overseeing the nursing home arm of Medicare’s California QIN–QIO. I then became the chief medical officer overseeing the largest nursing home chain in California, becoming their CEO for fourteen months before resigning in November of 2018.

---

390 *https://www.nbcnews.com/health/health-news/coronavirus-nursing-homes-greatest-threat-years-here-s-what-the y-n1153181.*

391 *https://www.cbsnews.com/news/coronavirus-nursing-home-death/.*

From the moment that I heard about the outbreak at Life Care Center of Kirkland, my entire body of experiences informed me as to what was coming. I have been working ever since attempting to educate policy makers and government officials in order that they might have a better understanding of the nursing home industry in order to better protect residents and staff. My first articles published in March were focused on the need for effective infection prevention, including a focus on the front line staff.[392,393]

On February 29th, with the outbreak of COVID–19 in a Washington state nursing home, the experts in geriatrics and long term care medicine knew what was coming. Many of us did everything in our power to sound the alarm. Unfortunately, our voices were not heard in a timely fashion. We must all live with the dire consequences. We must also recognize and thank the incredible people who serve on the front lines in nursing homes. They are incredibly caring and compassionate human beings, many of whom don't even make a living wage. Media accounts of nursing home care all too often ignore their efforts. Too many have now given their lives unnecessarily due to the lack of immediate action to this pandemic on the part of the federal government, the state, the counties and the nursing home industry.

COVID–19 ultimately made its way into most nursing homes. There are those who use this fact to create a false narrative that there was little that could have been done to have significantly reduced the devastating impact of this virus on nursing home residents. Nothing could be further from the truth. There was a lot that could have been done, and we must honor those who have died by taking action to reimagine the nursing home industry. My comments will focus first on the pandemic response, as there are specific operational elements that should be reviewed and can not be ignored. However, these elements are only the beginning, and we have been fortunate to already have the beginning of a roadmap for the future put forth by the Coronavirus Commission on Safety and Quality in Nursing Homes, which I suggest should immediately be reconstituted in the form of a Federal Advisory Committee. Many of their recommendations should immediately be acted on. The dissenting opinion must not be ignored and needs additional work in order to achieve consensus. Those who have given their lives deserve this level of attention.

In April of 2020, CALTCM published our "Long Term Care Quadruple Aim for COVID–19 Response,"[394] the pillars of which have withstood the test of time and continue to reflect the key elements necessary to combat this deadly virus. CALTCM's Quadruple Aim was developed and shared with the California Department of Public Health (CDPH) in March, and with CMS in April, and was posted on the CALTCM website on April 17th. It starts with the need for every nursing home to have an abundance of Personal Protective Equipment (PPE). Pandemic supply chain dynamics made procuring PPE challenging. The state, counties and facilities did not have the wherewithal to transcend this challenge in order to obtain PPE for every nursing home. As we know, the federal government, through the DPA process, had the ability to surmount this challenge and should have immediately done so. Additionally, and pertinent to reimagining nursing homes, real estate owners and REIT's behind the nursing home industry had the ability to leverage their assets to acquire PPE, and generally chose not to intervene. As a clinician, I don't care who takes responsibility for the acquisition of PPE, it just has to happen. Without PPE, COVID–19 can't be stopped. While everyone was complaining

---

[392] *https://www.mcknights.com/blogs/a-mantra-in-wake-of-coronavirus-stay-home-and-save-a-life/.*

[393] *https://www.linkedin.com/in/mike-wasserman-8535676/detail/recent-activity/posts/.*

[394] *https://www.caltcm.org/assets/CALTCM%20COVID19%20QUADRUPLE%20AIM%20FI NAL.pdf.*

about the lack of PPE and the inability to acquire it, nursing home residents were infected with the virus and died. Even today, according to Mr. Dicken's testimony, ten percent of nursing homes still struggle to have adequate PPE. This is unacceptable. The single most important intervention (prior to the availability of a vaccine) in nursing homes, assisted living facilities and group homes is an abundance of PPE. In the future, the government and the industry must transcend all obstacles and assure that a lack of PPE will never again get in the way of protecting vulnerable older adults.

The second element of the Quadruple Aim is readily available testing. Nursing home staff were the main vector for transmission of the virus. CALTCM convened a group of experts who developed recommendations related to testing.[395] Testing of all staff was critical to protecting both the residents and the staff themselves. Telling nursing homes to come up with their own plans for testing was never the answer. The federal government should have used its clout and resources to assure that testing was performed and that labs prioritized the processing of the tests. The nursing home industry should similarly have supported testing by actions rather than words. In the coming months and years, we will hear many stories of where this did not happen due to fundamental weaknesses in both our government and the industry. What is truly unfortunate is that even today our country's testing capabilities are not state of the art.

Stellar infection prevention is the third element of the Quadruple Aim. The Centers for Disease Control and Prevention, and countless Departments of Public Health across the country worked tirelessly to provide nursing facilities with infection control training. Unfortunately, that approach was always going to be insufficient if the nursing home industry wasn't fully on board with embracing the role of infection preventionist's to their fullest extent. The worst kept secret in the nursing home industry is the fact that the infection preventionist (IP) is not allotted the time necessary to do an effective job. Furthermore, the key reason for requiring a full-time IP is the need to literally "hot-wire" the nursing home chain of command. Most nursing home administrators are focused on their census, and also lack expertise in clinical areas. One of the immediate *solutions* to the COVID–19 pandemic that we developed was the concept of a virtual centralized support and guidance center that could provide expertise to individual nursing homes on a daily basis. Such a support and guidance center could have been used to support COVID–19 positive nursing homes. CALTCM published a white paper on this in April,[396] and a paper on the concept in July.[397] We also shared this concept with CDPH and CMS in March and April, respectively. The need to specifically engage the IP was one element of our recommended approach. In fact, on March 13th, CALTCM proposed that every nursing home in California be mandated to require their designated infection preventionist (IP) be full-time. It took nearly 3 months for the CDPH to make this recommendation part of every nursing home's mitigation plan. In the fall, Governor Newsom signed AB 2644, making it a requirement that every nursing home in California have a full-time infection preventionist. The recommendation requiring the need for full-time infection preventionists was also made to

[395] Wasserman M, Ouslander JG, Lam A, et al. Editorial: Diagnostic Testing for SARS-Coronavirus-2 in the Nursing Facility: Recommendations of a Delphi Panel of Long-Term Care Clinicians. *J Nutr Health Aging.* 2020;24(6): 538–443. doi:10.1007/s12603–020–1401–9.

[396] *https://www.caltcm.org/assets/WHITE%20PAPER%20A%20Plan%20to%20Protect%20Our%20Nursing%20Home%20Residents%20.pdf.*

[397] Wasserman M, Wolk AJ, Lam A. *Jour Nursing Home Res,* 2020;6:24–29. An Aspirational Approach to Nursing Home Operations During the COVID–19 Pandemic. *http://dx.doi.org/10.14283/jnhrs.2020.6, https://www.jnursinghomeresearch.com/2263-an-aspirational-approach-to-nursing-home-operations-during-the-covid-19-pandemic.html.*

CMS in April, countering previously watered down guidance in the nursing home regulations. We must do everything possible to support the role of the facility IP. Doing this early in the pandemic would have improved the success of the federal and state governmental efforts. Effectively impacting the operations of nursing homes requires a paradigm shift with a focus on the improved delivery of clinical care. The requirement of a full-time IP is a necessary, but not sufficient, step in the right direction.

The fourth and final element of the Quadruple Aim is that nursing homes must operate in their emergency preparedness mode. This is essentially a proxy for excellent leadership and management. If COVID–19 has shone a light on one thing, it's the inherent weaknesses in the management structure of nursing homes. Nursing homes are complex small businesses, delivering care to frail older adults with multiple chronic illnesses. They are literally mini-hospitals, but with far fewer resources. Nursing home administrators are not prepared to run a hospital, and should not be expected to have the skills necessary to manage a facility during a pandemic. More importantly, running a "mini-hospital" should require the full engagement of physicians competent in the care of complex, frail, older adults. A significant number of the nursing home deaths brought on by this virus were preventable. If there is an overarching message from the COVID–19 pandemic, it's the need to actively engage experts in geriatrics and long term care medicine in the policy and decision making processes that impact the lives of older adults. To the clinical experts this pandemic has never been about control, money or power. It's been about saving lives. Despite the Herculean efforts of experts in geriatrics and long term care medicine, we've literally had to beg for table scraps to weigh in on policies with county, state and federal government officials, much less the nursing home industry itself. Some have had a greater impact than others, but this never should have been this way. We must learn from this experience.

The evolution of nursing homes from post-war rest homes to today's "mini-hospitals" began with implementation of the hospital DRG system in 1983. There was a brief period in which hospitals purchased nursing homes. They quickly realized that they could discharge patients to nursing homes without taking responsibility or accountability for the outcomes. Meanwhile, nursing home investors learned how to make substantial profits from Medicare and Medicaid without regard to quality of care. COVID–19 has unmasked a deeply flawed industry. The existing oversight of the nursing home industry has not worked to protect residents or staff during this pandemic. The survey process as implemented today does not work. It is time to lead the way in developing an effective oversight and quality improvement process. Surveys often worsen staff morale and have not been shown to have significant demonstrable benefit. The focus of surveys must be on improving the delivery of care and protecting the quality of life of the residents. We support active oversight, and believe that it is critical for CMS to engage experts in geriatrics and long term care, as well as resident advocates, in developing a new and more effective process for carrying out federally mandated surveys. An AMDA Task Force published a paper regarding this in the fall, and those of us who have served on the front line of nursing home care over the past few decades are ready and willing to engage in improving this important process.[398]

---

[398] Nazir A, Steinberg K, Wasserman M, et al., *JAMDA,* Time for an Upgrade in the Nursing Home Survey Process: A Position Statement From the Society of Post-Acute and Long-Term Care Medicine. 2020, ISSN 1525–8610, *https://doi.org/10.1016/j.jamda.2020.09.022.*

Where does this leave us? This past summer the Coronavirus Commission on Safety and Quality in Nursing Homes met and produced a list of recommendations that settled on ten themes. Unfortunately, instead of acting on these recommendations, CMS leadership at the time chose to act as if they had already been following the recommendations. Nothing could have been further from the truth, which was alluded to in Mr. Dicken's testimony. I will proceed to review these recommendations as they form an excellent framework for how we might reimagine the nursing home industry as we go forward.

Testing and screening was "Theme 1" of the report. While the worst of the pandemic is over, and we now have vaccines, testing is still a critical issue, especially in regards to variants. A DPA level approach to testing should have been taken, and we still need that type of approach. With the ongoing growth of variants, it is essential that we aggressively sequence variants that are being found in nursing homes. From the beginning of this pandemic, it was essential to provide rapid turnaround of Pcr testing. Ideally, we should have point of care Pcr testing by now. It is unconscionable that all Pcr testing provided to nursing homes does not have less than 24 hour turnaround. In lieu of Pcr testing, antigen testing has provided an alternative approach to point of care testing. There are opportunities to provide home antigen tests to nursing home staff. The testing doesn't have to start and end with COVID–19. Similar tests are available for influenza and other viruses. We need to take advantage of what we've learned during this pandemic to reduce the impact of other deadly viruses that have plagued nursing homes in the past. There are continued opportunities to reduce both false negatives and positives.

Equipment and personal protective equipment were in "Theme 2" of the report. Every nursing home in the country MUST have an abundant supply of PPE. This is critical not only for COVID–19, but for other communicable diseases. Furthermore, N95s are essential, and no nursing home should ever be at risk of running out. There is a critical need to address supply chain issues so that they never occur again. There is also the need to assure that any financial support is effectively put towards PPE and testing equipment.

Cohorting was covered in "Theme 3" of the report. We have the opportunity to learn from our COVID–19 pandemic experience to evaluate the best ways to balance resident and staff safety with infection prevention and control. During the early months of the pandemic, the waiving of resident transfer and discharge requirements had many unintended consequences. For this reason, it is critical that evidence and science drive cohorting guidance.

Visitation was addressed in "Theme 4" of the report. While the decision to restrict visitation made immediate sense due to the lethal nature of COVID–19, it also contributed to social isolation. The consequences of social isolation have been found to have been significant. With the advent of fully vaccinated nursing home residents and the increasing percentage of staff vaccinations, we have turned a corner. But there is still a lot of work to be done in order to maximize safety when allowing visits to and from friends and family. Visitation is a vital resident right and nowhere is the collaboration between the CDC and CMS more critical. The term person-centered care is bandied about, but in order to make the care of nursing home residents truly person-centered we must fully engage experts in geriatrics and long term care medicine in developing the most effective approaches. CALTCM has used a modified Delphi process to make visitation recommendations,[399] but in order to create expert driven guidance

[399] Bergman C, Stall NM, Haimowitz D, Aronson L, Lynn J, Steinberg K, Wasserman M. Recommendations for Welcoming Back Nursing Home Visitors During the COVID–19 Pandemic: Results of a Delphi Panel. *J Am Med*

to fully address the risks and benefits of these approaches, CMS should convene similar groups of experts to assist in developing future guidance.

Communications was "Theme 5" of the report. Throughout the pandemic ineffective communications have challenged the implementation of programs and guidance to nursing homes across the country. There needs to be increased specificity and expansion of guidance in regards to communications. While the concept of heath literacy is normally thought of in relation to interacting with patients, it also pertains to how we communicate with nursing home staff and the families of residents. In addition to effective guidance and communication with nursing homes, how the CDC and CMS communicate with each other also matters. Improving communications can be facilitated by fully engaging the QIN–QIOs.

The workforce ecosystem was "Theme 6" of the report. There are people in our society who are unable to be cared for at home. Older adults and younger disabled individuals requiring a nursing home level of care often have complex medical needs. Many have cognitive impairment or dementia. Most persons living in nursing homes need assistance with activities of daily living, whether it be for toileting and bathing, or for transferring out of a bed or chair. Meeting the needs of these residents requires an educated and well trained staff. The literature prior to and throughout the pandemic has been clear in relation to the need for appropriate levels of staff. A CMS study in 2001 established the importance of having a minimum of 0.75 registered nurse (RN) hours per resident day (hprd), 0.55 licensed nurse (LVN/LPN) hprd, and 2.8 (to 3.0) certified nursing assistant (CNA) hprd, for a total of 4.1 nursing hprd to prevent harm or jeopardy to residents.[400] As part of this study, a simulation model of direct care workers (CNAs) established the minimum number of staff necessary to provide five basic aspects of daily care in a facility with different levels of resident acuity. A more recent study shows that for the highest acuity nursing homes, CNA staffing should be 3.6 hprd.[401] For the lowest resident workloads, this converts to 1 CNA for every 7 residents on the day and evening shifts and 1 CNA to 11 residents at night. For the heaviest resident workloads, 3.6 CNA hprd converts to 1 CNA for 5.5 residents on days and evenings and 1 CNA for every 11 residents on nights.

A number of organizations have endorsed the minimum of 4.1 hprd standard, and have suggested that at least 30 percent of hours should be provided by RNs and LVNs/LPNs and facilities should have 24-hour RN care.[402,403,404] Some experts have recommended even higher staffing standards (a total of 4.55 hprd) to improve the quality of nursing home care, with higher adjustments for higher resident acuity.[405] These numbers can not be a ceiling, but must become the floor. Efforts must be taken to ensure that nursing homes provide greater levels of staffing

---

Dir Assoc. 2020 Dec;21(12):1759–1766. doi: 10.1016/j.jamda.2020.09.036. Epub 2020 Oct 7. PMID: 33256956; PMCID: PMC7539058.

[400] Centers for Medicare and Medicaid Services. Report to Congress: Appropriateness of Minimum Nurse Staffing Ratios in Nursing Homes Phase II Final Report. Baltimore, MD: Centers for Medicare and Medicaid Services; 2001.

[401] Schnelle JF, Schroyer LD, Saraf AA, Simmons SF. Determining nurse aide staffing requirements to provide care based on resident workload: A discrete event simulation model. *JAMDA.* 2016; 17:970–977.

[402] Institute of Medicine. Keeping patients safe: transforming the work environment of nurses. Washington, DC: National Academy of Medicine, 2004.

[403] American Nurses' Association. Nursing staffing requirements to meet the demands of today's long term care consumer recommendations from the Coalition of Geriatric Nursing Organizations (CGNO). Position Statement 11/12/14, *www.nursingworld.org.*

[404] Coalition of Geriatric Nursing Organizations (CGNO). Nursing staffing requirements to meet the demands of today's long-term care consumer recommendations, 2013.

[405] Harrington C, Kovner C, Kayser-Jones J, Berger S, Mohler M, Burke R. et al. Experts recommend minimum nurse staffing standards for nursing facilities in the United States. *Gerontologist.* 2000; 40 (1):1–12.

as appropriate based on acuity. The other issue that begs clear direction from CMS is in relation to having full-time Infection Preventionists. There should be a minimum of one full-time IP for all facilities with greater than 40 beds, and the number of full-time equivalents should increase proportionally for facilities with greater than 100 beds. There also needs to be clear training guidelines and consideration of certification requirements for this position.

Workforce systems were "Theme 7" of the report. There has been a lot of discussion prior to and during the pandemic around a lack of interest for working in nursing homes. We clearly must address wages and benefits if we are to catalyze interest in becoming CNAs or having nurses work in nursing homes. It is time to overhaul the entire workforce ecosystem. The Commission recommended convening a LTC workforce commission. I concur with this recommendation, and would suggest that such a commission be tasked with quickly making actionable recommendations that can be implemented in the near future. There is also evidence that certified medical directors are associated with an increase in nursing home quality[406] and there are many anecdotal reports of engaged medical directors making a difference during the pandemic. The average 99-bed nursing home is an approximately $10 million per year complex business. Local nursing home leaders are rarely prepared to run such a complex business. The nursing home administrator is essentially the CEO of the business. What training is required to be a nursing home administrator? What about the director of nursing? They are the chief operating officer, managing and leading an inadequately trained and often poorly paid clinical workforce to provide care for some of the most complex persons in our history. A hospital organizational chart includes physicians at the highest levels. Where is such physician engagement in today's nursing homes? Effective teamwork and leadership from Medical Directors, NH administrators, and Directors of Nursing are critical for nursing homes, particularly in a pandemic, and ineffective teaming signals a critical need for leadership training.[407,408] Variation in leadership style and high levels of turnover also impede the establishment of stable leadership in nursing homes.[409] This then impacts staff turnover and quality of care.[410] Enhancing leadership and management training for nursing home leadership teams is a key area that hasn't been fully discussed and desperately needs attention.

Historically, physicians have been engaged by nursing homes with the express purpose of helping to fill beds, or to satisfy a specific regulatory requirement. It is highly unusual for physicians to be engaged in facility leadership and operations. This concept would be anathema in the hospital setting, but has been readily accepted in the nursing home industry. AMDA, now called the Society for Post Acute and Long Term Care Medicine, was founded in 1977 and two years ago passed a resolution to the effect that the role of the nursing home medical director should have nothing to do with referrals.[411]

---

406 Rowland FN, Cowles M, Dickstein C, Katz PR. Impact of medical director certification on nursing home quality of care. *J Am Med Dir Assoc.* 2009 Jul;10(6):431–5.

407 *https://onlinelibrary.wiley.com/doi/full/10.1111/jgs.16513.*

408 Maas ML, Specht JP, Buckwalter KC, Gittler J, and Bechen K. (2008). Nursing home staffing and training recommendations for promoting older adults' quality of care and life: Part 2. Increasing nurse staffing and training. *Research in Gerontological Nursing,* 1(2), 134–152.

409 Williams G, Wood EV, and Ibram F. (2015). From medical doctor to medical director: Leadership style matters. *British Journal of Hospital Medicine,* 76(7), 420–422.

410 Donoghue C, and Castle NG. (2009). Leadership styles of nursing home administrators and their association with staff turnover. *The Gerontologist,* 49(2), 166–174).

411 *https://paltc.org/amda-white-papers-and-resolution-position-statements/policy-e19a-medical-director-compensated.*

The American Board of Post-Acute and Long-Term Care Medicine provides a certification for nursing home medical directors. There are 1240 nursing homes in California and only 125 certified medical directors. This percentage is similar nationally. The vast majority of medical directors in nursing homes around the country are not fully engaged with their facility leadership team. This has a negative impact on quality during normal times, but the impact has been amplified during the pandemic. Whether in dealing with COVID–19, or trying to provide quality care in the future, it is essential that the clinical experts be actively involved in the day to day operations of nursing homes. It is important that medical directors be allowed to perform their duties without undue influence from nursing home ownership. There should be no quid pro quo related to admissions, and medical directors should feel free to provide leadership and make recommendations regarding the delivery of care without fear of losing their position. One of my colleagues lost their medical director position early in the pandemic in order to be replaced by hospitalists who were perceived as providing a source of admissions to the facility. The best way to avoid such behavior would be to require certification for all nursing home medical directors. In California, Assemblyman Nazarian has introduced AB 749, requiring certified medical directors for every nursing home in the state. Until this happens at a national level, The Society for Post Acute and Long Term Care Medicine (AMDA) has requested that CMS create a registry of all medical directors in the country, so that we might directly communicate with them and offer resources and support for this vital role.

Technical assistance and quality improvement were "Theme 8" of the report. We must increase the availability of onsite collaborative, data-driven support. The QIN– QIOs must be effectively engaged. This means eliminating the need for QIN–QIOs to "recruit" nursing homes and to require them to participate. It is also necessary to reduce the QIN–QIO's administrative burden. Too much time and energy is spent with needless reports, when that time could be better spent with on-site training.

Facilities were "Theme 9" of the report. It is time for facility design enhancement. This includes addressing ventilation, space, capital incentives. It means considering approaches such as the Green House model.

Nursing home data was "Theme 10" of the report. There must be a comprehensive retrospective look at COVID–19 data beginning in January 2020. We must capture the deaths related to COVID–19 (residents and staff), regardless of location at the time of death. There must also be an accounting of adverse events secondary to social isolation such as functional decline, weight Loss, pressure ulcers, and behavioral symptoms. Retrospective COVID–19 data must include a look at Pcr testing data (residents and staff), to include turnaround time, as well as an analysis of screening with and without outbreaks. Similarly, antigen testing data (residents and staff) must be similarly analyzed. Prospective data analysis must focus on genetic sequencing of variants and the value of both PCR and antigen testing (staff and residents) in fully vaccinated nursing homes.

There is little disagreement regarding the fact that the financial structure of nursing homes is not conducive to maximizing scarce resources while providing quality care to residents. The separation of real estate, operations and management is a contrivance that leads to unmanageable pressures. The additional pressure from liability insurance costs compounds these pressures. It is time to bring transparent change to the ownership maze and consolidate nursing home ownership so that the full focus can be on delivering care to the residents. This is a complex topic that in and of itself is worthy of an entire tome. As someone who was the CEO over-seeing the largest nursing home chain in California, it would be my privilege to testify before this committee on this topic. In the meantime, I would make a recommendation to help take the pressure off of nursing home operators during this challenging time. I suggest that nursing homes be exempted from paying rent and liability insurance premiums for the next six months. The costs of this would obviously be borne by the real estate owners and the insurance companies. I believe that it's time for them to do their part while we figure out how the nursing home industry can survive and come out stronger than it was before.

In order to imagine the future of nursing homes, picture a three-legged stool. If the three legs aren't equal, the stool will fall over. The legs represent Finance, Operations and Clinical Services. Rarely at the facility level or the corporate level of a large chain, are these treated equally. One will almost never find Clinical Services being given the same attention as Finance and Operations. This is the fundamental, and in the case of COVID–19, the fatal flaw in how today's nursing homes operate. If clinical services are not treated equally, the nursing home industry cannot, and I might say should not, survive.

Effectively providing care for a complex group of individuals requires competencies at every level of the organizational chart. Aside from having an appropriate level of staffing, nursing homes require properly prepared, highly skilled leadership teams that can balance the financial, operational and clinical aspects of this incredibly complex business. Which brings us to a specific roadblock that has prevented us from advancing beyond the status quo.

A recent study demonstrated higher mortality and higher taxpayer expenditures related to private equity in the nursing home industry.[412] This study puts the impact of the pandemic in stark perspective. Today's nursing home industry attracts investors primarily because of its real estate and "related party" potential.[413,414] As long as real estate is the primary driver of financial success, and related parties are allowed to siphon money away from operations, the nursing home industry as a whole will continue to fail to provide value and quality. The COVID–19 pandemic has demonstrated the importance of having immediate access to financial reserves, but those potential funds have been converted into real estate capital and private equity. That capital could have been effectively leveraged to provide for abundant PPE and testing as well as for additional staff. Instead, for the most part, that capital either sat on the sidelines or was leveraged for other purposes such as buying more real estate. If we are going to reimagine nursing homes, the clinical operations must have access to these funds.

The Medicare Payment Advisory Commission produces highly precise reports of nursing home profitability that are based on the same illusion about the structure of nursing home finances. As the Government Accounting Office has demonstrated time and again, our government's attempts to secure quality and value from its investment have been outmaneuvered by private sector accountants and attorneys. We must illuminate and address the structural dynamics that successfully sustain the substandard status quo. In a recent *Health Affairs* Blog,[415] we published a set of recommendations to address transparency. The tentacles of related parties have a negative impact on facility finances and operations. One of the unseen

---

[412] Gupta A, Howell ST, Yannelis C. Does Private Equity Investment in Healthcare Benefit Patients? Evidence from Nursing Homes. National Bureau of Economic Research Working Paper Series, No. 28474, February 2021. 10.3386/w28474, *http://www.nber.org/papers/w28474.*

[413] Harrington C, Ross L, Kang T. Hidden Owners, Hidden Profits, and Poor Nursing Home Care: A Case Study. *Int J Health Serv.* 2015;45(4):779–800. doi: 10.1177/0020731415594772. Epub 2015 Jul 9. PMID: 26159173.

[414] *https://www.washingtonpost.com/business/2020/12/31/brius-nursing-home/.*

[415] *https://www.healthaffairs.org/do/10.1377/hblog20210208.597573/full/.*

consequences of the existing related party structure is the upward pressure on costs that not only impacts for-profit nursing homes, but non-profits as well.

Oversight and enforcement are catch-all phrases that policymakers wield as solutions to poor quality in nursing homes. The government deploys its oversight strategies based upon an illusion that nursing home operators constitute the industry, ignoring the role of the real estate, related party owners and private equity. Applying penalties to the operations of nursing homes has not generally been shown to be an effective means for improving quality. The largest owners appeal and delay payments, sometimes for years, while non-profits and "mom and pop" nursing homes struggle under the weight of hefty penalties that may be misguided and don't support quality improvement. I recently participated in, and co-authored a paper making recommendations for upgrading the survey process.[416] In my opinion, the only way to address this issue is to convene a Commission composed primarily of clinical experts, regulatory experts and advocates.

Nursing homes are also weighed down by liability insurance costs that are compounded by this sector's perpetual quality issues. The insurance industry has little incentive to reduce premiums. Ironically, both plaintiffs' and defense attorneys have little incentive to see a change in the system. Nursing home liability must be thoughtfully reformed.

The nursing home industry and the government must also fully engage experts in geriatrics, post-acute and long-term care medicine, geriatric psychiatry, as well as experts in the care of the growing younger population of nursing home residents with disabilities and psychiatric conditions. Nursing home policy cannot be effectively imagined or implemented without these experts' active involvement.

The more subtle threats to the nursing home industry come from ignorance and arrogance. Ignorance related to the lack of understanding of how a geriatrics-focused, team-based approach to care is essential. Arrogance related to the fact that we can no longer keep running nursing homes as we have for the past four decades. If we are to reimagine nursing homes, we must be certain that the clinical focus is never allowed to be subservient to the finances. The entire industry must be reimagined. We must start by assuring appropriate staffing. The staff must be trained and must earn a living wage with corresponding benefits, and turnover must be reduced. Leadership teams must set their primary focus on providing quality care. We cannot afford money being siphoned out of facilities toward excessive real estate, related party and insurance industry profit. The residents we care for deserve to be prioritized. After nearly a year of hell, where all have been cut off from their loved ones, and many have lost their lives, we owe them that much.

I want to close by reiterating the fact that experts in geriatrics across the country would relish the opportunity to assist in the development of policy related to the health and well-being of frail older adults. This is what we've spent our lives training for. Many of us were inconsolable as the federal government, the Departments of Public Health and many counties made decisions without the full input of the clinical experts throughout this pandemic. It is time to learn from these mistakes and develop a structure that allows for the development of expert-driven policy. I plead with you to find a way to encourage the direct involvement of the experts

---

[416] Nazir A, Steinberg K, Wasserman M, et al., *JAMDA*, Time for an Upgrade in the Nursing Home Survey Process: A Position Statement From the Society of Post-Acute and Long-Term Care Medicine. 2020, ISSN 1525–8610, *https://doi.org/10.1016/j.jamda.2020.09.022*.

as we move forward. If such a process had already been in place, a significant number of lives would have been saved.

Letter Submitted by Rachel Winters

Dear esteemed representatives:

I am a registered voter in Pennsylvania (Westmoreland County) and I am writing to share my story, like others across the Commonwealth, who have family in assisted living/long term care facilities. The restrictions during the COVID pandemic placed on these facilities by the Pennsylvania Department of Health, CDC, and Centers for Medicare and Medicaid have adversely affected the quality of life for the constituents that rely on these facilities for their care.

My father, Herbert Henderson, is a veteran of the United States Air Force and proudly served his country in Vietnam. In November of 2019, my father had a series of strokes that impaired his speech and mobility. He was in and out of hospitals and rehabilitation facilities spending a total of 14 days at home since November 26, 2019. We placed him at Saint Anne's Home in Greensburg, PA on March 8, 2020 for further physical and occupational therapy. Saint Anne's was shut down on March 13, 2020 because of the COVID–19 outbreak. My family decided to let my father complete his therapy at Saint Anne's and wait to see if we could witness his progress to determine if my 75 year old mother could care for him at home. That opportunity never came.

We had to send my father to the hospital twice during the COVID pandemic, once in May for congestive heart failure and again in July for colitis and C. Diff. Each time we had to weigh the decision to send him out knowing that he would be in quarantine for 10–14 days upon returning to Saint Anne's. Each time he had to quarantine after a hospitalization was excruciating. He would become agitated, his speech was slurred and difficult to understand, and the last hospitalization he lost the ability to feed himself with utensils.

The first time my father was able to go outside was for a table visit in August, 3 months after arriving to Saint Anne's. The facility is hard pressed to retain staff given the current health crises, so there isn't enough people to get him outside to enjoy the sunshine on his face or hear the birds in the trees. This is something we did with him every time we visited for the short period we were allowed in the building. We went up every day, for two hours and made sure he got outside in one of Saint Anne's beautiful gardens. My dad loves to be outside.

My family and I have followed every protocol and abided by every changing rule and regulation sent down by the state and the CDC. We were allowed 2 compassionate care visits with my dad and 13 table visits which were 20 minutes in length, with an 8 foot table separating us.

Despite the frequent COVID tests of staff, not seeing family/friends, and the severe reduction in social activities, my father contracted COVID–19 the end of November 2020. He was isolated in his room for 3 weeks with the door shut and covered in plastic. The only view he had was to an interior courtyard, which meant that we could not visit. The ventilation system in his room that was to circulate air and prevent the virus from getting into the building made it impossible for him to hear us on the phone. Not only could we not see him, we couldn't talk to him either. The only interaction he had was with the nurses and aides who worked at Saint

Anne's, many whom were unfamiliar to him because his usual care staff had also contracted COVID. He spent Thanksgiving alone in his room. When he was finally released from isolation, he was a shell of a man. My mom and I went up for our usual window visit and he wouldn't speak to us, just staring out into space.

The lack of stimulation via activities, communal dining, and personal contact is taking a toll on all residents in personal care/long-term care facilities. These individuals haven't committed any crimes and yet they are being punished for getting old, frail and sick. These homes are understaffed and overwhelmed trying to keep up with the regulations and rules placed upon them. It is an extreme disservice to the people in these facilities, their families, and the staff that we are over a year into this pandemic and there is no end in sight. The COVID pandemic is killing off the elderly not by contracting the virus, but by disengaging them for everyday life. They are sitting in their rooms in front of a TV waiting to die.

In December, we were notified that my father isn't doing well. He hadn't eaten anything for 3 weeks; he ripped out the IV meant to provide him hydration; he was refusing blood work and his medications; he was telling everyone at Saint Anne's that he wants to die. We were advised to sign him up for hospice because he is in the twilight of his life. We were allowed two compassionate care visits and one tent visit when his conditioned worsened. Then the infection rate in Westmoreland County increased and based on the regulations we are not allowed in Saint Anne's to see my dad. We got to watch him slowly deteriorate through a pane of glass.

My mom and I have been up at my dad's window at 3-5 days a week since the lockdown for at least an hour. We were sitting out there in the rain, snow, and freezing temperatures. We want him to know that he is not forgotten. He doesn't understand why we can't come in there and sit next to him on his bed or hold his hand.

Countless birthdays, holidays, and anniversaries were spent either looking at my father through a closed window or separated by an 8 foot long table with a Plexiglas barrier. No touch. No physical contact. An entire year has gone by without being able to take my dad outside to one of the courtyards to hear the birds sing or walk him up and down the halls of the facility. My parents have been married 57 years. This is the longest that they have not been physically together since my dad was in the Air Force and deployed.

When he was admitted to Saint Anne's he was walking with a walker, able to feed himself, and called us on his cellphone. Now a year later, he requires two people and a lift to get him in and out of bed. He no longer remembers how to answer his phone, let alone call us to talk. His fine motor abilities have declined. I take him finger foods and watching him trying to pick up his food is painful. He has lost 40 pounds this year. His speech also suffered. He is hard to understand, even on his best days.

Thankfully he has improved since December. Saint Anne's started to lift some restrictions based on the new CMS guidelines. We were scheduled to see him in his room March 17 and 19, but a staff member tested positive for COVID and we were no longer allowed in the building. We instead had 2 tent visits scheduled for 30 minutes.

Would have things been different if we were allowed to be with him all this time? Has he given up the will to live because of the current circumstances or is it just a progression of his illness? We may never know, but these questions will linger with us for a lifetime.

My family may not personally benefit from any efforts made by you on our behalf, but I don't want other families to go through this. The last year has been pure hell. I was hoping with the vaccine things might change.

These protocols and regulations may have looked good on paper to prolong life and decrease infection in residential facilities, but the realities are something all together different. While the protocols may have prolonged the quantity of life, they has drastically impacted the quality of life.

I'm sure there will be another virus or health crisis in the future. It's inevitable. This can not happen again. The complete closure of these facilities and lack of access to loved ones is cruel and unusual punishment. Our seniors deserve better.

Sincerely yours,

Rachel Winters

Chapter 2

COVID-19 Had a Devastating Impact on Medicare Beneficiaries in Nursing Homes During 2020*

U.S. Department of Health and Human Services

Key Takeaways

- 2 in 5 Medicare beneficiaries in nursing homes were diagnosed with either COVID-19 or likely COVID-19 in 2020.
- Almost 1,000 more beneficiaries died per day in April 2020 than in April 2019.
- Overall mortality in nursing homes increased to 22 percent in 2020 from 17 percent in 2019.
- About half of Black, Hispanic, and Asian beneficiaries in nursing homes had or likely had COVID-19, and 41 percent of White beneficiaries did.
- Understanding the pandemic's effects on nursing home residents is necessary if tragedies like this are to be averted.

Why These Data Are Important

The COVID-19 pandemic has presented extraordinary challenges for the Nation's health care system. Nursing home residents have been particularly affected by the disease, as they are predominately elderly, tend to have underlying conditions, and live in close quarters.

The media have chronicled the fear, loneliness, and isolation residents have endured, as well as the grief they have felt watching so many peers die. However, data on the number of nursing home residents who were diagnosed with COVID-19 or likely COVID-19 have not been readily available, particularly for early in the pandemic. Nursing homes are not required to report cases and deaths that occurred before May 8, 2020. It is important that we understand the extent of the outbreaks in nursing homes, including increases in deaths, to not only acknowledge the pandemic's toll, but to improve efforts to mitigate the damage of the continuing pandemic, and better prepare for future public health emergencies.

---

* This is an edited, reformatted and augmented version of U.S. Department of Health and Human Services, Office of Inspector General Data Snapshot Publication No. OEI-02-20-00490, dated June 2021.

In: The Significance of the COVID Pandemic in Nursing Homes
Editor: John S. Gill
ISBN: 979-8-88697-660-1

This data snapshot provides objective, standardized data based on Medicare claims for all Medicare beneficiaries in nursing homes throughout the country.[a] This snapshot is part of an Office of Inspector General (OIG) initiative focusing on COVID-19 and nursing homes.[1] Recent work examined infection control and complaint surveys conducted during the early months of the pandemic.[2] Upcoming work will focus on strategies nursing homes have used to combat the pandemic.[3] The goal of this body of work is to help protect the health and safety of the vulnerable nursing home population.

Understanding how many beneficiaries in nursing homes were affected, who they were, and what characteristics may have put some at greater risk can help prevent future tragedies. This data snapshot aims to inform public health and contribute to the body of knowledge needed to combat this pandemic and protect vulnerable seniors as well as the general population. As this pandemic has shown, hardships faced in nursing homes can quickly spread across the rest of the Nation.

Diagnoses and Overall Deaths

2 in 5 Medicare beneficiaries in nursing homes were diagnosed with COVID-19 or likely COVID-19 in 2020. About 3.1 million Medicare beneficiaries resided in nursing homes in 2020. Forty-two percent of them—1.3 million beneficiaries—had or likely had COVID-19, according to diagnoses on their Medicare claims. For context, about 6 percent of the Nation's population were reported to have been infected by the end of December.[4] Of the 1.3 million Medicare beneficiaries residing in nursing homes who had or likely had COVID-19, 762,594 were confirmed to have COVID-19 and 532,901 were diagnosed as likely having it, meaning COVID-19 was suspected but not confirmed by a positive test result.

This analysis includes all beneficiaries who were enrolled in Medicare and resided in a nursing facility or skilled nursing facility— collectively referred to here as nursing homes— during 2020. It determines the number of beneficiaries who were diagnosed with COVID-19 or likely COVID- 19 in a nursing home as well as those diagnosed in the hospital or other care settings after being transferred from the nursing home. It also provides the overall number of

---

[a] This data snapshot provides new information and is not equivalent to other previously reported data on nursing home COVID-19 cases and deaths. Our analysis is based on Medicare claims data and does not include nursing home residents who are not Medicare beneficiaries. Further, our findings include Medicare residents diagnosed with "likely COVID" and describe trends in overall mortality of Medicare nursing home residents, not just those with COVID-19.

[1] OIG, *COVID-19 Portal.* Accessed at https://oig.hhs.gov/coronavirus/index.asp. U.S. Department of Health and Human Services, Office of Inspector General, *Operation CARE: Caring, Awareness, & Resources for Our Elders.* Accessed at https://oig.hhs.gov/ fraud/care/index.asp on March 11, 2021.

[2] OIG, *Onsite Surveys of Nursing Homes During the COVID-19 Pandemic: March 23–May 30, 2020*, OEI-01-20-00430, December 2020.

[3] OIG Work Plan, *Meeting the Challenges Presented by COVID-19: Nursing Homes.* Accessed at https://oig.hhs.gov/ reports-and-publications/workplan/summary/wp-summary-0000474. asp on January 29, 2021.

[4] The COVID Tracking Project at The Atlantic, *National Data: Cases.* Accessed at https://covidtracking.com/ data/national/cases on March 18, 2021. The total confirmed and probable cases for the total population as of December 31, 2020 is reported as 19,864,374. United States Census Bureau, *2020 Census Apportionment Results*, "Table 2. Resident Population for the 50 States, the District of Columbia, and Puerto Rico: 2020 Census." Accessed at https://www.census.gov/data/tables/2020/dec/2020-apportionment-data.html on May 6, 2021. The United States population, including Puerto Rico, in 2020 as determined by the U.S. Census was 334,735,155.

deaths; it does not attribute cause of death. See Methodology for more detailed information on nursing home residency and diagnosis codes.

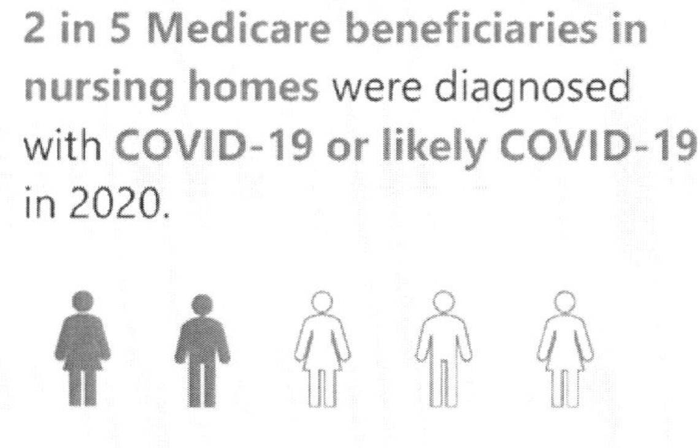

The number of infected beneficiaries in nursing homes grew exponentially in the spring of 2020. The country's first confirmed case of COVID-19 was in January 2020.[5] Over the course of a few weeks in the spring, the number of beneficiaries in nursing homes who had or likely had COVID-19 increased dramatically. In March, 492 Medicare beneficiaries in nursing homes per day were diagnosed as having or likely having COVID-19. That increased almost tenfold in April, which averaged more than 4,700 new cases per day.

In total, just over 21,000 Medicare beneficiaries were diagnosed as having or likely having COVID-19 from January through March 2020. By the end of June, there were almost 419,000 overall.

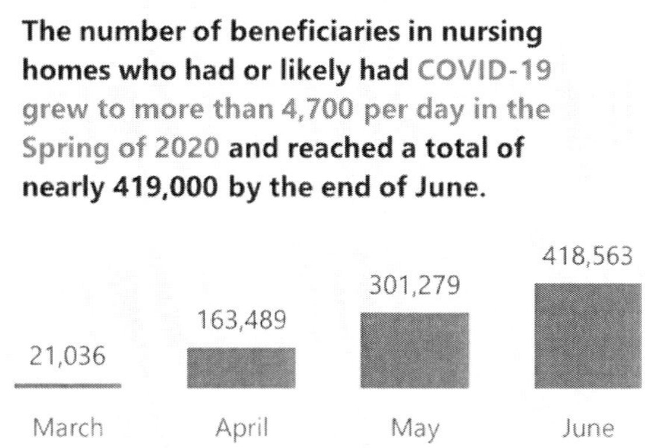

Source: OIG analysis of Medicare data, 2021.

The number of new COVID-19 and likely COVID-19 cases grew even higher at the end of the year. On average, more than 5,800 Medicare beneficiaries in nursing homes were being diagnosed each day in November. In December, the number topped 6,600 per day. By the end of December, the total number of cases (1.3 million) was about 62 times more than it had been at the end of March.

[5] Holshe, M.L., et al. (2020). First Case of 2019 Novel Coronavirus in the United States. *New England Journal of Medicine*, 382, 929-936.

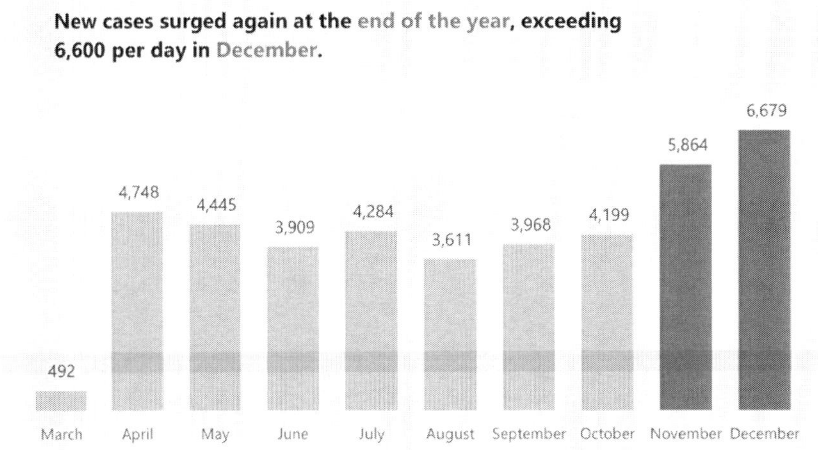

Source: OIG analysis of Medicare data, 2021.

Some states were impacted more than others. By the end of June, more than a quarter of the Medicare beneficiaries in nursing homes in each of 11 States had or likely had COVID-19. These States—Connecticut, Delaware, District of Columbia, Georgia, Illinois, Louisiana, Maryland, Massachusetts, New Jersey, New York, and Pennsylvania—were also some of the hardest hit in terms of percentage of their general population that contracted the disease during that time.[6] By the end of December, more than half the Medicare beneficiaries in nursing homes in each of four States—Connecticut, Illinois, Louisiana, and New Jersey—had or likely had COVID-19.

The overall mortality rate in nursing homes rose 32 percent in 2020. The pandemic had far- reaching implications for all nursing home beneficiaries, beyond those who had or likely had COVID-19. Among all Medicare beneficiaries in nursing homes, 22.5 percent died in 2020, which is an increase of one-third from 2019 when 17.0 percent of Medicare beneficiaries in nursing homes died. This 32-percent increase amounts to 169,291 more deaths in 2020 than if the mortality rate had remained the same as in 2019. Each month of 2020 had a higher mortality rate than the corresponding month a year earlier.

Almost 1,000 more beneficiaries died per day in April 2020 than in the previous year. In April 2020 alone, a total of 81,484 Medicare beneficiaries in nursing homes died. This is almost 30,000 more deaths—an average of about 1,000 per day—compared to the previous year. This increase in number occurred even though the nursing home population was smaller in April 2020. Overall, Medicare beneficiaries in nursing homes were almost twice as likely to die in April 2020 than in April 2019. In April 2020, 6.3 percent of all Medicare beneficiaries in nursing homes died, whereas 3.5 percent died in April 2019.

The mortality rates also rose at the end of 2020. In November, 5.1 percent of all Medicare beneficiaries in nursing homes died, and in December that increased to 6.2 percent. Again,

[6] The COVID Tracking Project at The Atlantic, *The Data: Data by State*, "Cases: Historical Data." Accessed at https://covidtracking.com/data on March 11, 2021. United States Census Bureau, *2020 Census Apportionment Results*, "Table 2. Resident Population for the 50 States, the District of Columbia, and Puerto Rico: 2020 Census." Accessed at https://www.census.gov/data/tables/2020/dec/2020-apportionment-data.html on May 6, 2021. The percentage of each State's population that had contracted COVID-19 was calculated using confirmed and probable case totals as of June 30, 2020, and the state population results of the 2020 Census.

these rates are markedly higher than the previous year. In November 2019, 3.6 percent of all Medicare beneficiaries in nursing homes died, and, in December 2019, 3.8 percent did.

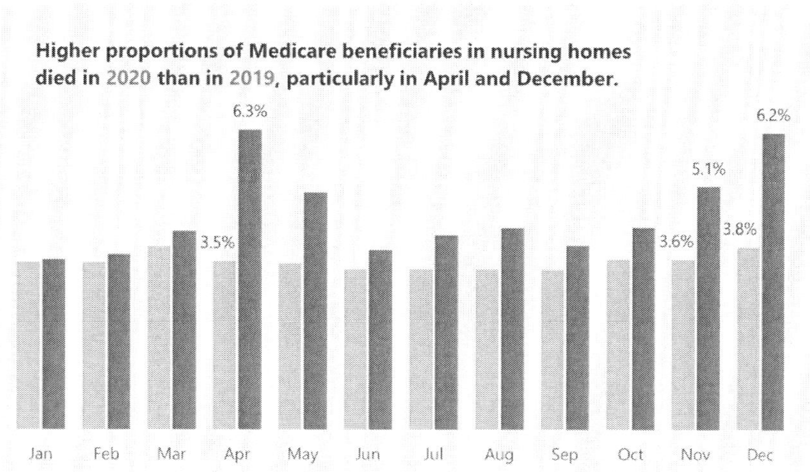

Source: OIG analysis of Medicare data, 2021.

Medicare Beneficiary Characteristics

About half of Black, Hispanic, and Asian beneficiaries in nursing homes had or likely had COVID-19 in 2020. About half of Black beneficiaries, Hispanic[7] beneficiaries, and Asian beneficiaries in nursing homes had or likely had COVID-19 in 2020. Other research has similarly found that Black individuals and Hispanic individuals experience higher rates of COVID-19.[8]

Each of these groups was more likely than White beneficiaries to have or likely have COVID-19.

Forty-one percent of White beneficiaries in nursing homes had or likely had COVID-19 in 2020. See appendix for more detailed information for each group.

The mortality rates for each of these four groups increased in 2020, but to different extents. Asian beneficiaries in nursing homes had the greatest increase, with 27 percent dying in 2020 compared with 17 percent the previous year. The mortality rates for Hispanic beneficiaries in nursing homes and Black beneficiaries in nursing homes both reached 23 percent in 2020, up from 15 percent in 2019. The mortality rate of White beneficiaries grew less relatively, increasing to 24 percent in 2020 from 18 percent the previous year.

---

[7] Hispanic refers to beneficiaries identified as Hispanic or Latino.

[8] For example, CMS found that Black Medicare beneficiaries and Hispanic Medicare beneficiaries have experienced higher rates of COVID-19 compared to White beneficiaries. See CMS, *Preliminary Medicare COVID-19 Data Snapshot*. Accessed at https://www.cms.gov/research-statistics-data-systems/preliminary-medicare-covid-19-data-snapshot on May 13, 2021. Likewise, a recent review examining the association between COVID-19 infections, hospitalization, and mortality and race and ethnicity in the general population concluded that Black individuals and Hispanic individuals experienced disproportionately higher rates of COVID-19 compared to White individuals. See Mackey, K., et al. (2021). Racial and Ethnic Disparities in COVID-19-Related Infections, Hospitalizations, and Deaths. *Annals of Internal Medicine,* 174(3), 362-373.

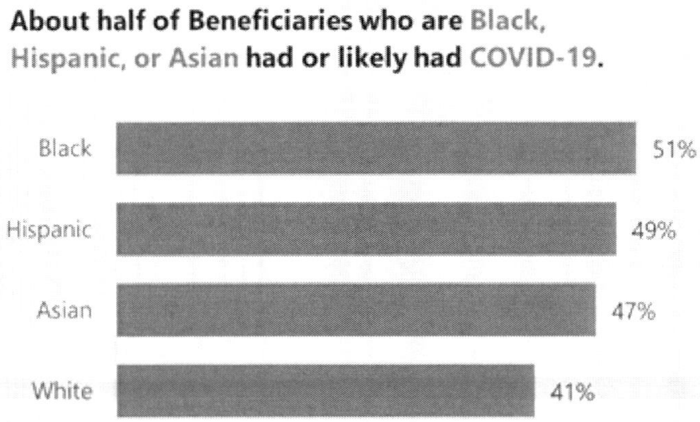

Source: OIG analysis of Medicare data, 2021.

Note: These categories are based on data from nursing home assessments, which combine race and ethnicity in one question. This information is intended to be self-reported, but a caregiver or staff may respond if the beneficiary cannot.

For beneficiaries in nursing homes, age does not appear to be a factor in rates of COVID- 19 infections. All age groups of Medicare beneficiaries in nursing homes had similar infection rates in 2020. Just over 2 in 5 beneficiaries in each age group—under 65 years, 65 to 74 years, 75 to 84 years, and 85 years and older—had or likely had COVID-19. See appendix for more detailed information for each group.

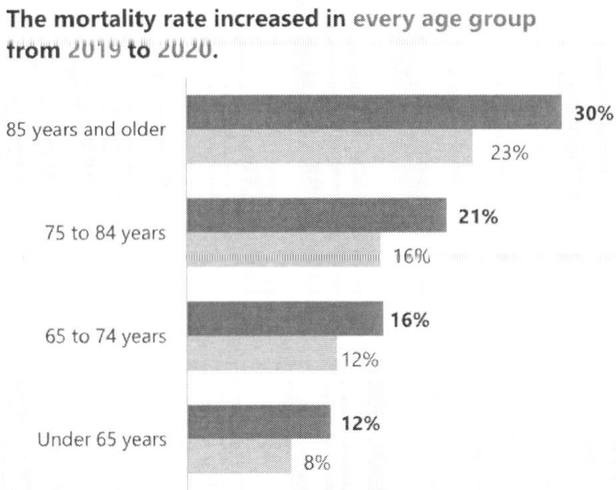

Source: OIG analysis of Medicare data, 2021.

Mortality rates were different across the age groups, but all increased during the pandemic. In 2020, the mortality rates ranged from 12 percent in the youngest group to 30 percent of the oldest. Before the pandemic, mortality ranged from 8 percent to 23 percent.

Gender also does not appear to be a factor in rates of COVID-19 infections. Forty-three percent of female Medicare beneficiaries in nursing homes had or likely had COVID-19 in 2020. The rate was similar for male beneficiaries—41 percent.

Again, mortality rose for both females and males during the pandemic. In 2020, the mortality rate for female beneficiaries in nursing homes reached 21 percent, up from the pre-pandemic rate in 2019 of 16 percent. The mortality rate for male beneficiaries increased to 24 percent from 19 percent.

Dually eligible beneficiaries—those enrolled in both Medicare and Medicaid—were much more likely than Medicare-only beneficiaries to contract COVID-19. Fifty-six percent of dually eligible beneficiaries in nursing homes had or likely had COVID-19 in 2020, compared to 29 percent of Medicare-only beneficiaries.

Although each group's mortality rate rose during the pandemic, the increase was greater for dually eligible beneficiaries. Specifically, 26 percent of dually eligible beneficiaries in nursing homes died in 2020, up from 19 percent the previous year. Meanwhile, the mortality rate for their Medicare-only counterparts grew to 19 percent from 16 percent. Previous research has shown that dually eligible beneficiaries are generally poorer and sicker—having low-incomes and multiple chronic conditions to manage—compared to other Medicare beneficiaries.[9]

Conclusion

The COVID-19 pandemic has been devastating for Medicare beneficiaries in nursing homes. Two in five Medicare beneficiaries in nursing homes either had or likely had the disease in 2020. From March through June, and again in November and December, the number of cases grew dramatically. Some Medicare beneficiaries in nursing homes seemed to be at greater risk than others. Specifically, Black beneficiaries, Hispanic beneficiaries, and Asian beneficiaries were more likely than White beneficiaries to have or likely have COVID-19. Further, dually eligible beneficiaries had significantly higher rates of COVID-19 infections than Medicare-only beneficiaries. In addition, overall mortality for Medicare beneficiaries in nursing homes increased by almost a third in 2020. Each month in 2020 had a higher mortality rate than the corresponding month in 2019.

The toll that the COVID pandemic has taken on Medicare beneficiaries in nursing homes demonstrates the need for increased action to mitigate the effects of the ongoing pandemic and to avert such tragedies from occurring in the future. OIG is committed to understanding and helping to protect nursing home residents from the impacts of COVID-19. We recognize that CMS is also committed to protecting nursing home residents.

Additional data analysis may help CMS in its efforts. The analyses in this report demonstrate the value of using Medicare data to understand the extent to which nursing home residents nationwide have been affected by the pandemic, who they were, and what characteristics are associated with greater risk. CMS currently relies on data from the CDC's National Healthcare Safety Network (NHSN) Long-Term Care Facility COVID-19 module,

---

[9] CMS, *People Dually Eligible for Medicare and Medicaid.* Accessed at https://www.cms. gov/Medicare-Medicaid-Coordination/Medicare-and-Medicaid-Coordination/Medicare-Medicaid-Coordination-Office/Downloads/MMCO_Factsheet.pdf on December 17, 2020. CMS, *Medicare-Medicaid Coordination Office FY 2019 Report to Congress.* Accessed at https://www.cms.gov/files/document/mmco-report-cong ress.pdf on December 17, 2020. Medicare Payment Advisory Commission, *Data book: Beneficiaries dually eligible for Medicare and Medicaid—January 2018*, p. 3. Accessed at http://medpac.gov/docs/default-source/data-book/jan18_medpac_ macpac_dualsdata book_sec.pdf on December 17, 2020.

which are self-reported by nursing homes. Adding Medicare claims data could strengthen and broaden CMS's analyses.

Unlike the NHSN, claims data cover the entire year and include demographic information about each beneficiary as well as information about the beneficiary's conditions and care needs. These data are important to understanding the effects of the pandemic and, moving forward, could play an integral part in understanding health disparities within the nursing home population and preparing for and dealing with future public health crises.

Methodology

We based this study on an analysis of data from several sources including: (1) the Minimum Data Set (MDS); (2) the Medicare Enrollment Database; and (3) Medicare Parts A, B, and C claims. We obtained the data from CMS's Integrated Data Repository and focused our analysis on Medicare beneficiaries residing in nursing homes in 2020.

Identification of Medicare Beneficiaries Residing in Nursing Homes

We used the MDS to identify individuals who resided in nursing homes.[10] The MDS includes assessments completed by the nursing home for each individual residing in these facilities. Nursing homes must complete these assessments periodically for all residents—including beneficiaries receiving Medicare or Medicaid. Using each resident's unique identifier, we matched the data from the MDS to the Medicare Enrollment Database to identify the residents who were enrolled in Medicare.[11] Next, we identified the Parts A, B, and C claims for these Medicare beneficiaries.

We considered a beneficiary a nursing home resident starting from the date of the first MDS assessment at the facility until the date that the beneficiary leaves the facility to go home or dies. Therefore, a beneficiary who resided in a nursing home and entered a hospital for treatment is still considered a nursing home resident during the time spent in the hospital.[12]

Analysis of Beneficiaries Who Had or Likely Had COVID-19

We determined the extent to which Medicare beneficiaries residing in nursing homes were diagnosed as having or likely having COVID-19 in 2020.

---

[10] We also used the Medicare Parts A and C Skilled Nursing Facility claims to identify additional beneficiaries residing in nursing homes, typically for beneficiaries in swing-bed hospital stays when MDS assessments were not readily accessible.

[11] We matched the unique identifier for each resident from the MDS along with the resident's name, sex, and date of birth to the Medicare Enrollment Database to confirm the identity of the nursing home resident and identify those who were enrolled in Medicare.

[12] For our analysis, if 150 days elapsed since the last MDS assessment and a discharge or date of death was not noted, a beneficiary is assumed to have been discharged home and is no longer considered a nursing home resident. CMS considers that, if a resident has not had a MDS transaction for 150 days, the resident is assumed to have been discharged. See CMS, *MDS 3.0 Frequency Report*. Accessed at https://www.cms.gov/Research-Statistics-Data-and- Systems/Computer-Data-and-Systems/Minimum-Data-Set-3-0-Public-Reports/ Minimum-Data-Set-3-0-Frequency- Report on April 21, 2021.

We considered a beneficiary who had a diagnosis code of B97.29 or U07.1 on a claim to have a diagnosis of COVID-19. The CDC designated B97.29 as an interim code to identify confirmed cases of COVID-19 prior to April 1, 2020.[13] It later established U07.1 as the unique code to identify confirmed cases of the disease effective April 1. Further, we considered a beneficiary who had a diagnosis code of Z20.828 on a claim to likely have COVID-19. The CDC designated Z20.828 to report "suspected," "possible," or "probable" cases of COVID-19 prior to April and onward.[14]

We calculated the total number of Medicare beneficiaries in nursing homes who had or likely had COVID-19 in 2020. These counts include the beneficiaries who were diagnosed with COVID-19 or likely COVID-19 in a nursing home as well as those diagnosed in other care settings after being transferred from the nursing home. For each Medicare beneficiary in a nursing home, we determined if the beneficiary was diagnosed with COVID-19, likely COVID-19, or neither. If a beneficiary is diagnosed at one point with likely COVID-19 and later diagnosed with COVID-19, we considered that beneficiary to be diagnosed with COVID-19 as opposed to likely COVID-19.

We also calculated the total number of Medicare beneficiaries residing in nursing homes who died during this period. These counts include the beneficiaries who died in the nursing home as well as those who died in the hospital or other health care settings, such as hospice, after being transferred from the nursing home. We calculated for each month the number of Medicare beneficiaries diagnosed as having or likely having COVID-19. We also calculated the number of Medicare beneficiaries residing in nursing homes who died. We used the date of death from the Social Security Administration, which is contained in the Medicare Enrollment Database, to identify those beneficiaries who died.

Next, we compared the number of all Medicare beneficiaries in nursing homes in 2019 and the number of all Medicare beneficiaries in nursing homes who died in 2019. We did the same for 2020. We also calculated similar statistics per month to identify any trends.

Analysis of Beneficiary Characteristics

We described the Medicare beneficiaries residing in nursing homes who had or likely had COVID-19 in 2020. To do so, we analyzed the information on age, gender, and Medicare

[13] CDC, *ICD-10-CM Official Coding Guidelines–Supplement Coding encounters related to COVID-19 Coronavirus Outbreak* (February 20, 2020–March 31, 2020). Accessed at https://www.cdc.gov/nchs/data/icd/interim-coding-advice-coronavirus-March-2020-final.pdf on July 20, 2020. See also, American Health Information Management Association (AHIMA), *AHIMA and AHA FAQ: ICD-10-CM/PCS Coding for COVID-19.* Accessed at https://journal.ahima.org/ahima-and-aha-faq-on-icd-10-cm-coding-for-covid-19/ on December 15, 2020. Since this code was not exclusive to the coronavirus responsible for COVID-19, providers were urged to limit the assignment of B97.29 to confirmed cases of COVID-19. See also CDC, *ICD-10-CM Official Coding and Reporting Guidelines* (April 1, 2020, through September 30, 2020). Accessed at https://www.cdc.gov/nchs/data/icd/COVID-19-guidelines-final.pdf on July 20, 2020.

[14] CDC, *ICD-10-CM Official Coding Guidelines–Supplement Coding encounters related to COVID-19 Coronavirus Outbreak* (February 20, 2020-March 31, 2020). Accessed at https://www.cdc.gov/nchs/data/icd/interim-coding-advice-coronavirus-March-2020-final.pdf on July 20, 2020. See also CDC, *ICD-10-CM Official Coding and Reporting Guidelines* (April 1, 2020, through September 30, 2020). Accessed at https://www.cdc.gov/nchs/data/icd/COVID-19-guidelines-final.pdf on July 20, 2020.

eligibility (e.g., Medicare-only, dually eligible for Medicare and Medicaid) from the Medicare Enrollment Database. We analyzed race and ethnicity information from the MDS.[15]

For each characteristic, we determined the extent to which Medicare beneficiaries in nursing homes who had or likely had COVID-19 differed from other Medicare beneficiaries in nursing homes. In addition, for each characteristic, we compared the percentage of Medicare beneficiaries in nursing homes who died in 2020 to those who died in the 2019.

Limitations

This study determines the number of Medicare beneficiaries residing in nursing homes who had or likely had COVID-19 based on Medicare claims data; it does not include a review of medical records. It also determines the number of Medicare beneficiaries who died; it does not include a review of death certificates nor determinations about whether COVID-19 was the cause of death for these beneficiaries. The race and ethnicity categories used in this report are based on data from nursing home assessments, which combine race and ethnicity in one question. This information is intended to be self-reported, but a caregiver or staff may respond if the beneficiary cannot.

Standards

We conducted this study in accordance with the *Quality Standards for Inspection and Evaluation* issued by the Council of the Inspectors General on Integrity and Efficiency.

Appendix A

Beneficiary Characteristics

Exhibit A-1. COVID-19 rates by race and ethnicity of nursing home beneficiaries

Race/Ethnicity	Number of Beneficiaries in Nursing Homes	Percentage Who Had or Likely Had COVID-19	Percentage Who Died*
Asian	48,691	47%	27%
Black	354,241	51%	23%
Hispanic	139,995	49%	23%
White	2,241,441	41%	24%

Source: OIG analysis of Medicare data, 2021.

* This refers to the percentage of Medicare beneficiaries in nursing homes who died from any cause.

These categories are based on data from nursing home assessments, which combine race and ethnicity in one question. This information is intended to be self-reported, but a caregiver or staff may respond if the beneficiary cannot.

[15] During MDS assessment, nursing home residents (or their representative, if residents are unable to respond) select one or more categories from six race and ethnicity options—American Indian or Alaska Native, Asian, Black or African American, Native Hawaiian or Other Pacific Islander, White, and Hispanic or Latino. See Office of Management and Budget, *Revisions to the Standards for the Classification of Federal Data on Race and Ethnicity*, Federal Register Vol. 62, No. 210, October 30, 1997. Accessed at https://www.govinfo.gov/content/pkg/FR-1997-10-30/pdf/97-28653.pdf on December 3, 2020.

Exhibit A-2. COVID-19 rates by age of nursing home beneficiaries

Age	Number of Beneficiaries in Nursing Homes	Percentage Who Had or Likely Had COVID-19	Percentage Who Died*
Under 65 years	282,397	44%	12%
65 to 74 years	709,973	42%	16%
75 to 84 years	956,507	42%	21%
85 years and older	1,127,874	42%	30%

Source: OIG analysis of Medicare data, 2021.

* This refers to the percentage of Medicare beneficiaries in nursing homes who died from any cause.

Index

A

B

C

D

H

I

J

L

M

N

O

P

Q

R

S